T0258516

UNDERSTANDING HEALTH POLICY
A Clinical Approach

NINTH EDITION

Thomas Bodenheimer, MD
Professor Emeritus
Department of Family & Community Medicine
University of California, San Francisco

Kevin Grumbach, MD
Professor
Department of Family & Community Medicine
University of California, San Francisco

Rachel Willard-Grace, MPH
Director, Center for Excellence in Primary Care
Associate Professor
Department of Family & Community Medicine
University of California, San Francisco

Mc
Graw
Hill

New York   Chicago   San Francisco   Athens   London   Madrid   Mexico City
New Delhi   Milan   Singapore   Sydney   Toronto

Understanding Health Policy: A Clinical Approach, Ninth Edition

1 2 3 4 5 6 7 8 9 LCR 28 27 26 25 24 23

ISBN 978-1-265-90502-6
MHID 1-265-90502-9
ISSN 1080-9465

Notice

Medicine is an ever-changing science. As new research and clinical experience broaden our knowledge, changes in treatment and drug therapy are required. The authors and the publisher of this work have checked with sources believed to be reliable in their efforts to provide information that is complete and generally in accord with the standards accepted at the time of publication. However, in view of the possibility of human error or changes in medical sciences, neither the authors nor the publisher nor any other party who has been involved in the preparation or publication of this work warrants that the information contained herein is in every respect accurate or complete, and they disclaim all responsibility for any errors or omissions or for the results obtained from use of the information contained in this work. Readers are encouraged to confirm the information contained herein with other sources. For example, and in particular, readers are advised to check the product information sheet included in the package of each drug they plan to administer to be certain that the information contained in this work is accurate and that changes have not been made in the recommended dose or in the contraindications for administration. This recommendation is of particular importance in connection with new or infrequently used drugs.

This book was set in Minion Pro by MPS Limited.
The editors were Kay Conerly, Sylvia Choi, and Jennifer Bernstein.
The production supervisor was Catherine Saggese.
Project management was provided by Monika Chaudhari, MPS Limited.

This book is printed on acid-free paper.

Names: Bodenheimer, Thomas, author. | Grumbach, Kevin, author. | Willard-Grace, Rachel, author.
Title: Understanding health policy : a clinical approach / Thomas Bodenheimer, Kevin Grumbach, Rachel Willard-Grace.
Description: Ninth edition. | New York : McGraw Hill, [2024] | "A Lange medical book." | Includes bibliographical references and index. | Summary: "This is a book about health policy as well as individual patients and caregivers and how they interact with each other and with the overall health system. When treating a patient's illness, health expenditures as a percentage of gross domestic product or variations in surgical rates between one city and another seem remote if not irrelevant—but they are neither remote nor irrelevant. Health policy affects the patients we see on a daily basis. Managed care referral rules determine which specialist will see a patient; coverage gaps in the Medicare benefit package affects access to care for the elderly. Understanding Health Policy hopes to bridge the gap separating the microworld of individual patient care and the macrouniverse of health policy"— Provided by publisher.
Identifiers: LCCN 2023030436 | ISBN 9781265905026 (paperback ; alk. paper)
 | ISBN 9781265905514 (ebook)
Subjects: MESH: Health Policy | Health Care Costs | Health Care Rationing |
 Health Care Reform | Health Equity | National Health Insurance, United States | United States
Classification: LCC RA418 | NLM WA 540 AA1 | DDC 362.1—dc23/eng/20230727
LC record available at https://lccn.loc.gov/2023030436

McGraw Hill books are available at special quantity discounts to use as premiums and sales promotions, or for use in corporate training programs. To contact a representative, please visit the Contact Us pages at www.mhprofessional.com

Contents

Section V: The Political Economy of Health Care 183

Section VI: Conclusion and Study Guide 223

Preface

Since its first edition in 1998, *Understanding Health Policy: A Clinical Approach* has illuminated the workings of the US health care system. For this ninth edition, we are happy to welcome a third author, Rachel Willard-Grace, a health services researcher focused on building better teams to improve health care delivery. As a former medical assistant, pharmacy tech, and health care administrator, Rachel brings a new perspective on how health care is organized and delivered.

This is a book about health policy as well as individual patients and caregivers and how they interact with each other and with the overall health system. We, the authors, have taken care of patients and are also health care analysts. In one sense, these two sides of our lives seem quite separate. When treating a patient's illness, health expenditures as a percentage of gross domestic product or variations in surgical rates between one city and another seem remote if not irrelevant—but they are neither remote nor irrelevant. Health policy affects the patients we see on a daily basis. Managed care referral rules determine which specialist will see a patient; coverage gaps in the Medicare benefit package affects access to care for older adults. *Understanding Health Policy* hopes to bridge the gap separating the microworld of individual patient care and the macrouniverse of health policy.

THE AUDIENCE

The book is primarily written for health professions students and practitioners—physicians, nurses, nurse practitioners, physician assistants, pharmacists, social workers, community health workers, public health experts, and others—who will benefit from understanding the complex environment in which they work. Physicians feature prominently in the text, but in the actual world of clinical medicine, patients' encounters with other health care providers are an essential part of their health care experience. Physicians would be unable to function without the many other members of the health care team. Patients seldom appreciate the contributions made to their well-being by public health personnel, research scientists, educators, and many other health-related professionals. We hope that the many nonphysician members of the clinical care, public health, and health professions education teams as well as students aspiring to join these teams will find the book useful. Nothing can be accomplished without the combined efforts of everyone working in the health care field.

THE GOAL OF THE BOOK

Understanding Health Policy attempts to explain how the health care system works. We focus on basic principles of health policy in hopes that the reader will come away with a clearer, more systematic way of thinking about health care in the United States, its problems, and the alternatives for managing these problems.

Given the public's intense concerns about health care in the United States, we call out the failings as well as the successes of the US approach to financing and organizing care. Only by recognizing the difficulties of the system can we begin to fix its problems. The goal of this book, then, is to help all of us understand the health care system so that we can better work in the system and change what needs to be changed.

CLINICAL VIGNETTES

In our attempt to unify the overlapping spheres of health policy and individual health care encounters, we use clinical vignettes as a central feature of the book. These short descriptions of patients, physicians, and other caregivers interacting with the health care system are based on our own experiences, the experiences of colleagues, or cases reported in the medical literature or popular press. Most of the people and institutions presented in the vignettes have been given fictitious names to protect privacy. Some names used are emblematic of the occupations, health problems, or attitudes portrayed in the vignettes; most do not have special significance.

OUR OPINIONS

In exploring controversial issues of health policy, our own opinions inevitably color and shade the words we use and the conclusions we reach. We present several of our most fundamental values and perspectives here.

THE RIGHT TO HEALTH CARE

We believe that health care should be a right enjoyed equally by everyone. Certain things in life are considered essential. Society is not outraged if someone is turned away from a movie or concert because he or she cannot afford a ticket. But sick people who are turned away from a medical practice can make headlines, and rightly so. All people should have equal access to a reasonable level of appropriate, high-quality health services, regardless of ability to pay.

In 2009, the United States entered into a fierce debate over whether health care should be a right. The debate focused on President Barack Obama's campaign to enact universal health insurance. Following a year of public ferment, Congress passed the Affordable Care Act, which moves in the direction of guaranteeing health care as a right. Yet, at the time of writing this edition of *Understanding Health Policy,* the controversy continues.

THE CENTRALITY OF HEALTH EQUITY

We recognize the serious, persistent inequities in the health and health care of the US population. Study after study find that socially marginalized groups suffer poorer health than groups with greater social privilege and power. These disparities are shaped by deeply rooted forces such as racism, sexism, poverty, and rural isolation. Improving the health care system requires eliminating these inequities.

THE IMPERATIVE TO CONTAIN COSTS

We believe that limits must be placed on the costs of health care. Rising costs make health services and health insurance unaffordable. Many companies are shifting more health care costs onto their employees. As government health budgets balloon, cutbacks are inevitable, generally hurting older adults and people in low-income brackets. Individuals with no health insurance or inadequate coverage have a far harder time paying for care as costs go up. As a general rule, when costs go up, access goes down.

We believe that cost controls can be imposed in a manner that does relatively little harm to the health of the public. Scientific advances that spawn new, expensive technologies may benefit some patients but are often inappropriately used for patients whom they do not benefit. The accelerating cost of administering the health care system wastes money that could be reinvested in clinical and public health programs that promote health. Eliminating medical services that produce no benefit and cutting administrative waste are examples of a path to "painless" cost control.

THE NEED FOR POPULATION-BASED HEALTH CARE

Most physicians, nurses, and other health professionals are trained to provide clinical care to individuals. Yet clinical care is not the only determinant of health status; standard of living and public health measures have an even greater influence on the health of a population. Health care, then, should have another dimension: concern for the population as a whole. Individual clinicians may be first-rate in caring for their patients' heart attacks, but may not worry enough about the prevalence of smoking, uncontrolled diabetes, and substance use, or about nieghborhoods that are "food deserts" or lack safe spaces for exercise, affecting the health of the group of patients enrolled in their practices and the broader community. The COVID-19 pandemic starkly revealed the need for greater integration of public health and clinical medicine. We believe that health care providers should be trained to add a population orientation to their current role of caring for individuals.

ACKNOWLEDGMENTS

We could not have written this book by ourselves. The circumstances encountered by hundreds of our patients and dozens of our colleagues provided the insights we needed to understand and describe the health care system. Any inaccuracies in the book are entirely our responsibility. Our warmest thanks go to our families, who have provided both encouragement and patience.

Earlier versions of Chapters 2, 4, 7, 11, 12, and 17 were published serially as articles in the *Journal of the American Medical Association* (1994;272:634–639, 1994;272:971–977, 1994;272:1458–1464, 1995;273:160–167, 1995;274:85–90, and 1996;276:1025–1031) and are published here with permission (copyright, 1994, 1995, and 1996, American Medical Association).

CONCLUSION

This is a book about health policy. As such, we will cite technical studies and will make cross-national generalizations. As health care practitioners, however, we are daily reminded of the human realities of health policy. *Understanding Health Policy: A Clinical Approach* is fundamentally about the people we care for: the underinsured janitor with high-deductible insurance enduring the pain of recurrent gallstone attacks because surgery might be unaffordable, or the retired university professor who sustains a stroke and whose life savings are disappearing in nursing home bills uncovered by her Medicare or private insurance plans.

Almost every person, whether a parent struggling to pay rent, a young college graduate navigating a first job, a well-to-do physician, or a millionaire insurance executive, will someday become ill, and all of us will die. Everyone stands to benefit from a system in which health care for all people is accessible, affordable, equitable, appropriate in its use of resources, and of high quality.

Thomas Bodenheimer
Kevin Grumbach
Rachel Willard-Grace
San Francisco, California

Introduction: The Strengths and Weaknesses of US Health Care

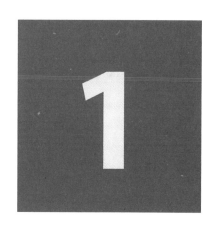

Louise Brown was an accountant with a 25-year history of diabetes. Her physician taught her to monitor her glucose at home, and her health coach helped her follow a healthy diet. Her diabetes was brought under good control. Diabetic retinopathy was discovered at yearly eye examinations, and periodic laser treatments of her retina prevented loss of vision. Ms. Brown lived to the age of 92, a success story of the US health care system.

Angela Martini grew up in a low-income urban neighborhood with underfunded schools, became pregnant as a teenager, and has been on public assistance while caring for her four children. Her Medicaid coverage pays for yearly preventive care visits with her family physician at no cost to Angela. A mammogram ordered by her physician detected a suspicious lesion, found to be cancer on biopsy. She was referred to a surgical breast specialist, underwent a mastectomy, was treated with a hormonal medication, and has been healthy for the past 15 years.

For people with private or public insurance who have access to health care services, the melding of high-quality primary and preventive care with appropriate specialty treatment can produce the best medical care in the world. The United States is blessed with thousands of well-trained physicians, nurses, pharmacists, and other caregivers who compassionately and skillfully provide health services to patients who seek their assistance. This is the face of the health care system in which we can take pride. Success stories, however, are only part of the reality of health care in the United States. Some persons receive too little care because they are uninsured or inadequately insured. Others are subjected to unnecessary treatments.

James Jackson was recently unemployed but unable to qualify for Medicaid because his state did not expand Medicaid under the 2010 Patient Protection and Affordable Care Act. At age 34, he developed abdominal pain but did not seek care for 10 days because he had no insurance and feared the cost of treatment. He began to vomit, became weak, and was finally taken to an emergency room by his cousin. The physician diagnosed a perforated ulcer with peritonitis and septic shock. The illness had gone on too long; Mr. Jackson died on the operating table. Had he received prompt medical attention, his illness would likely have been cured.

Betty Yee was a 68-year-old woman with angina, high blood pressure, and diabetes. Her total bill for medications, only partly covered by Medicare, came to $150 per month. She was unable to afford the medications, her blood pressure went out of control, and she suffered a stroke. Ms. Yee's final lonely years were spent in a nursing home; she was paralyzed on her right side and unable to speak.

Consuelo Gonzalez had moderate pain in her back relieved by over-the-counter acetaminophen. She went to an orthopedic surgeon who ordered an MRI, which showed a small disc protrusion. The doctor recommended surgery, after which Ms. Gonzalez' pain became much worse. She consulted a general internist who told her that the MRI abnormality was not serious, that the surgery had been unnecessary, and that physical therapy might help. After a year of physical therapy, the pain partially subsided.

SPENDING TOO MUCH AND GETTING TOO LITTLE

The United States is spending too much money on health care and getting too little health. Health care spending per person is far higher than in other high-income countries. Yet the United States is the only one of those countries that does not have universal health coverage. The United States has the lowest life expectancy at birth, the highest death rates for avoidable or treatable conditions, and the highest maternal and infant mortality among high income nations—health statistics comparable to much less economically developed nations. Racial and ethnic inequities abound in the United States; for example, average life expectancy in 2019 for Black Americans and American Indians or Alaska Natives was 4 and 7 years lower, respectively, than for White Americans (Commonwealth Fund, 2023).

The mirror image of these deficiencies is that many Americans, like Consuelo Gonzalez, receive too much health care and end up in worse health. Studies suggest that perhaps one-fourth of hospital days, one-fourth of procedures, and two-fifths of medications are unnecessary (Brook, 1989). Waste is estimated to account for 25% of total US health care spending (Shrank et al., 2019).

THE PUBLIC'S VIEW OF THE HEALTH CARE SYSTEM

Health care in the United States encompasses a wide spectrum, ranging from the highest-quality, most compassionate treatment of those with complex illnesses, to the turning away of the very ill because of lack of ability to pay; from well-designed protocols for prevention of illness to inappropriate high-risk surgical procedures performed on uninformed patients. While the past decades have witnessed major upheavals in health care, one fundamental truth remains: the United States has the least universal, most costly health care system in the industrialized world.

Many people view the high costs of care, the lack of universal access, and pervasive health inequities as indicators of serious failings in the health care system. A 2022 Gallup poll found that only 38% of people in the United States had confidence in the health care system; 78% worry about the availability and affordability of health care.

WHAT TO EXPECT FROM THIS BOOK

To correct the weaknesses of the health care system while building on its strengths, it is necessary to understand how the system works. To promote that understanding, the book is organized into 5 sections: Financing and Payment; Equity and Resource Allocation; the Organization of Health Care; Cost, Quality, and Value; and the Political Economy of Health Care. Section One describes how money moves in the health care system. Why do we start by focusing on money? Although money is largely a means to the end of delivering health services to meet the needs of the public, much of health policymaking focuses on financing and payment as key levers for influencing health system performance. Chapters 2 and 3 discuss private and public models of health insurance, the growing problem of underinsurance (high out-of-pocket costs for many people who have health insurance), and how insurance coverage affects access to care. Chapter 4 focuses on how money moves from health insurance plans to the people and organizations delivering care and the different ways of paying health care providers.

Section Two picks up on the theme of health access by providing a conceptual framework for understanding health equity. Chapter 5 examines health and health care inequities based on race-ethnicity, gender, sexual orientation, and other factors, and how systemic and interpersonal racism and other forms of oppression of marginalized groups contribute to these inequities. Chapter 6 adds the framework of medical ethics for understanding social justice in health care, including issues of resource allocation.

Section Three turns to the organization of health care. Chapter 7 provides a conceptual overview, grouping services and providers into primary, secondary, and tertiary care sectors. Chapter 8 then reviews the history of different organizational models in the United States from the independent physician offices and community hospitals of the twentieth century to the large vertically and horizontally integrated delivery systems prevalent in the twenty-first century. Central to the organization of care is the people working in the health care system, the topic of Chapter 9. Section Three closes by shining a light on an often-neglected component of the health care system: long-term care for people living with disabilities who need ongoing assistance in activities of daily living.

Section Four covers cost, quality, and value. Value in health care is defined as the quality of care achieved for a given cost. This framework is used in Chapter 11 to describe how controlling costs may be painful to patients' health, or painless, depending on whether the approach increases value. Specific cost control mechanisms are reviewed in Chapter 12 and quality improvement strategies are discussed in Chapter 13. Prevention and public health interventions are often high-value approaches; these are covered in Chapter 14.

Section Five addresses the political economy of health care. We begin by describing the ways in which four other nations (Germany, Canada, the United Kingdom, and Japan) approach health care financing, payment, and organization and the lessons of these models for the United States. We then review more than 100 years of efforts in the United States to achieve universal health coverage, leading up to enactment of the Affordable Care Act in 2010. The section closes with a critical examination of the business of US health care in an era in which investor-owned, for-profit enterprises are consolidating into huge conglomerates with tremendous economic power in the US health care market.

To improve health policy, one must first understand the basic concepts, terms, and workings of health care. To chart a better future for health care in the United States, one must understand the health system's current performance, how we got to where we are, and the forces driving this ever-evolving story. Better understanding is the goal of this book.

REFERENCES

Brook RH. Practice guidelines and practicing medicine. *JAMA*. 1989;262:3027–3030.

Commonwealth Fund. U.S. Health Care from a Global Perspective, 2022: Accelerating Spending, Worsening Outcomes. Issue Brief, January 31, 2023. https://www.commonwealthfund.org/publications/issue-briefs/2023/jan/us-health-care-global-perspective-2022.

Shrank WH, Rogstad TL, Parekh N. Waste in the US health care system. *JAMA*. 2019;322:1501–1509.

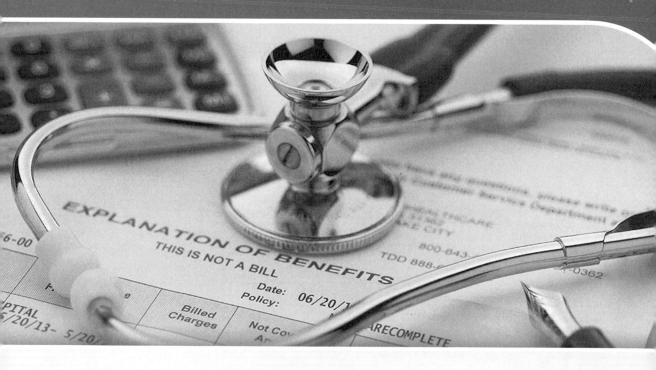

FINANCING AND PAYMENT– HOW MONEY MOVES

Paying for Health Care

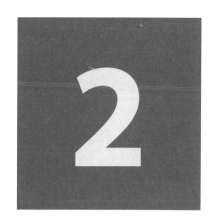

Health care is not free. Someone must pay. But how? Does each person pay when receiving care? Do people contribute regular amounts in advance so that their care will be paid for when they need it? When a person contributes in advance, might the contribution be used for care given to someone else? If so, who should pay how much? Should people's spending on health care differ based on their health care needs or level of income?

Health care financing in the United States evolved to its current state through a series of social interventions. Each intervention solved a problem but in turn created its own problems requiring further intervention. This chapter will use an historical framework to discuss the evolution of health care financing, tracing the development of private insurance as well as major government programs such as Medicare and the Patient Protection and Affordable Care Act (ACA).

MODES OF PAYING FOR HEALTH CARE

The four basic modes of paying for health care are out-of-pocket payment, individual private insurance, employment-based group private insurance, and government financing (Table 2–1). These four modes can be viewed both as an historical progression and as a categorization of current health care financing.

▷ Out-of-Pocket Payments

Fred Farmer broke his leg in 1919. His son ran 4 miles to get the doctor, who came to the farm to splint the leg. Fred gave the doctor a couple of chickens to pay for the visit. His great-grandson, Ted, who

was uninsured, broke his leg in 2019. He was driven to the emergency department, where the physician ordered an x-ray and called in an orthopedist who placed a cast on the leg. The cost was $11,800.

One hundred years ago, people like Fred Farmer paid physicians and other health care practitioners in cash or through barter. In the first half of the twentieth century, out-of-pocket cash payment was the most common method of payment. This is the simplest mode of financing—direct purchase by the consumer of goods and services (Fig. 2–1).

People in the United States purchase most consumer items and services, from haircuts to gourmet restaurant dinners, through direct out-of-pocket payments. This is not the case with health care (Arrow, 1963; Evans, 1984), and one may ask why health care is not considered a typical consumer item.

Need Versus Luxury

Whereas a gourmet dinner is a luxury, health care is regarded as a basic human need by most people.

For 2 weeks, Marina Perez has had vaginal bleeding and has felt dizzy. She has no insurance and is terrified that medical care might eat up her $500 in savings. She scrapes together $100 to see her doctor, who finds that her blood pressure falls to 90/50 mm Hg upon standing and that her hematocrit is 26%. The doctor calls Marina's sister Juanita to drive her to the hospital. Marina gets into the car and tells Juanita to take her home.

Table 2–1. Health care financing in 2020

Type of Payment	Percentage of National Health Expenditures, 2020
Out-of-pocket payment	10%
Individual private insurance	9%
Employment-based private insurance	29%[a]
Government financing	42%
Other	10%
Total	100%

Principal Source of Coverage	Percentage of Population, 2020[b]
Uninsured	9%
Individual private insurance	10%
Employment-based private insurance	49%
Government financing	32%
Total	100%

Sources: Data extracted from U.S. Census Bureau: *Health Insurance Coverage* in the United States: 2020, September 2021. https://www.census.gov/content/dam/Census/library/publications/2021/demo/p60-274.pdf; Hartman M, Martin AB, Washington B, Catlin A. National health care spending in 2020: growth driven by federal spending in response to the COVID-19 pandemic. *Health Aff (Millwood).* 2022;41:13–25.
[a]Because private insurance tends to cover healthier people, the percentage of expenditures is less than the percentage of population covered. Public expenditures are higher than the percent of the population covered because older adults and persons with disabilities are concentrated in the public Medicare and Medicaid programs.
[b]Because many people have more than one source of coverage, these numbers are estimates.

If health care is a basic human right, then people who are unable to afford health care must have a payment mechanism available that is not reliant on out-of-pocket payments.

Unpredictability of Need and Cost

Whereas the purchase of a gourmet meal is a matter of choice and the price is shown to the buyer, the need for and cost of health care services are unpredictable. Most people do not know if or when they may become severely ill or injured or what the cost of care will be.

Jake has a headache and visits the doctor, but he does not know whether the headache will cost $100 for a physician visit plus the price of a bottle of ibuprofen, $1,400 for an MRI, or $900,000 for surgery and irradiation for brain cancer.

The unpredictability of many health care needs makes it difficult to plan for these expenses. The medical costs associated with serious illness or injury exceed a middle-class family's savings.

Patients Need to Rely on Physician Recommendations

Unlike the purchaser of a gourmet meal, a person in need of health care may have little knowledge of what he or she is buying at the time when care is needed.

Jenny develops acute abdominal pain and goes to the hospital to purchase a remedy for her pain. The physician tells her that she has acute cholecystitis or a perforated ulcer and recommends hospitalization, an abdominal CT scan, and upper endoscopic studies. Will Jenny, lying on a gurney in the emergency room and clutching her abdomen with one hand, use her other hand to leaf through a textbook of internal medicine to determine whether she really needs these services, and should she have brought along a copy of Consumer Reports to learn where to purchase them at the cheapest price?

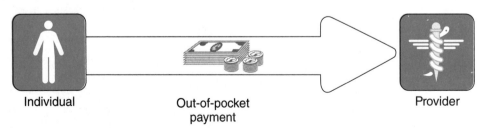

Individual   Out-of-pocket payment   Provider

▲ **Figure 2–1.** Out-of-pocket payment is made directly from patient to provider.

Health care is the foremost example of asymmetry of information between providers and consumers (Evans, 1984). A patient with abdominal pain is in a poor position to question a physician who is ordering laboratory tests, x-rays, or surgery. When health care is elective, patients can weigh the pros and cons of different treatment options, but even so, recommendations may be filtered through the biases of the physician providing the information. Compared with the voluntary demand for gourmet meals, the demand for health services is partially involuntary and is often physician rather than consumer-driven.

For these reasons among others, out-of-pocket payments are flawed as a method of paying for health care services. Because the direct purchase of health services became increasingly difficult for consumers and was not meeting the needs of hospitals and physicians to be reliably paid, health insurance came into being.

Individual Private Insurance

In 2012, Brian Carpenter was self-employed. To pay the $800 monthly premium for his individual health insurance policy, he had to work extra jobs on weekends, and the $5,000 deductible meant he would still have to pay quite a bit of his family's medical costs out of pocket. Mr. Carpenter preferred to pay these costs rather than take the risk of spending the money saved for his children's college education on a major illness. When he became ill with leukemia and the hospital bill reached $280,000, Mr. Carpenter appreciated the value of health insurance. Nonetheless he had to feel disgruntled when

he read a newspaper story listing his insurance company among those that paid out on average less than 65 cents for health services for every dollar collected in premiums.

With private health insurance, a third party, the insurer, is added to the patient and health care provider, who are the two basic parties of the health care arrangement. While the out-of-pocket mode of payment is limited to a single financial transaction, private insurance requires two transactions—a premium payment from the individual to an insurance plan (also called a health plan), and a payment from the insurance plan to the provider (Fig. 2–2). Most insurance plans require patients to pay out-of-pocket for the first portion of their health expenses each year before insurance coverage kicks in; these deductibles may be on the order of $2,000 or more per year. In addition, insurance plans often require patients to pay part of the cost of each service as coinsurance (e.g., patients pay 20% of the cost of a physician visit), or copayment (e.g., patients pay $20 for each visit or prescription).

In nineteenth-century Europe, voluntary benefit funds were set up by guilds, industries, and mutual societies. In return for paying a monthly sum, people received assistance in case of illness. This early form of private health insurance was slow to develop in the United States. In the early twentieth century, European immigrants set up some small benevolent societies in US cities to provide sickness benefits for their members. In the early twentieth century, two commercial insurance companies, Metropolitan Life and Prudential, collected 10 to 25 cents per week from workers for life insurance policies that also paid for funerals and the expenses of

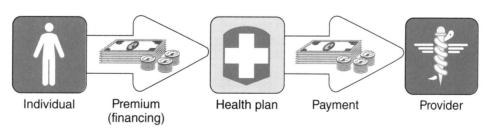

Individual   Premium   Health plan   Payment   Provider
                   (financing)

▲ Figure 2–2. Individual private insurance. A third party, the insurance plan (health plan), is added, dividing payment into a financing component and a payment component. The ACA added a federal subsidy to help individuals pay the insurance premium.

a final illness. The policies were paid for by individuals on a weekly basis, so large numbers of insurance agents had to visit their clients to collect the premiums as soon after payday as possible. Because of the huge administrative costs, individual health insurance remained a minor method of paying for health care in the twentieth century (Starr, 1982). Insurance plans also began charging much higher premiums to people with high medical needs than to healthy people, making individual insurance unaffordable for the people who needed it the most (a practice known as "experience rating," which is discussed more at the end of the chapter).

In 2014, Brian Carpenter signed up for individual insurance for his family of four through Covered California, the state exchange set up under the Affordable Care Act. Because his family income was 200% of the federal poverty level, he received a subsidy of $1,373 per month, meaning that his premium would be only $252 per month for a silver plan. His deductible was $2,000. Insurance companies were no longer allowed to deny coverage for his preexisting leukemia.

The ACA, enacted in 2010 and implemented in 2014, resuscitated the long dormant financing method of individual insurance. To attract people who were otherwise uninsured to purchase individual private insurance, the ACA provides federal subsidies, like the one Brian Carpenter enjoyed, to obtain individual private health insurance through federal or state health insurance exchanges (Kaiser Family Foundation, 2013). Subsidies became available for individuals and families with incomes between 100% and 400% of the federal poverty level ($27,750 to $111,000 for a family of four in 2022). The American Rescue Plan Act of 2021 and the Inflation Reduction Act of 2022, enacted during the COVID-19 pandemic, temporarily added subsidies for many middle-income individuals and families with incomes above 400% of the federal policy level and made the subsidies more generous for people at all income levels. The ACA established federal and state-based insurance exchanges to assist people seeking individual coverage to shop for insurance plans meeting the federal standards, simplifying the process of comparing plans for consumers. The ACA also prohibited insurance companies from denying coverage for medical conditions that existed prior to the purchase of

the insurance. The benefit packages offered by plans in the exchanges vary depending on whether individuals purchase a low-premium bronze plan with high out-of-pocket costs, a high-premium platinum plan with lower out-of-pocket costs, or intermediate silver or gold plans (Table 2–2). In addition to providing a "carrot" for people to purchase individual insurance, the ACA also initially had a "stick." The ACA required all US citizens and legal residents to have insurance coverage with generous benefits. To ensure that healthy people formed part of the market pool so as to "spread risk," those who failed to purchase individual insurance and did not have employer-sponsored insurance, or did not qualify for

Table 2–2. Summary of the individual health insurance provisions of the Affordable Care Act (ACA), 2022

As enacted in 2010, US citizens and legal residents were required to have health coverage with exemptions available for such issues as financial hardship. Those who chose to go without coverage paid a tax penalty. In 2017, the tax penalty was reduced to $0, essentially eliminating the original individual mandate (the requirement that people without health insurance purchase an individual insurance plan).

Tax credits, which help pay for health insurance premiums, increase for families with incomes from 100% to 400% of the Federal Poverty Level. In addition cost-sharing subsidies reduce the amount of out-of-pocket costs individuals and families must pay; the amount of subsidy varies by income.

Uninsured individuals and families purchase individual insurance though insurance marketplaces called health insurance exchanges. Seventeen states have elected to set up their own exchanges and the remainder of states are covered by the federal exchange, Healthcare.gov.

The American Rescue Plan of 2021 increased the dollar amounts of the subsidies and extended subsidies above 400% of the Federal Poverty Level for 2021 and 2022. The Inflation Reduction Act of 2022 further extended these changes through 2025.

Insurance companies marketing their plans through the exchanges offer four benefit categories:
- Bronze plans have low premiums but higher out-of-pocket costs
- Silver plans have fewer out-of-pocket costs and higher premiums
- Gold plans have low out-of-pocket costs and high premiums
- Platinum plans have very low out-of-pocket costs and very high premiums

Under the American Rescue Plan, about 5 million people can purchase a Silver plan for no premium and average yearly deductibles of $177, because subsidies increased markedly under this legislation.

Source: Kaiser Family Foundation. Explaining health care reform: questions about health insurance subsidies. Issue brief. November 2018. https://www.kff.org/health-reform/issue-brief/explaining-health-care-reform-questions. Kaiser Family Foundation. How the American Rescue Plan Affects Subsidies for Marketplace Shoppers and People Who Are Uninsured. March 25, 2021. https://www.kff.org/health-reform/issue-brief/how-the-american-rescue-plan-act-affects-subsidies-for-marketplace-shoppers-and-people-who-are-uninsured/.

Medicaid, Medicare, or veteran's health care benefits, had to pay a tax penalty. In 2017, the tax penalty was repealed. The legislative history and contentious politics of the ACA are discussed in Chapter 16.

Employment-Based Private Insurance

Betty Lerner and her schoolteacher colleagues each paid $6 per year to Prepaid Hospital in 1929. Ms. Lerner suffered a heart attack and was hospitalized at no cost. The following year Prepaid Hospital built a new wing and raised the teachers' prepayment to $12.

Rose Riveter retired in 1961. Her health insurance premium for hospital and physician care, formerly paid by her employer, had been $25 per month. When she called the insurance company to obtain individual coverage, she was told that premiums at age 65 cost $70 per month. She could not afford the insurance and wondered what would happen if she became ill.

A different approach to private health insurance in the United States was impelled by the increasing effectiveness and rising costs of hospital care at a time when few people had individual insurance. Hospitals became places not only in which to die, but also in which to get well. However, many patients were unable to pay for hospital care, and this meant that hospitals were unable to attract "customers."

In 1929, Baylor University Hospital agreed to provide up to 21 days of hospital care to 1,500 Dallas schoolteachers such as Betty Lerner if they paid the hospital $6 per person per year. As the Great Depression deepened and private hospital occupancy in 1931 fell to 62%, similar hospital-centered private insurance plans spread. These plans (anticipating "narrow network" managed care plans), restricted care to a particular hospital. The American Hospital Association built on this prepayment movement and established statewide Blue Cross hospital insurance plans allowing free choice of hospital. By 1940, 39 Blue Cross plans controlled by the private hospital industry had enrolled over 6 million people. The Great Depression reduced the amount patients could pay physicians out of pocket, and in 1939, the California Medical Association set up the first Blue Shield plan to cover physician services. These plans, controlled by state medical societies, followed Blue Cross in spreading across the nation (Starr, 1982; Fein, 1986).

In contrast to the consumer-driven development of health insurance in European nations, coverage in the United States was initiated by health care providers seeking a steady source of income. Hospital and physician control over the "Blues," a major sector of the health insurance industry, guaranteed that payment would be generous and that cost control would remain on the back burner (Law, 1974; Starr, 1982).

The rapid growth of employment-based private insurance was spurred by an accident of history. During World War II, wage and price controls prevented companies from granting wage increases, but allowed the growth of fringe benefits. With a labor shortage, companies competing for workers began to offer health insurance to employees such as Rose Riveter as a fringe benefit. After the war, unions picked up on this trend and negotiated for health benefits. The results were dramatic: Enrollment in group hospital insurance plans grew from 12 million in 1940 to 142 million in 1988.

With employment-based health insurance, employers pay a portion of the premium that purchases health insurance for their employees (Fig. 2–3). However, this flow of money is not as simple as it looks. The federal government views employer premium payments as a

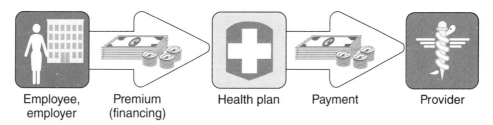

| Employee, employer | Premium (financing) | Health plan | Payment | Provider |

▲ Figure 2–3. Employment-based private insurance. In addition to the direct employer subsidy, indirect government subsidies occur through the tax-free status of employer contributions for health insurance benefits.

tax-deductible business expense. The government does not treat the health insurance fringe benefit as taxable income to the employee, even though the payment of premiums could be interpreted as a form of employee income. Because each premium dollar of employer-sponsored health insurance results in a reduction in taxes collected, the government is in essence subsidizing employer-sponsored health insurance. This subsidy is enormous, estimated at $316 billion in 2022.

The growth of employment-based health insurance attracted commercial insurance companies to the health care field to compete with the Blues for customers. The commercial insurers changed the entire dynamic of health insurance. The new dynamic was called **experience rating**. (The following discussion of experience rating applies to individual as well as employment-based private insurance.)

Healthy Insurance Company insures three groups of people—a young healthy group of bank managers, an older healthy group of truck drivers, and an older group of coal miners with a high rate of chronic illness. Under experience rating, Healthy sets its premiums according to the experience of each group in using health services. Because the bank managers rarely use health care, each pays a premium of $600 per month. Because the truck drivers are older, their risk of illness is higher, and their premium is $800 per month. The miners, who have high rates of black lung disease, are charged a premium of $1,000 per month. The average premium income to Healthy is $800 per member per month.

Blue Cross insures the same three groups and needs the same $800 per member per month to cover health care plus administrative costs for these groups. Blue Cross sets its premiums by the principle of community rating. For a given health insurance policy, all subscribers in a community pay the same premium. The bank managers, truck drivers, and mine workers all pay $800 per month.

Health insurance provides a mechanism to distribute health care more in accordance with human need rather than exclusively on the basis of ability to pay. To achieve this goal, funds are redistributed from the healthy to the sick, a subsidy that helps pay the costs of those unable to purchase services on their own.

Community rating achieves this redistribution in two ways:

1. Within each group (bank managers, truck drivers, and mine workers), people who become ill receive benefits in excess of the premiums they pay, while people who remain healthy pay premiums while receiving few or no health benefits.
2. Among the three groups, the bank managers, who use less health care than their premiums are worth, help pay for the miners, who use more health care than their premiums could buy.

Experience rating is less redistributive than community rating. Within each group, those who become ill are subsidized by those who remain well, but among the different groups, healthier groups (bank managers) do not subsidize high-risk groups (mine workers). Thus the principle of health insurance, which is to distribute health care more in accordance with human need rather than exclusively on the ability to pay, is weakened by experience rating (Light, 1992).

In the early years, Blue Cross plans set insurance premiums by the principle of community rating, whereas commercial insurers used experience rating as a "weapon" to compete with the Blues (Fein, 1986). Commercial insurers such as Healthy Insurance Company could offer cheaper premiums to low-risk employee groups such as bank managers, who would naturally choose a Healthy commercial plan at $600 over a Blue Cross plan at $800. Experience rating helped commercial insurers overtake the Blues in the private health insurance market. Moreover, many commercial insurers would not market employment-based or individual policies to such high-risk groups as mine workers, leaving Blue Cross with high-risk patients who were paying relatively low premiums. To survive the competition from the commercial insurers, many Blue Cross and Blue Shield plans switched to experience rating. As community rating withered, people who were older or sicker became less and less able to afford health insurance.

From the perspective of older adults and those with chronic illness, experience rating is discriminatory. Healthy persons, however, might have another viewpoint and might ask why they should voluntarily transfer their wealth to sicker people through the insurance subsidy. The answer lies in the unpredictability of health care needs. When purchasing health insurance, an individual does not know if he or she will suddenly change from a state of good health to one of illness. Thus, *within a group*, people are willing to risk paying for health insurance, even though they may not use it until later in their lives. *Among different groups*, however, healthy people have no economic incentive to voluntarily pay for community rating and subsidize another group of sicker people. This is why community rating cannot survive alongside experience rating in a market-driven competitive private insurance system (Aaron, 1991).

In a major reform contained within the ACA, insurers are now severely limited in using experience rating to set premiums; they can only vary premiums based on family size, geographic location, age, and smoking status, and limits are placed on how much premiums can differ between older and younger individuals (HealthCare.gov). The ACA restricts variation in premium costs and also prohibits the most extreme form of experience rating—complete denial of coverage based on preexisting conditions.

The most positive aspect of health insurance—that it assists people with serious illness to pay for their care—has also become one of its main drawbacks—the difficulty in controlling costs in an insurance environment. With direct purchase, the "invisible hand" of each individual's ability to pay holds down the price and quantity of health care. However, if a patient is well insured and the cost of care causes no immediate fiscal pain, the patient will use more services than someone who must pay for care out of pocket. In addition, particularly before the advent of regulation of fees by insurance plans, health care providers could increase fees more easily if a third party was available to foot the bill.

Thus, health insurance was originally an attempt by society to solve the problem of unaffordable health care under an out-of-pocket payment system, but its very capacity to make health care more affordable created a new problem. If people no longer had to pay out of their own pockets for health care, they would use more health care; and if health care providers could charge insurers rather than patients, they could more easily raise prices, especially during the era when the major insurers (the Blues) were controlled by hospitals and physicians. The solution of insurance fueled the problem of rising costs. As private insurance in the latter portion of the twentieth century became largely experience rated and employment based, persons who had low incomes, who were chronically ill, or who were older found it increasingly difficult to pay for care out-of-pocket or afford individual insurance.

▶ Government Financing

In 1984 at age 74 Rose Riveter developed colon cancer. She was now covered by Medicare, which had been enacted in 1965. Even so, her Medicare premium, hospital deductible expenses, physician copayments, short nursing home stay, and uncovered prescriptions cost her $2,700 the year she became ill with cancer.

Employment-based private health insurance grew rapidly in the 1950s, helping working people and their families to afford health care. But two groups in the population received little or no benefit: people in low-income brackets and older adults. People in low-income brackets were usually unemployed or employed in jobs without the fringe benefit of health insurance; they could not afford insurance premiums. Older adults, who needed health care the most and whose premiums had been partially subsidized by community rating, were hard hit by the trend toward experience rating. In the late 1950s, fewer than 15% of older adults had any health insurance (Harris, 1966). Only one program could provide affordable care for these two groups: tax-financed government health insurance.

Government entered the health care financing arena long before the 1960s through direct public provision of care such as the Indian Health Service, state-operated mental hospitals, and municipal hospitals. But only with the 1965 enactment of Medicare (for older adults and for some people with disabilities) and Medicaid (for people in low-income brackets) did public insurance payments for privately operated health services become a major feature of health care in the United States. Medicare Part A (Table 2–3) covers hospital care and is financed largely through social security taxes from employers and employees. Medicare Part B (Table 2–4) covers physician services and is paid for by federal taxes and monthly premiums from beneficiaries. Medicare Part D, enacted in 2003, offers prescription drug coverage and is financed by

Table 2–3. Summary of Medicare Part A, 2023

Who is eligible?

Upon reaching the age of 65 years, people who are eligible for Social Security are automatically enrolled in Medicare Part A whether or not they are retired. A person who has paid into the Social Security system for 10 years and that person's spouse are eligible for Social Security. People who are not eligible for Social Security can enroll in Medicare Part A by paying a monthly premium.

People under the age of 65 years who are totally and permanently disabled may enroll in Medicare Part A after they have been receiving Social Security disability benefits for 24 months. People with amyotrophic lateral sclerosis (ALS) or end-stage renal disease requiring dialysis or a transplant are also eligible for Medicare Part A without a 2-year waiting period.

How is it financed?

Financing is through the Social Security system. Employers and employees each pay to Medicare 1.45% of wages and salaries. Self-employed people pay 2.9%. The 2010 Affordable Care Act increased the employee rate for higher-income taxpayers (incomes greater than $200,000 for individuals or $250,000 for couples) from 1.45% to 2.35%.

What services are covered?[a]

Services	Benefit	Medicare Pays
Hospitalization	First 60 days period[b] 61st to 90th day[b] 91st day and beyond with lifetime reserve days[c] Beyond 90 days if lifetime reserve days are used up	All but a $1,600 deductible per benefit period All but $400/day All but $800/day Nothing
Skilled nursing facility	First 20 days 21st to 100th day Beyond 100 days	All All but $200/day Nothing
Home health care	Medically necessary care for homebound people, provided by professionals such as nurses, physical/occupational/speech therapists, medical social workers, but not for custodial or personal care such as help with meals, cleaning, shopping	100% for skilled care as defined by Medicare regulations
Hospice care	As long as a doctor certifies person suffers from a terminal illness	100% for most services, copays for outpatient drugs and 5% coinsurance for inpatient respite care
Unskilled nursing home care	Care that is mainly custodial is not covered	Nothing

[a]For patients in Medicare Advantage plans, covered services and patient responsibility for payment changes based on the specifics of each Medicare Advantage plan.
[b]Part A benefits are provided by each benefit period rather than for each year. A benefit period begins when a beneficiary enters a hospital and ends 60 days after discharge from the hospital or from a skilled nursing facility.
[c]Beyond 90 days, Medicare pays for 60 additional days only once in a lifetime ("lifetime reserve days").

federal taxes and monthly premiums from beneficiaries. Medicaid is a program run by the states that is funded by federal and state taxes, which pays for the care of millions of low-income people. In 2020, Medicare and Medicaid expenditures totaled $830 and $671 billion, respectively (Hartman et al., 2022).

Medicare

In 2022, Medicare served 59 million people. With its large deductibles, copayments, and gaps in coverage, Medicare beneficiaries are in need of additional insurance. Many purchase supplemental private insurance or have retiree coverage from their previous employment. About 20% of Medicare beneficiaries also receive Medicaid coverage, which serves as secondary insurance and covers many costs not paid by Medicare. The 10% of beneficiaries with no additional coverage paid an average of $7,473 in out-of-pocket costs in 2016 (Kaiser Family Foundation, 2019).

The Medicare Modernization Act (MMA) of 2003 made two major changes in the Medicare program: the the establishment of a prescription drug benefit (Part D) and expansion of the role of private health plans (the Medicare Advantage program, Part C).

Table 2–4. Summary of Medicare Part B, 2023

Who is eligible?
People who are eligible for Medicare Part A who elect to pay the Medicare Part B premium of $164.90 per month. Some low-income persons can receive financial assistance with the premium and the Part B deductible. Higher-income beneficiaries (over $97,000 for individual, $194,000 for couple) have higher premiums related to income.

How is it financed?
Financing is in part by general federal revenues (personal income and other federal taxes) and in part by Part B monthly premiums.

What services are covered?[a]

Services	Benefit	Medicare Pays
Medical expenses Physician services Physical, occupational, and speech therapy Medical equipment Diagnostic tests (no coinsurance for laboratory services)	All medically necessary services	80% of approved amount after a $226 annual deductible
Preventive care	Pap smears; mammograms; colorectal/prostate cancer, cardiovascular and diabetes screening; pneumococcal and influenza vaccinations; yearly physical examinations	Included in medical expenses, and for some services the deductible and 20% copayment are waived
Outpatient medications	Partially covered under Medicare Part D	All except for premium, deductible, and coinsurance
Eye refractions, hearing aids, dental services	Not covered	Nothing

[a]For patients in Medicare Advantage plans, covered services and patient responsibility for payment change based on the specifics of each Medicare Advantage plan.

Medicare Drug Benefit One of the glaring omissions in the original enactment of Medicare was the failure to include coverage for medications, unless administered as part of a hospital stay. Medicare Part D provides partial coverage for prescription drugs, administered by private insurance companies, with 73% of the premiums for these Part D plans financed through government revenues and the rest from premiums paid directly by beneficiaries. In 2021, 77% of Medicare beneficiaries were enrolled in Part D plans. The average 2022 premium was $33 per month with some plans charging over $100 per month. The standard Part D deductible in 2019 was $480, but plans can set their deductible lower. Beneficiary cost-sharing also varies by plan, and copayments are greater for more expensive drugs (Kaiser Family Foundation, 2021b).

Part D has been criticized for the substantial out-of-pocket payments that beneficiaries still must pay for medications, and for the decision to contract drug coverage through a proliferation of private drug plans, each with their own different and changing formularies of covered medications which create confusion for beneficiaries. Moreover, the MMA prohibited government from negotiating with pharmaceutical companies for lower drug prices. The Inflation Reduction Act of 2022 assists Part D beneficiaries by imposing a $2,000 per year cap on drug out-of-pocket costs for beneficiaries starting in 2025 and by limiting increases in Part D premiums from 2024 to 2030. In addition, Medicare will be allowed to negotiate prices with drug manufacturers for 10 drugs in 2026 and more drugs thereafter (Kaiser Family Foundation, 2022c).

Medicare Advantage Under the Medicare Advantage program, a beneficiary can elect to enroll in a private managed care health plan contracting with Medicare. Medicare subsidizes the premium for that private health plan and the health plan pays physicians, hospitals, and other providers. Beneficiaries' out-of-pocket costs are lower if they receive care from entities contracting with their Medicare Advantage plan, and most plans include the Medicare Part D drug benefit and often some additional benefits, giving beneficiaries a financial incentive to join a Medicare Advantage plan. In 2022, almost half of Medicare beneficiaries were enrolled in a Medicare Advantage plan. Two for-profit health insurance companies—UnitedHealthcare and Humana—account for 46% of the Medicare Advantage market (Kaiser Family Foundation, 2022a). Two-thirds of Medicare Advantage enrollees pay no additional premium to enroll in a Medicare Advantage plan, other than their usual Medicare Part B premium (Kaiser Family Foundation, 2022b).

To channel more patients into Medicare Advantage plans, the MMA provided generous payments to those plans. In 2019, Medicare paid $321 more per beneficiary for Medicare Advantage enrollees than for those in traditional Medicare (Kaiser Family Foundation, 2021a) even though Medicare Advantage enrollees are overall healthier (Weil, 2019). The plans receive higher federal payments for patients who have a greater disease burden score, and plans commonly up-code diagnoses to inappropriately raise their scores and thereby inflate their payments. Audits of 37 plans found that all but two plans were overpaid, costing the Medicare program tens of billions of dollars (Schulte, 2019). These findings have challenged the notion of Medicare Advantage being a "better value" option for Medicare.

In summary, Medicare is a complex program. Although a type of government insurance, with the majority of program costs financed through taxes, a growing proportion of its benefits are channeled through an array of private insurance plans. Critics of this trend argue that the program would be far simpler and less costly if the government maintained direct control over payments to physicians, hospitals, and pharmaceutical suppliers.

Medicaid

The Medicaid program is jointly administered by the federal and state governments. Initially, the federal government contributed between 50% and 76% of total Medicaid costs, with the federal contribution being greater for states with lower per capita incomes. Although designed for low-income Americans, not all people in low-income brackets have traditionally been eligible for Medicaid. Until enactment of the ACA, Medicaid required that people not only be in low-income brackets but also meet "categorical" eligibility

criteria such as being a young child, pregnant, older adult, or person with disabilities.

The ACA eliminated the categorical eligibility criteria and required that beginning in 2014, states offer the program to all citizens and legal residents with income at or below 138% of the Federal Poverty Level—$18,754 for an individual or $38,295 for a family of four in 2022. The ACA intended that all states expand Medicaid eligibility and provided states an incentive for expansion by having the federal government pay almost all the cost of the increased Medicaid enrollment. However, in June 2012, the Supreme Court ruled that the ACA's Medicaid expansion was optional for states. In 2023, 40 states plus the District of Columbia had expanded Medicaid.

In 2022, Medicaid covered 82 million people, making it the single largest health insurance program in the nation. In response to the COVID-19 pandemic, the Federal Government relaxed Medicaid eligibility resulting in a 17 million increase in Medicaid recipients between February 2020 (just before the pandemic) and April 2022. When the expansion of eligibility ends in 2023, between 5 and 14 million people may be disenrolled from Medicaid.

Since 1981, the federal government has ceded to states enhanced control over Medicaid programs through Medicaid waivers, which may allow states to increase or reduce the scope of covered services, require Medicaid recipients to pay part of their costs, and obligate Medicaid recipients to enroll in managed care plans (see Chapter 4). In 2022, 69% of Medicaid recipients were enrolled in managed care plans. Because Medicaid paid primary care physicians an average of 72% of Medicare fees in 2019 (in some states below 60%), many physicians limit the number of Medicaid patients they will see, especially in states with low Medicaid payment rates and in states with more Medicaid managed care (Holgash & Heberlein, 2019; Zuckerman et al., 2021).

In 1997, the federal government created the Children's Health Insurance Program (CHIP), a companion program to Medicaid, to cover children in low-income families with earnings above Medicaid eligibility. CHIP plans covered 7 million children in 2022. Although undocumented immigrants are generally not eligible for Medicaid, the Federal Government allows states to include coverage of prenatal care for undocumented immigrants under CHIP. In 2022,

18 states included this benefit for undocumented immigrants (Kaiser Family Foundation, 2022d).

Government health insurance for people in low-income brackets and older adults added a new factor to the health care financing equation: the taxpayer (Fig. 2–4). With government-financed health plans, the taxpayer can interact with the health care consumer in two distinct ways:

1. The social insurance model, exemplified by Medicare, allows only those who have paid a certain amount of social security taxes to be eligible for Part A and only those who pay a monthly premium to receive benefits from Parts B and D. As with private insurance, social insurance requires people to make a contribution in order to receive benefits.
2. The contrasting model is the Medicaid public assistance model, in which eligibility is not linked to an individual's personal tax payments and many of those who contribute (taxpayers) may not be eligible for benefits (Bodenheimer & Grumbach, 1992).

It must be remembered that private insurance contains a subsidy: redistribution of funds from the healthy to the sick. Tax-funded insurance has the same subsidy and usually adds another: redistribution of funds from upper- to lower-income groups. Under this double subsidy, exemplified by Medicare and Medicaid, healthy middle-income employees generally pay more in social security payments and other taxes than they receive in health services, whereas unemployed, disabled, and lower-income older adults tend to receive more in health services than they contribute in taxes.

Like employment-based private insurance, the advent of government financing improved financial access to care for some people, but, in turn, aggravated the problem of rising costs.

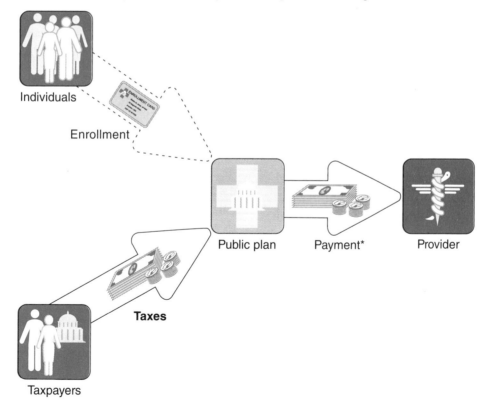

Individuals

Enrollment

Public plan   Payment*   Provider

Taxes

Taxpayers

▲ **Figure 2–4.** Government-financed insurance. Under the social insurance model (e.g., Medicare Part A), only individuals paying taxes into the public plan are eligible for benefits. In other models (e.g., Medicaid), an individual's eligibility for benefits may not be directly linked to payment of taxes into the plan.
*Some public plans, for example Medicare Advantage, pay a private insurance intermediary that in turn pays providers.

THE BURDEN OF FINANCING HEALTH CARE

Different methods of financing health care place different burdens on the various income levels of society. Payments are classified as **progressive** if they take a rising percentage of income as income increases, **regressive** if they take a falling percentage of income as income increases, and **proportional** if the ratio of payment to income is the same for all income classes (Pechman, 1985).

What principle should underlie the choice of revenue source for health care? A central purpose of the health care system is to maintain and improve the health of the nation's population. As discussed in Chapter 5, rates of mortality and disability are far higher for low-income people than for the wealthy. Burdening families who are in low-income brackets with high payments for health care (i.e., regressive payments) reduces their disposable income, amplifies ill effects of poverty, and thereby worsens their health. It makes little sense to finance a health care system—the purpose of which is to improve health—with payments that worsen health. Thus, regressive payments could be considered "unhealthy."

> *Rita earns $15,000 per year for her family of four. She develops pneumonia, and her out-of-pocket health costs come to $1,500, 10% of her family income.*

> *Cathy earns $150,000 per year for her family of four. She develops pneumonia, and her out-of-pocket health costs come to $1,500, 1% of her family income.*

Out-of-pocket payments are a regressive mode of financing. As a percent of their income, US households in the lowest-income quintile spend about 10 times more in out-of-pocket payments than households in the highest-income quintile (Carman et al., 2020). Aggravating the regressivity of out-of-pocket payments is the fact that lower-income people, who tend to be exposed to more health hazards and have access to fewer supports for health, tend to be sicker and thus have more out-of-pocket payments than the wealthier and healthier. Many economists and health policy experts would consider this regressive burden of payment as unfair.

> *Jim Hale is a young, healthy, self-employed accountant whose monthly income is $12,000, with a health insurance premium of $600, or 5% of his income.*

> *Jack Hurt is a sporadically employed construction worker. His income is $2,700 per month, of which $900 (33%) goes for his health insurance. His experience-rated insurance premium is higher because he is in poor health.*

Experience-rated private health insurance is a particularly regressive method of financing health care because it saddles people with a higher burden of illness, who are often low income, with highest costs. If Jim Hale and Jack Hurt were enrolled in a community-rated plan, each with a premium of $600, they would respectively pay 5% and 22% of their incomes for health insurance. With community rating, the burden of payment is still regressive, but less so than with experience rating.

Most private insurance is not individually purchased but rather obtained through employment. How is the burden of employment-linked health insurance premiums distributed?

> *Jill is an assistant hospital administrator. To attract her to the job, the hospital offered her a package of salary plus health insurance of $8,600 per month: $8,000 in salary and $600 for her health insurance.*

> *Bill is a nurse's aide, whose union negotiated with the hospital for a total package of $4,600 per month; of this amount $4,000 is salary and $600 pays his health insurance premium.*

Do Jill and Bill pay nothing for their health insurance? Not exactly. Employers generally agree on a total package of wages and fringe benefits; if Jill and Bill did not receive health insurance, their pay would probably go up by nearly $600 per month. That is why employer-paid health insurance premiums are generally considered deductions from wages or salary; the cost is borne by the employee (Blumberg et al., 2007). For Jill, health insurance amounts to only 7% of her income, but for Bill it is 13%. In 2012, employer-sponsored health insurance premiums represented 58% of family income for the bottom 40% of American families compared with 4% for the top 5% (Blumenthal & Squires, 2014).

> *Larry Lowe earns $20,000 in adjustable gross income, and pays $2,000 in federal and state income taxes, or 10% of his income.*

> *Harold High earns $200,000 and pays $35,700 in income taxes, or 18% of his income.*

Both Larry and Harold pay 1.45% of their incomes, or $290 and $2,900, respectively, in an additional tax earmarked for Medicare Part A. (Their employers also pay a matching 1.45% Medicare tax.)

A variety of taxes fund government health programs such as Medicare and Medicaid. One major source of financing is the income tax, which is overall a progressive tax (notwithstanding the gaming of tax-loopholes by some of the very rich). The Medicare payroll tax is a proportionate tax, in that both Larry and Harold pay the same percentage of their income. The combined burden of all taxes that finance health care is slightly progressive, with households in the highest 40% of incomes paying 10% of their income on health taxes compared with 7% of income paid by households in the lowest 60% of incomes (Carman et al., 2020).

Accounting for all sources of payment for health services, the sum total of health care financing is regressive. In 2015, households in the lowest-income quintile spent 33.9% of their income to finance health care, compared with 16.0% of income contributed by households in the highest-income quintile (Carman et al., 2022). Although people in the United States benefit from having health insurance even when regressively financed, the US health care system is overall financed in a manner that is unhealthy.

CONCLUSION

Neither Fred Farmer nor his great-grandson Ted had health insurance, but the modern-day Mr. Farmer's predicament differs dramatically from that of his ancestor. Third-party financing of health care has fueled an expansive health care system that offers treatments unimaginable a century ago, but at tremendous expense.

Each of the four modes of financing health care developed historically as a solution to the inadequacy of the previous modes. Private insurance provided protection to patients against the unpredictable costs of medical care, as well as protection to providers of care against the unpredictable ability of patients to pay. But the private insurance solution created three new, interrelated problems:

1. The opportunity for health care providers to increase fees to insurers caused health services to become increasingly unaffordable for those with inadequate insurance or no insurance.
2. The employment-based nature of group insurance placed people who were unemployed, retired, or working part-time at a disadvantage for the purchase of insurance.
3. Competition inherent in a deregulated private insurance market gave rise to the practice of experience rating, which made insurance premiums unaffordable for many older adults and other medically needy groups.

To solve these problems, government financing was required, but government financing fueled an even greater inflation in health care costs.

As each "solution" was introduced, health care financing improved for a time. But rising costs have made services unaffordable even for people who are insured (Chapter 3). The problems of each financing mode and the problems created by each successive solution have accumulated into a complex crisis characterized by inadequate access for some and high costs for everyone.

REFERENCES

Aaron HJ. *Serious and Unstable Condition: Financing America's Health Care*. Washington, DC: Brookings Institution; 1991.

Arrow KJ. Uncertainty and the welfare economics of medical care. *Am Econ Rev*. 1963;53:941.

Blumberg LJ, Holahan J, Hadley J, Nordahl K. Setting a standard of affordability for health insurance coverage. *Health Aff (Millwood)*. 2007;26:w463–w473.

Blumenthal D, Squires D. Do health care costs fuel economic inequality in the United States? The Commonwealth Fund Blog, September 9, 2014. www.commonwealthfund.org/publications/blog/2014/sep/do-health-costs-fuel-inequality.

Bodenheimer T, Grumbach K. Financing universal health insurance: taxes, premiums, and the lessons of social insurance. *J Health Polit Policy Law*. 1992;17:439–462.

Carman KG, Liu J, White C. Accounting for the burden and redistribution of health care costs: Who uses care and who pays for it. *Health Serv Res*. 2020;55(2):224–231.

Evans RG. *Strained Mercy*. Toronto: Butterworths; 1984.

Fein R. *Medical Care, Medical Costs*. Cambridge, MA: Harvard University Press; 1986.

Harris R. *A Sacred Trust*. New York, NY: New American Library; 1966.

Hartman M, Martin AB, Washington B, Catlin A. National health care spending in 2020: growth driven by federal spending in response to the COVID-19 pandemic. *Health Aff (Millwood)*. 2022;41:13–25.

Holgash K, Heberlein M. Physician acceptance of new Medicaid patients. Medicaid and CHIP Payment and Access Commission (MACPAC), January 24, 2019. https://www.macpac.gov/wp-content/uploads/2019/01/Physician-Acceptance-of-New-Medicaid-Patients.pdf.

Kaiser Family Foundation. Summary of the Affordable Care Act. 2013. http://kff.org/health-reform/fact-sheet/summary-of-the-affordable-care-act.

Kaiser Family Foundation. How Much do Medicare Beneficiaries Spend Out-of-Pocket on Health Care? November 4, 2019. https://www.kff.org/report-section/how-much-do-medicare-beneficiaries-spend-out-of-pocket-on-health-care-issue-brief/.

Kaiser Family Foundation. Higher and Faster Growing Spending Per Medicare Advantage Enrollee Adds to Medicare's Solvency and Affordability Challenges, August 17, 2021a. https://www.kff.org/medicare/issue-brief/higher-and-faster-growing-spending-per-medicare-advantage-enrollee-adds-to-medicares-solvency-and-affordability-challenges.

Kaiser Family Foundation. An Overview of the Medicare Part D Prescription Drug Benefit. October 13, 2021b. https://www.kff.org/medicare/fact-sheet/an-overview-of-the-medicare-part-d-prescription-drug-benefit/.

Kaiser Family Foundation. Medicare Advantage in 2022: Enrollment Update and Key Trends. August 25, 2022a. https://www.kff.org/medicare/issue-brief/medicare-advantage-in-2022-enrollment-update-and-key-trends.

Kaiser Family Foundation. Medicare Advantage in 2022: Premiums, Out-of Pocket Limits, Cost Sharing, Supplemental Benefits, Prior Authorizations, and Star Ratings. August 25, 2022b. https://www.kff.org/medicare/issue-brief/medicare-advantage-in-2022-premiums-out-of-pocket-limits-cost-sharing-supplemental-benefits-prior-authorization-and-star-ratings.

Kaiser Family Foundation. How Will the Prescription Drug Provisions in the Inflation Reduction Act Affect Medicare Beneficiaries? August 18, 2022c. https://www.kff.org/medicare/issue-brief/how-will-the-prescription-drug-provisions-in-the-inflation-reduction-act-affect-medicare-beneficiaries.

Kaiser Family Foundation. Health Coverage of Immigrants. April 6, 2022d. https://www.kff.org/racial-equity-and-health-policy/fact-sheet/health-coverage-of-immigrants/.

Law SA. *Blue Cross: What Went Wrong?* New Haven, CT: Yale University Press; 1974.

Light DW. The practice and ethics of risk-rated health insurance. *JAMA*. 1992;267:2503–2508.

Pechman JA. *Who Paid the Taxes, 1966–1985*. Washington, DC: Brookings Institution; 1985.

Schulte F. Medicare Advantage audits reveal pervasive overcharges. Updated 2019. https://publicintegrity.org/2016/08/29/20148/medicare-advantage-audits-reveal-pervasive-overcharges.

Starr P. *The Social Transformation of American Medicine*. New York, NY: Basic Books; 1982.

Weil AR. Physicians, Medicare, and more. *Health Aff (Millwood)*. 2019;38:519.

Zuckerman S, Skopec L, Aarons J. Medicaid physician fees remained substantially below fees paid by Medicare in 2019. *Health Aff (Millwood)*. 2021;40:343–348.

Health Insurance and Access to Health Care

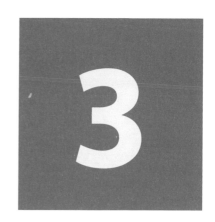

Access to health care is the ability to obtain health services when needed. Lack of adequate access for millions of people is a crisis in the United States.

Access to health care has many components. One of the most influential "enabling" components is the ability to pay (Aday & Andersen, 1974). Because of the high cost of health services, insurance coverage is instrumental in determining a person's ability to afford care. This chapter focuses on financial barriers to care, specifically the access challenges faced by the *uninsured* and the *underinsured*. Chapter 5 addresses other enabling factors for access to care, such as the availability of health care personnel and facilities and linguistically and culturally congruent care, and provides a broader framework for understanding health equity.

LACK OF INSURANCE

In 2015, Dan Coverless noticed that he was urinating a lot and feeling weak. He lived in South Carolina and earned $12,500 per year working part-time as a construction worker. Because South Carolina did not elect to participate in the Affordable Care Act's Medicaid expansion, Mr. Coverless was not eligible for Medicaid despite his low income. He also did not qualify for federal tax subsidies to purchase private insurance. His friend told him that his symptoms might mean that he had diabetes and that he should go see a doctor, but lacking health insurance, Mr. Coverless was afraid of the cost. Eight days later, his friend found him in a coma. He was hospitalized for diabetic ketoacidosis.

Health insurance coverage, whether public or private, is a key factor in making health care accessible. Despite gains in insurance coverage since the Affordable Care Act (ACA) was passed in 2010, 27 million people in the United States in 2021 had no health insurance whatsoever (Fig. 3–1). Table 3–1 shows sources of health insurance for the US population.

For many people in the United States, who do not have insurance, the unaffordability of health care is an insurmountable barrier. People lacking health insurance receive less care and have worse health outcomes than those with insurance. In 2021, 47% of uninsured adults reported not seeing a doctor or health care professional in the past 12 months compared to 18% with private insurance and 13% with public coverage. Twenty-one percent of adults without coverage went without needed care in the past year because of cost compared to 5% of adults with private coverage and 6% of adults with public coverage. Part of the reason for poor access among the uninsured is that 41% have no regular place to go when they are sick. Uninsured adults were 2.5 times as likely as adults with private coverage to delay filling or forgo a needed prescription drug due to cost. In addition, hospitals frequently charge uninsured patients much higher rates than those paid by private health insurers and public programs. Uninsured adults are more likely to use up savings, have difficulty paying for necessities, borrow money, or have medical bills sent to collections resulting in medical debt (Kaiser Family Foundation, 2022a).

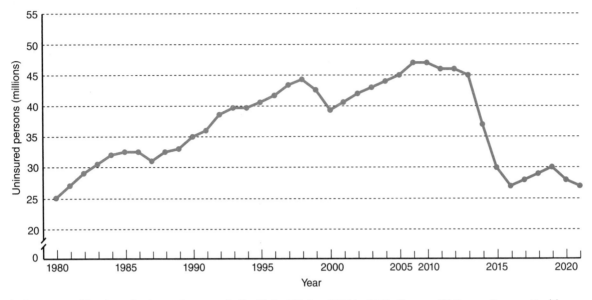

▲ **Figure 3–1.** Number of uninsured persons in the United States, 1980 to 2021. (Source: US Census Bureau. Health Insurance Coverage in the United States: 2021, September 2022. https://www.census.gov/content/dam/Census/library/publications/2022/demo/p60-278.pdf.)

Table 3–1. Sources of health insurance, 2021[a]

	Number of People (millions)
Medicare	60
Medicaid	63
Employment-based private insurance	179
Individual private insurance	33
Uninsured	27

[a]The number of people exceeds the US population of 332 million because millions of people have more than one source of health insurance, for example, those on Medicare plus Medicaid and those on Medicare plus private insurance.
Source: Data extracted from U.S. Census Bureau: *Health Insurance Coverage* in the United States, 2021, https://www.census.gov/content/dam/Census/library/publications/2022/demo/p60-278.pdf.

Compared with insured persons, the uninsured like Mr. Coverless have more avoidable hospitalizations, tend to be diagnosed at later stages of life-threatening illnesses, and are more seriously ill when hospitalized. Higher rates of cervical cancer and lower survival rates for breast cancer among the uninsured, compared with those with insurance, are associated with less access to cancer screenings (Ayanian et al., 2000). People without insurance have greater rates of uncontrolled hypertension, diabetes, and elevated cholesterol than those with insurance (Wilper et al., 2009). Most significantly, people who lack health insurance suffer a higher overall mortality rate than those with insurance (Woolhandler & Himmelstein, 2017). After adjusting for age, sex, education, poorer initial health status, and smoking, lack of insurance itself increases the risk of dying by 40% (Wilper et al., 2009).

▶ Medicaid and Access to Care

Medicaid, the federal and state public insurance plan, has made great strides in improving access to care for many low-income people.

When Maria Buenasuerte became pregnant, her sister told her that she was eligible for Medicaid. She lived near a community health center and made an appointment the same week with a certified nurse midwife. She had an uncomplicated pregnancy and delivered a healthy baby attended by her midwife and obstetrician at the local community hospital.

Concepcion Ortiz lived in a town of 25,000 persons. When she became pregnant, she enrolled in Medicaid. She called each private obstetrician in town, but none would take Medicaid patients. The nearest community health center accepting Medicaid was 75 miles away and no one in Concepcion's family had a car. When she reached her sixth month, she became desperate.

Compared with uninsured people, those with Medicaid are more likely to have a regular source of medical care and are less likely to report delays in receiving care. Adults with Medicaid, although less likely than uninsured adults to report delays in seeking care, are still about twice as likely as privately insured adults to report delays (Kaiser Commission on Medicaid and the Uninsured, 2015). An access barrier faced by Medicaid recipients is finding a physician. In most states, Medicaid pays physicians far less than does Medicare or private insurance with the result that many physicians limit the number of Medicaid patients they accept. Medicaid patients such as Maria Buenasuerte and Conception Ortiz often depend on community health centers for their care.

Similarly, when comparing specific services such as rates of immunizations, screening for breast and cervical cancer, hypertension and diabetes control, and timeliness of prenatal care, rates for people on Medicaid tend to fall between those of the uninsured and people with private insurance (Landon et al., 2007). Counties in states that expanded Medicaid under the ACA have significantly lower mortality than counties in nonexpansion states (Allen & Sommers, 2019).

Who Are the Uninsured and Why Are They Uninsured?

Norris, a shipyard worker in Miami, was laid off in 2018 at age 55 and was unable to get another job. When he became unemployed and lost his employer-sponsored private insurance, he was ineligible for Medicaid because Florida had not expanded eligibility under the ACA. Because his income was below the Federal Poverty Level, he was not eligible for ACA private insurance subsidies and is uninsured.

Morris works full-time for a corner grocery store in Jacksonville, Florida that employs five people.

Morris once asked the owner whether the employees could receive health insurance, but the owner said it was too expensive. Morris was excited when the ACA passed and his family would be eligible for tax-subsidized private insurance in 2014. His excitement turned to chagrin when he found out that even with the subsidy, it would cost him $1,500 per month in premiums to enroll in a health plan that had a deductible below $5,000 per year. He remained uninsured.

Morris's nephew Boris is an undocumented immigrant who delivers groceries at the same store. He is not eligible for ACA private insurance subsidies or Florida's Medicaid program.

The uninsured include many low-income individuals living in states not participating in Medicaid expansion, individuals opting out of ACA coverage due to excessive premiums or deductibles, individuals not enrolling in Medicaid even when eligible, and undocumented immigrants remaining ineligible for Medicaid and insurance subsidies. Responding to the COVID-19 pandemic, the American Rescue Plan of 2021 temporarily reduced ACA premiums and deductibles, provisions that have been extended to 2025. This legislation led to a reduction in the number of uninsured.

In 2021, 70% of the uninsured had one or more full-time workers in the family. These employed uninsured tend to be lower-wage workers at small firms like Morris. The unemployed uninsured like Norris often have incomes below the poverty line but are ineligible for Medicaid in several states (Kaiser Family Foundation, 2022a).

Insurance coverage differs widely by race-ethnicity and socioeconomic status. In 2021, 8% of non-Latino Whites were uninsured, compared with 13% of African Americans and 25% of Latinos (Fig. 3–2). Seventeen percent of individuals with annual household incomes below the Federal Poverty Level were uninsured, compared with 3.4% of those with incomes above 400% of poverty (Fig. 3–3) (US Census Bureau, 2022).

UNDERINSURANCE

Insurance coverage makes a difference for access to care. But many people with insurance are underinsured, which means that their health insurance coverage has

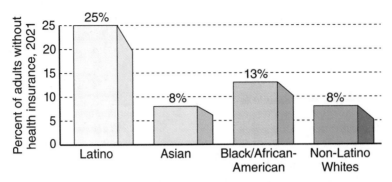

▲ **Figure 3–2.** Lack of health insurance by race and ethnicity in 2021. (Source: US Census Bureau. Health Insurance Coverage in the United States: 2021, September 2022. https://www.census.gov/content/dam/Census/library/publications/2022/demo/p60-278.pdf.)

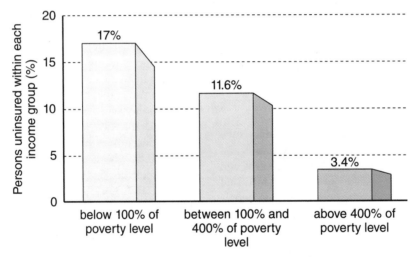

▲ **Figure 3–3.** Lack of health insurance by income in 2020. (Source: US Census Bureau. Health Insurance Coverage in the United States: 2021, September 2022. https://www.census.gov/content/dam/Census/library/publications/2022/demo/p60-278.pdf.)

limitations that expose them to large out-of-pocket payments that discourage access to needed services and saddle individuals with large medical bills. In a survey of bankruptcy filings from 2013 to 2016, close to 60% reported that medical expenses contributed to their bankruptcy (Himmelstein et al., 2019). Medical debt affects both uninsured and insured people; a 2022 national poll found that 61% of insured people had incurred medical debt (Levey, 2022).

A person who is insured for an entire year and meets any of the following three criteria is considered underinsured: (1) out-of-pocket costs, excluding share of insurance premiums, equal 10% or more of income; (2) out-of-pocket costs, excluding premiums, equal 5% or more of income if low-income (<200% of poverty); or (3) deductibles equal 5% or more of income. Based on this definition, in the first half of 2020, before the COVID pandemic, 41 million adults ages 19–64 were underinsured. Half of underinsured people reported problems paying medical bills or incurring medical debt. Forty-three percent of the underinsured reported going without needed care in the past year because of cost (Commonwealth Fund, 2020).

Table 3–2. Categories of underinsurance

1. Uncovered services
   Long-term care under Medicare
   Durable medical equipment under some insurance plans
   Caps on coverage such as limited physical therapy visits
   Restricted benefits from "limited benefits" insurance plans exempted
       from ACA requirements
2. Insurance deductibles and copayments

Two main reasons why insured people face high out-of-pocket expenses are: (1) uncovered services, and (2) high cost-sharing in the form of deductibles and copayments for covered services (Table 3–2).

Uncovered Services

Victoria and Gus Pappas had $100,000 in the bank when Gus had a stroke. After his hospitalization, he was paralyzed on the right side and unable to speak or swallow. After 12 months in the nursing home, most of the $100,000 was gone. At that point, Medicaid picked up the nursing home costs.

A glaring example of an uncovered service is the extremely limited benefits under Medicare for nursing home care and other long-term care expenses. As noted in Chapter 2, Medicare pays for a short duration of rehabilitative services at a long-term care facility following an acute hospitalization but does not cover extended care. As a result, many older families spend their life savings on long-term care, qualifying for Medicaid only after becoming impoverished (see Chapter 10).

Historically, private insurance varied widely from policy to policy in what services were covered, with some policies excluding maternity benefits, preventive care, mental health services, or other categories of services. Many plans also had a lifetime limit on the amount of total payments per insured person, exposing individuals and families to the entire costs of care after exhausting their insurance benefits. The ACA contained measures to limit many of these restrictions of covered services by private health plans, including prohibiting lifetime caps on payments. The ACA also required all private plans to meet a national standard for covered benefits which includes maternity care, family planning, and preventive services, among others. However, some limited plans are being sold that are not ACA compliant. Moreover, not all insurance plans cover equipment needed by people with permanent or temporary disabilities, such as wheelchairs, hospital beds, or oxygen equipment.

Insurance Deductibles and Copayments

The terms deductible, copayment, and coinsurance were defined in Chapter 2 as different forms of cost-sharing. Cost-sharing is a prominent element of employment-based private insurance, the ACA, and Medicare.

Individual Private Insurance

Jim Underwood is a self-employed painter with diabetes and hypertension who purchased individual insurance on the Colorado ACA marketplace in 2015. Because he received a government subsidy for his premiums he was able to afford a silver plan, but his annual deductible was $4,000 with a $20 copay for doctor visits and medications. He tried to take his four daily medications faithfully, but some months he lacked the funds to purchase refills. In 2021 with the American Rescue Plan, Jim's premiums and deductibles were temporarily reduced.

Although the ACA reduced uncovered services, it had the opposite effect on cost-sharing by institutionalizing high deductible plans in the individual insurance market. People buying individual coverage choose among bronze, silver, gold, and platinum plans. At one end of the spectrum, bronze plans have lower premiums and higher out-of-pocket costs, while at the other, platinum plans have higher premiums and lower out-of-pocket costs. The 2018 average Silver plan deductible was $4,000 for an individual and $8,000 for a family, with a copay around $30 for primary care and $60 for a specialist visit. While individuals and families enrolling in ACA individual insurance were no longer *un*insured, most, like Jim Underwood, found themselves seriously *under*insured due to the high out-of-pocket costs required in Bronze and Silver plans. The assistance provided by the American Rescue Plan will end by 2025.

Employment-Based Private Insurance

For people receiving health insurance from their employer, 88% must pay an annual deductible; the average

2022 deductible for a single employee working at a large firm was $1,493 and $2,543 for workers at small firms (Fig. 3–4). Most employed workers also pay an average of 20% of the cost of a hospital admission and a $27 copay for a primary care visit ($44 for a specialist visit). In addition, purchasing medications requires a copay (Claxton et al., 2022). These are costs over and above the employee's share of the insurance premium, which averaged 28% for family coverage. The average premium for employed workers has increased 43% since 2012. As a result, nearly 30% of people with employer-sponsored health insurance were considered underinsured in 2022.

Heidi Bauer worked at a bakery which offered employees and their families only a high-deductible health plan with a savings option. The employer paid $21,000 for the premium and $1,200 for a medical savings account that Heidi and her family could use to assist with medical expenses. Heidi paid $6,000 for her portion of the premium and faced a deductible of $8,000 plus 40% of physician fees when she needed health care. She could use the $1,200 in the savings account to help with those out-of-pocket costs.

In 2022, 29% of covered workers were enrolled in a high-deductible plan with a savings option. For small businesses like Heidi's, 49% of these plans had a deductible of $6,000 or more. The medical savings accounts that accompany these plans are funded by the employer; the average savings account in 2022 was $1,100 with 32% of firms paying nothing (Kaiser Family Foundation, 2022b).

Medicare

Ferdinand Foote was covered by Medicare and had no supplemental private "Medigap" insurance or Medicaid coverage. He was hospitalized for peripheral vascular disease caused by diabetes and a non-healing infected foot ulcer. He spent 4 days in the acute hospital and 1 month in the skilled nursing facility and made weekly physician visits following his discharge. The costs of illness not covered by Medicare included a $1,600 deductible for acute hospital care, a $200 per day copayment for days 21 to 30 of the skilled nursing facility stay, a $226 physician deductible, and a 20% ($20) physician copayment per visit for 12 visits. The total came to $4,066, not including Mr. Foote's copayments under his Medicare Part D drug plan for the medications he was prescribed to take after leaving the hospital.

In 2016, the average Medicare beneficiary paid $5,460 in out-of-pocket spending. These out-of-pocket expenses include premiums, deductibles, copayments,

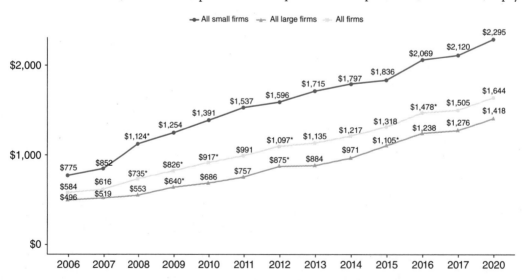

▲ **Figure 3–4.** Average general annual health plan deductible for single coverage, by firm size, 2006 to 2020. Reproduced with permission from Gary Claxton, Matthew Rae et al., Employer Health Benefits: 2020 Annual Survey, KFF, 2020. https://files.kff.org/attachment/Report-Employer-Health-Benefits-2020-Annual-Survey.pdf.)

and uncovered services. Half of Medicare beneficiaries in 2016 had an income below $26,200 (Kaiser Family Foundation, 2019).

The Effects of Underinsurance

Does underinsurance represent a serious barrier to the receipt of medical care? The Rand Health Insurance Experiment compared adults who had health insurance plans with no out-of-pocket costs and those who had plans with patient cost-sharing (deductibles or copayments). The study found that cost-sharing reduces the rate of ambulatory care use, especially among people in low-income brackets, and that patients with cost-sharing plans demonstrate a reduction in both appropriate and inappropriate medical visits. For low-income adults, the cost-sharing groups received Pap smears 65% as often as the free-care group. Hypertensive adults in the cost-sharing groups had higher diastolic pressures, and children had higher rates of anemia and lower rates of immunization (Brook et al., 1983; Lohr et al., 1986; Lurie et al., 1987). In 2020, 43% of underinsured adults had at least one cost-related access problem, for example not seeing a doctor when sick; skipping a recommended test, treatment, or follow-up; not getting needed specialist care; or not filling a prescription (Commonwealth Fund, 2020). In 2018, 17% of Medicare beneficiaries experienced at least one cost-related access problem (Kaiser Family Foundation, 2021). Underinsured adolescents have lower rates of vaccination coverage than the fully insured (Smith et al., 2009). In summary, lack of comprehensive insurance reduces access to health care and may contribute to poorer health outcomes.

TRENDS IN INSURANCE COVERAGE IN THE UNITED STATES

Historically, trends in health insurance coverage in the United States can be divided into three phases. The first phase, between the 1930s and mid-1970s, saw a large increase in the proportion of Americans with health insurance due to the growth of employment-based private health insurance and the 1965 passage of Medicare and Medicaid. The second phase marks a reversal of this trend; between 1980 and 2010, the number of uninsured people in the United States grew from 25 to about 50 million due to a sharp decrease in the number of people with private insurance. The number of uninsured peaked in 2010—the year the ACA was signed into law—signifying the onset of the third phase (Fig. 3–1). With the ACA, the number of uninsured decreased from 50 to 27 million between 2010 and 2021.

Two key factors—increasing health care costs and a changing labor force—explain the rise in the number of uninsured that occurred in the second phase and gave impetus to the ACA. From 2000 to 2022, average employer-sponsored family health insurance premiums rose from $6,500 to $22,463. For individual employee coverage, the increase went from $2,500 to $7,900. Most employers shifted more of the cost of health insurance premiums and health services onto their employees, resulting in employees dropping health coverage because of unaffordability. In 2018 the average employee paid 28% of the employer-sponsored family premium and 17% of an individual premium. Low-income workers have been hit especially hard by the combination of rising insurance costs and declining employer contributions (Claxton et al., 2022).

Simultaneously, the economy in the United States has undergone a major transition. The number of highly paid, largely unionized, manufacturing workers with employer-sponsored health insurance has declined, and the workforce has shifted toward more low-wage, nonunionized service and clerical workers whose employers are less likely to provide insurance. Between 1960 and 2016, the percentage of workers in manufacturing decreased from 30% to 8% of all nonfarm workers while service sector employment rose from 65% to 80%. From 1957 to 2010, the percentage of workers with part-time jobs—generally without health benefits—increased from 12% to 20%.

These same factors have driven the growing prevalence of underinsurance. The rapidly rising cost of health insurance led employers to increase employee share of premium costs and to migrate to high deductible plans.

THE INSTABILITY OF HEALTH INSURANCE

Jean Irons worked for Bethlehem Steel as a clerk and her benefits included health insurance. Bethlehem Steel was bought by a global corporation and her plant moved to another country. In 2011 she found a job as a food service worker in a small restaurant. Her pay decreased by 35%, and the restaurant did not provide health insurance.

Sally Lewis worked as a receptionist in a physician's office. She received health insurance through her husband, who was a construction worker. They got divorced, she lost her health insurance, and her physician employer told her that he could not provide her with health insurance because of the cost.

John Childs was a single father caring for his 3-year-old daughter in Arkansas. The state told him he needed to work to keep his Medicaid benefits, but he was unable to find a job in town that paid enough that he could afford childcare. He lost his Medicaid and became uninsured.

Juana Pacheco was laid off from her job as a hotel front desk manager when COVID decimated the hotel industry in 2020. She lost the health insurance she had utilized for the previous 15 years.

Individuals cycle through periods of having and losing insurance. A distinguishing feature of the US approach to health care financing is not only the lack of universal coverage, but also the instability of coverage. The dependence of group private insurance on employment inevitably produces interruptions in coverage because of the unstable nature of employment. People who are laid off from their jobs or who leave jobs because of illness lose their insurance. Family members insured through the workplace of a spouse may lose their insurance in cases of divorce, job loss, or death of the working family member. Social upheavals can upset health coverage for entire populations; millions lost their jobs in 2020 due to the COVID pandemic, resulting in nearly 2.7 million people losing their health insurance that year. The net result is that many people cycle in and out of the ranks of the uninsured every month.

CONCLUSION

The United States is an outlier among wealthy nations, first in leaving so many of its residents uninsured due to lack of a universal health coverage program, and second in the extensive degree of underinsurance among insured people. Federal legislation such as Medicare and Medicaid in 1965 and the ACA in 2010 expanded coverage to many previously uninsured people but did not produce a seamless system of comprehensive coverage for all Americans. People in lower income groups and from marginalized racial-ethnic groups are disproportionately represented among the uninsured and underinsured, experiencing the most injurious health and financial consequences from lack of comprehensive coverage. Chapter 5 explores these variations in health coverage using a broader framework of health equity, discussing the many factors that create disparities in health and in access to care.

REFERENCES

Aday LA, Andersen R. A framework for the study of access to medical care. *Health Serv Res.* 1974;9:208–220.

Allen H, Sommers BD. Medicaid expansion and health. *JAMA.* 2019;322:1253-1254.

Ayanian JZ, Weissman JS, Schneider EC, Ginsburg JA, Zaslavsky AM. Unmet needs of uninsured adults in the United States. *JAMA.* 2000;284:2061–2069.

Brook RH, Ware JE Jr, Rogers WH, et al. Does free care improve adults' health? Results from a randomized controlled trial. *N Engl J Med.* 1983;309:1426–1434.

Claxton G, Rae M, Damico A, Wager E, Young G, Whitmore H. Health benefits in 2022. *Health Aff (Millwood).* 2022;41:1670–1680.

Commonwealth Fund. U.S. Health Insurance Coverage in 2020: a Looming Crisis in Affordability. Issue Brief, August 19, 2020. https://www.commonwealthfund.org/publications/issue-briefs/2020/aug/looming-crisis-health-coverage-2020-biennial.

Himmelstein DU, Lawless RM, Thorne D, Foohey P, Woolhandler S. Medical bankruptcy: still common despite the Affordable Care Act. *Am J Public Health.* 2019;109:431–433.

Kaiser Commission on Medicaid and the Uninsured. Medicaid Moving Forward. Kaiser Family Foundation; 2015. www.kff.org/health-reform/issue-brief/medicaid-moving-forward/.

Kaiser Family Foundation. How Much Do Medicare Beneficiaries Spend Out of Pocket on Health Care? November 4, 2019. https://www.kff.org/medicare/issue-brief/how-much-do-medicare-beneficiaries-spend-out-of-pocket-on-health-care/.

Kaiser Family Foundation. Cost-Related Problems Are Less Common Among Beneficiaries in Traditional Medicare Than in Medicare Advantage. June 25, 2021. https://www.kff.org/medicare/issue-brief/cost-related-problems-are-less-common-among-beneficiaries-in-traditional-medicare-than-in-medicare-advantage-mainly-due-to-supplemental-coverage/.

Kaiser Family Foundation. Key Facts About the Uninsured Population. December 19, 2022a. https://www.kff.org/uninsured/issue-brief/key-facts-about-the-uninsured-population/.

Kaiser Family Foundation. Employer Health Benefits Survey, October 27, 2022b. https://www.kff.org/report-section/ehbs-2022-section-8-high-deductible-health-plans-with-savings-option/.

Landon BE, Schneider EC, Normand SL, Scholle SH, Pawlson LG, Epstein AM. Quality of care in Medicaid managed care and commercial health plans. *JAMA*. 2007;298:1674–1681.

Levey NN. 100 million people in America are saddled with health care debt Kaiser Health News, June 16, 2022. https://khn.org/news/article/diagnosis-debt-investigation-100-million-americans-hidden-medical-debt/.

Lohr KN, Brook RH, Kamberg CJ, et al. Use of medical care in the Rand Health Insurance Experiment. Diagnosis and service-specific analyses in a randomized controlled trial. *Med Care*. 1986;24(suppl 9):S1–S87.

Lurie N, Manning WG, Peterson C, Goldberg GA, Phelps CA, Lillard L. Preventive care: Do we practice what we preach? *Am J Public Health*. 1987;77:801–804.

Smith PJ, Lindley MC, Shefer A, Rodewald LE. Underinsurance and adolescent immunization delivery in the United States. *Pediatrics*. 2009;124(suppl 5):S515–S521.

US Census Bureau. Health Insurance Coverage in the United States: 2021, September 2022. https://www.census.gov/content/dam/Census/library/publications/2022/demo/p60-278.pdf.

Wilper AP, Woolhandler S, Lasser KE, McCormick D, Bor DH, Himmelstein DU. Hypertension, diabetes, and elevated cholesterol among insured and uninsured U.S. adults. *Health Aff (Millwood)*. 2009;28:1151–1159.

Woolhandler S, Himmelstein DU. The relationship of health insurance and mortality: is lack of insurance deadly? *Ann Intern Med*. 2017;167:424–431.

Paying Health Care Providers

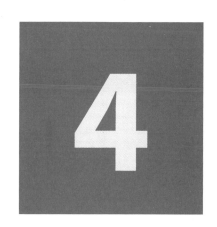

Chapter 2 described the different modes of financing health care: out-of-pocket payments, individual health insurance, employment-based health insurance, and government financing. Financing is only one part of the equation, however; the other part is paying the person or entity that actually provides a health care service. Whether a direct out-of-pocket payment from a patient or a payment from a third party insurance plan, a decision must be made about how that payment to a provider will be structured.

Dr. Mary Young has recently finished her family medicine residency and joined a small group practice, PrimaryCare. On her first day, she has the following experiences with health care payment: her first patient is insured by Blue Shield; PrimaryCare is paid a fee for the physician encounter and for the electrocardiogram (ECG) performed. Dr. Young's second patient requires the same services, for which PrimaryCare receives no payment but is forwarded $40 for each month that the patient is enrolled in the practice. In the afternoon, a hospital utilization review physician calls Dr. Young, explains the diagnosis-related group (DRG) payment system, and suggests that she send home a patient hospitalized with pneumonia. In the evening, she goes to the emergency department, where she has agreed to work two shifts per week for $200 per hour. She was also delighted to learn that her practice had received an extra payment for providing high-quality care for PrimaryCare patients.

During the course of a typical day, some physicians will be involved with four or five distinct types of payment. This chapter will describe the different ways in which physicians and hospitals are paid. Although payment has many facets, from the setting of prices to the processing of claims, this discussion will focus on one of its most basic elements: establishing the unit of payment. This basic principle must be grasped before one can understand the key concept of providers bearing financial risk for the costs of care.

UNITS OF PAYMENT

Methods of payment can be placed along a continuum that extends from the least to the most aggregated unit. The methods range from the simplest (one fee for one service rendered) to the most complex (one payment for many types of services rendered), with many variations in between (Table 4–1).

Definitions of Methods of Payment

Fee-for-Service Payment

The unit of payment is the visit or procedure. The physician or hospital is paid a fee for each office visit, ECG, intravenous medication, or other service or supply provided. This is the only form of payment that is based on individual components of health care. All other payment modes aggregate or group together several services into one unit of payment.

Table 4–1. Units of payment

	Least Aggregated: Procedure	Day	Episode of Illness	Patient	Most Aggregated: Time
Physician	Fee-for-service	—	Surgical or obstetric fee	Capitation	Salary
Hospital	Fee-for-service	Per diem	Hospital DRG	Capitation	Global budget

DRG, diagnosis-related group.

Episode-Based Payment

The physician or hospital is paid one sum for all services delivered during one illness or surgical procedure.

Per Diem Payments to Hospitals

The hospital is paid for all services delivered to a patient during 1 day in the hospital.

Capitation Payment

One payment is made for each patient's care during a month or year.

Payment for All Services Delivered to All Patients Within a Certain Time Period

This includes global budget payment of hospitals and salaried payment of physicians.

▶ Managed Care Plans

Traditionally physicians and hospitals have been paid on a fee-for-service basis. The development of managed care plans introduced changes in the methods by which hospitals and physicians are paid, largely for the purpose of controlling costs. Three major forms of managed care are: fee-for-service practice with utilization review, preferred provider organizations (PPOs), and health maintenance organizations (HMOs).

Fee-for-Service Payment with Utilization Review

This is the traditional type of payment, with the addition that the third-party payer (whether private insurance company or government agency) assumes the power to authorize or deny payment for expensive medical interventions such as hospital admissions, extra hospital days, and surgeries.

Preferred Provider Organization Payment

With PPO insurance products, insurers contract with a limited number of physicians and hospitals who agree to care for patients, usually on a discounted fee-for-service or, for hospitals, on a per diem basis, with utilization review (the insurer authorizing or denying payment for services deemed unnecessary). Patients with a PPO plan pay a much higher share of the cost when using physicians or hospitals outside the "preferred" network.

Health Maintenance Organization Payment

Patients with HMO insurance are required (except in emergencies) to receive their care from physicians and hospitals within that HMO. Point of service (POS) plans are HMOs that allow some flexibility in choice of provider. The types of HMOs are discussed in Chapter 8. Some HMOs pay physicians and hospitals using aggregated units of payment (e.g., capitation or salary).

METHODS OF PHYSICIAN PAYMENT

▶ Payment per Procedure: Fee-for-Service

Roy Singleton, a patient of Dr. Weisman, is seen for recent onset of diabetes. Dr. Weisman spends 20 minutes performing an examination, finger-stick blood glucose test, urinalysis, and ECG. Each service has a fee set by Dr. Weisman: $100 for a visit, $10 for a finger-stick glucose test, $20 for a urinalysis, and $60 for an ECG. Because Mr. Singleton is uninsured, Dr. Weisman reduces the total bill from $190 to $100.

In 2021, Dr. Lenz, an ophthalmologist, requested that Dr. Weisman do a medical consultation for Gertrude Rales, who developed congestive heart *failure and arrhythmias following cataract surgery. Dr. Weisman took 90 minutes to perform the consultation and was paid $132 by Medicare. Dr. Lenz had spent 90 minutes on the surgery plus pre- and postoperative care and received $680 from Medicare.*

Melissa High, a Medicaid recipient, makes three visits to Dr. Weisman for hypertension. He bills Medicaid $120 for one complex visit and $60 each for two follow-up visits. Under the state's Medicaid fee schedule he is paid $37 for the complex visit and $24 for each follow-up visit. Medicaid does not allow Dr. Weisman to bill Ms. High for the balance of his fees.

Dr. Weisman contracted with Blue Cross to care for its PPO patients at 70% of his normal fee. Rick Payne, a PPO patient, comes in with 2 weeks of new headaches and a normal neurologic exam. Dr. Weisman is paid $84 for a complex visit. Before a magnetic resonance imaging (MRI) scan can be ordered, the PPO must be asked for authorization.

Traditionally, private physicians have been paid by patients and insurers through the fee-for-service mechanism, as in these vignettes. Physicians may discount their fees for uninsured or other patients in financial need. Private insurers, as well as Medicare and Medicaid in the early years, usually paid physicians according to the usual, customary, and reasonable (UCR) system, which allowed physicians a great deal of latitude in setting fees. As cost containment became more of a priority, the UCR approach to fees was largely supplanted by payer-determined fee schedules. An example is Melissa High's three visits, which incurred charges of $240 of which Medicaid paid only $85.

In the early 1990s, Medicare moved to a fee schedule determined by a resource-based relative-value scale (RBRVS). With this system, fees (which vary by geographic area) are set for each service by estimating the time, mental effort and judgment, technical skill, physical effort, and stress typically related to that service (Bodenheimer et al., 2007). The RBRVS system pays surgical and other procedures at a far higher rate than primary care and cognitive services. In 2021, primary care physician (PCP) Dr. Weisman received $132 for 90 minutes of his time while specialist Dr. Lenz received $680 for 90 minutes.

PPO-managed care plans often pay contracted physicians on a discounted fee-for-service basis and require prior authorization for expensive procedures, as in the case of Rick Payne.

With fee-for-service payments, physicians have an economic incentive to perform more services because more services bring in more payments (see Chapter 13). The fee-for-service incentive to provide more services has contributed to the rapid rise in health care costs in the United States (National Commission on Physician Payment Reform, 2013). Despite reform efforts since the 1980s to move physician patient away from fee-for-service to more aggregated units, 70% of physician revenue remained fee-for-service in 2018 (Hunter et al., 2021).

Prior to the COVID-19 pandemic, physicians were rarely paid fees for phone visits, and few used video visits. With the explosion of these telehealth modalities in 2020, physicians could bill for both these types of "virtual" visits. As of late 2022, payments for phone visits are being phased out by many payers, limiting access to telemedicine visits to those patients and practices who have the resources and experience to conduct video visits.

Payment per Episode of Illness

Dr. Nick Belli removes Tom Stone's gallbladder and is paid $900 by Blue Cross. Besides performing the cholecystectomy, Dr. Belli sees Mr. Stone three times in the hospital and twice in his office for postoperative visits. Because surgery is paid by means of a global fee, Dr. Belli may not bill separately for the visits, which are included in his $900 cholecystectomy fee.

Surgeons usually receive a single payment for several services (the surgery itself and postoperative care) that have been grouped together, and obstetricians are paid in a similar manner for a delivery plus pre- and postnatal care. This bundling together of payments is often referred to as payment at the unit of the case or episode (Bundled payments, 2018).

With payment by episode, surgeons have an economic incentive to limit the number of postoperative visits because they do not receive extra payment for extra visits. On the other hand, they continue to have an incentive to perform more surgeries, as with the traditional fee-for-service system.

▶ The Important Concept of Risk

At this point, it is helpful to introduce the concept of risk. Risk refers to the potential to lose money, earn less money, or spend more time without additional payment on a transaction. Under fee-for-service, the party paying the bill (insurance company, government agency, or patient) absorbs all the risk; if Dr. Weisman sees Rick Payne 10 times rather than five times for his headaches, Blue Cross pays more money and Mr. Payne spends more in copayments. Bundling of services transfers a *portion* of the risk from the payer to the physician; if Dr. Belli sees Tom Stone 10 times rather than five times for follow-up after cholecystectomy, he does not receive additional money. However, Blue Cross is also partially at risk; if more Blue Cross enrollees require gallbladder surgery, Blue Cross is responsible for more $900 payments. As a general rule, the more services aggregated into one payment, the larger the share of financial risk that is shifted from payer to provider.

▶ Payment per Patient: Capitation

Capitation payments (per capita payments or payments "by the head") are monthly payments made to a physician for each patient signed up to receive care from that physician—generally a primary care physician. Under fee-for-service, patients who require expensive health services cost their health plan more than they pay the plan in insurance premiums; the insurer is at risk and loses money. Physicians and hospitals who provide the care earn more money for treating ill people. In a 180-degree role reversal, capitation shifts financial risk from insurance plan to providers. An HMO that pays physicians via capitation has little to fear in the short run from patients who become ill. The HMO pays a fixed sum per patient each month no matter how many services are provided. The providers, in contrast, earn no additional money yet spend a great deal of time and incur large office and hospital expenditures to care for people who are sick. On the other hand, providers may be financially disincentivized to accept care for patients who face severe illness or disability.

Certain methods have been developed to mitigate the financial risk associated with capitation payment. One method involves reintroducing fee-for-service payments for specified services. Such types of services provided but not covered within the capitation payment are called *carve-outs*; their payment is "carved out" of the capitation payment and paid separately. For example, immunizations and minor surgical procedures may be carved out and paid on a fee-for-service basis.

A common method of managing risk is called "risk-adjusted capitation." For physicians paid by capitation, patients with greater health care needs require a great deal more time without any additional payment, creating an incentive to sign up healthy patients and avoid those who are sick. Risk-adjusted capitation provides higher monthly payments for older patients, and for those with chronic illnesses or other characteristics predicting higher health care needs. Precisely how to risk-adjust is a topic of debate. In Chapter 2, we discussed how Medicare uses a risk score based on diagnoses coded on bills to adjust its capitation payments to Medicare Advantage plans, and the concern about plans "overcoding" for these diagnoses. These same issues apply to capitation payments to physicians. Alternative approaches put more emphasis on social factors that predict health needs, with the dual goals of promoting social equity in payment and reducing "gaming" of the risk adjustment measure (National Quality Forum, 2017; Phillips et al., 2021).

Capitation may control costs by providing an alternative to the inflationary tendencies of fee-for-service payment. In addition, capitation has been advocated for its potential beneficial influence on the organization of care. Capitation payments require patients to register with a physician or group of physicians. The clear enumeration of the population of patients in a primary care practice offers advantages for monitoring appropriate use of services and planning for these patients' needs. Capitation also allows for more flexibility at the practice level in how to most effectively and efficiently organize and deliver services. For example, fee-for-service typically only pays for an in-person visit with a physician or other licensed clinician such as a nurse practitioner; under capitation payment, a physician could delegate routine preventive care tasks to nurses or medical assistants in the practice, without experiencing a financial disincentive for these alternative ways of delivering care. Capitation also explicitly defines—in advance—the amount of money available to care for an enrolled population of patients, providing a better framework for rational allocation of resources and innovation in developing better modes of delivering services. For a large group of PCPs, the sheer size of the aggregated capitation payments provides clout and flexibility over how to best arrange ancillary and specialty services.

Capitation with Two-Tiered Structures

Jennifer is a young woman in England with strep throat; her general practitioner, Dr. Walter Liston, sees her and prescribes antibiotics. Jennifer pays no money at the time of the visit and receives no bill. Dr. Liston is paid the British equivalent of $15 per month to care for Jennifer, no matter how many times she requires care. When Jennifer develops appendicitis and requires an x-ray and surgical consultation, Dr. Liston sends her to the local hospital for these services; payment for these referral services is incorporated into the hospital's operating budget paid for separately by the National Health Service.

British System—Capitation payments to physicians in the United States are complicated, as will shortly be seen. But in the United Kingdom, they have traditionally been simple (see Chapter 15). Under the traditional British National Health Service, each person enrolls with a general practitioner. For each person on the general practitioner's list, the physician receives a monthly capitation payment. The more patients on the list, the more money the physician earns. Patients are required to route all nonemergency medical needs through the general practitioner "gatekeeper," who makes referrals for specialist services or hospital care. Patients can freely change from one general practitioner to another. This simple arrangement, illustrated in Fig. 4–1, is referred to as a two-tiered capitation structure. One tier is the health plan (the government in the case of the United Kingdom) and the other tier the individual PCP or several physicians in group practice.

US System—In the United States, capitation payment is associated with HMO plans and not with traditional or PPO insurance. A few HMO plans have two-tiered structures, with HMOs paying capitation fees directly to PCPs (Fig. 4–1). However, capitation payment in

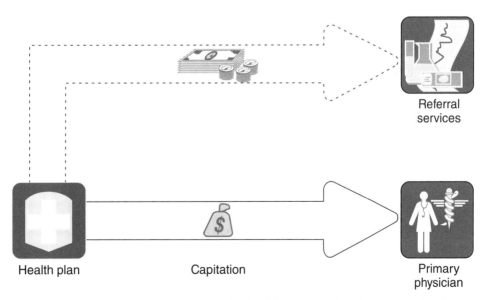

Referral
services

Health plan   Capitation   Primary
                                                              physician

▲ **Figure 4–1.** Two-tiered capitated payment structures. The health plan pays the primary care physician by capitation and pays for referral services (e.g., x-rays and specialist consultations) through a different payment stream.

US-managed care organizations often involves a three-tiered structure.

Capitation with Three-Tiered Structures

In three-tiered structures, HMOs do not pay capitation fees directly to individual physicians or small practices, but instead rely on an intermediary administrative structure for processing these payments (Robinson & Casalino, 1995). In one variety of such three-tiered structures (Fig. 4–2), physicians remain in their own private offices but join together into physician groups called independent practice associations (IPAs).

> *George is enrolled through his employer in SmartCare, an HMO plan of Smart Insurance Company. SmartCare has contracted with DoctorFriendly IPA and DoctorFriendly Multispecialty Group, which provide physician services for SmartCare's enrollees in the area where George lives. George has chosen to receive his care from Dr. Bunch, a PCP affiliated with DoctorFriendly IPA. SmartCare pays the IPA a $200 monthly capitation fee on George's behalf for all physician and related outpatient services. DoctorFriendly IPA in turn pays Dr. Bunch a $40 monthly capitation fee to serve as George's primary care physician.*
>
> *George develops symptoms of urinary obstruction consistent with benign prostatic hyperplasia. Dr. Bunch orders laboratory tests and refers George to a urologist for cystoscopy. The laboratory and the urologist bill the IPA on a fee-for-service basis. At the end of the year, the IPA has money left over in a diagnostic and specialist services risk pool and distributes some of this surplus revenue to its physicians as a bonus.*

Sorting out the flow of payments and nature of risk-sharing becomes difficult in this type of three-tiered capitation structure. In most three-tiered HMO plans, the financial risk for diagnostic and specialist services is borne by the overall IPA or multispecialty group and spread among the participating physicians. In the 1980s and 1990s, IPAs often provided financial incentives to PCPs to limit the use of diagnostic and specialist services by returning to these physicians any surplus funds that remain at the end of the year. This method of compensation was known as capitation-plus-bonus payment. The less frequent the use of diagnostic and specialist services, the higher the year-end bonus for IPA physician gatekeepers. This arrangement came under criticism as representing a conflict of interest for PCPs because their personal income was increased by denying diagnostic and specialty services to their patients (Rodwin, 1993). More recently, some managed care organizations have begun to tie bonus payments to quality measures—"pay for performance"—rather than to cost control (see Chapter 13).

▶ Payment per Time: Salary

> *Dr. Joyce Parto is employed as a salaried obstetrician-gynecologist by a large medical group affiliated with a local hospital. She considers the financial security and lack of business worries in her current work setting an improvement over the stresses she faced as a solo fee-for-service practitioner before joining the physician group. However,*

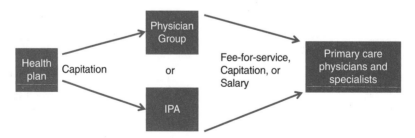

▲ **Figure 4–2.** Three-tiered capitation payment structures. The health plan pays a capitation payment to a physician group or independent practice association (IPA), which in turn pays primary care and specialist physicians fee-for-service, capitation, or salary.

she has some concerns that the other obstetricians are allowing the hospital's obstetric residents to manage most of the deliveries during the night, and wonders if the lack of financial incentives to attend deliveries may be partly to blame. She is also annoyed by the bureaucratic hoops she has to jump through to cancel an afternoon clinic to attend her son's school play.

In contrast with traditional private physicians, physicians in the public sector (municipal, Veterans Health Administration and military hospitals, state mental hospitals) and in community clinics are usually paid by salary (Fig. 4–3). Salaried practice aggregates payment for all services delivered during a month or year into one lump sum. The growth of physicians working as employees of medical groups, community health centers, and hospitals (see Chapter 8) has brought salaried practice to the private sector, sometimes with a salary-plus-bonus arrangement.

Physicians paid purely by salary bear little if any individual financial risk; the employer, whether a medical group or community health center, is at risk if expenses are too high. To manage risk, administrators may place constraints on their physician employees, such as scheduling them for a high volume of patient visits. Salaried physicians are at risk of not getting extra pay for extra work hours. For a physician paid an annual salary without allowances for overtime pay, a high volume of complex patient visits may turn an 8-hour day into a 12-hour day with no increase in income. Some organizations offer bonuses to salaried physicians if their patients receive high-quality, low-cost care (see pay-for-performance, below), or index a large portion of the salary to the physician's individual clinical productivity.

METHODS OF HOSPITAL PAYMENT

▶ Payment per Procedure: Fee-for-Service

Kwin Mock Wong is hospitalized for a bleeding ulcer. At the end of his 4-day stay, the hospital sends a $48,000 seven-page itemized hospital bill to Blue Cross, Mr. Wong's insurer.

In the past, insurance companies made fee-for-service payments to private hospitals based on the principle of "reasonable cost," a system under which hospitals had a great deal of influence in determining the level of payment. Because the American Hospital Association and Blue Cross played a large role in writing payment regulations for Medicare, that program initially paid hospitals according to a similar reasonable cost formula (Law, 1974). More recently, private and public payers negotiate lower payments or shift financial risk toward the hospitals by using per diem, DRG, or capitation payments.

▶ Payment per Day: Per Diem

John Johnson, a patient with PPO insurance with a severe headache and left leg weakness, is admitted to the hospital. During his 3-day stay, he undergoes MRI scanning, lumbar puncture, and cerebral arteriography, procedures that are all costly to the hospital in terms of personnel and supplies. The hospital receives $6,600, or $2,200 per day from the PPO plan; Mr. Johnson's stay costs the hospital $9,200 in expenses.

Tom Thompson, in the same PPO, is admitted for congestive heart failure. He receives intravenous furosemide for 3 days and his condition improves.

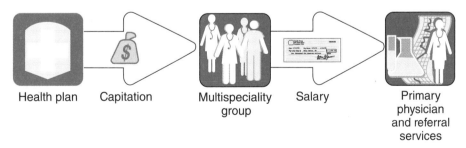

Health plan — Capitation — Multispeciality group — Salary — Primary physician and referral services

▲ **Figure 4–3.** Salaried payment. A physician group receives capitation payments from the health plan and then pays its physicians by salary.

Diagnostic testing is limited to a chest x-ray, ECG, and basic blood work. The hospital receives $6,600; the cost to the hospital is $5,600.

Many insurance companies and Medicaid plans contract with hospitals for per diem payments rather than paying a fee for each itemized service. The hospital receives a lump sum for each day the patient is in the hospital. The insurer may send a utilization review nurse to the hospital to review the charts of its patients, and if the nurse decides that a patient is not acutely ill, the insurance plan may stop paying for additional days.

Per diem payments represent a bundling of all services provided for one patient on a particular day into one payment. With traditional fee-for-service payment, if the hospital performs several expensive diagnostic studies, it makes more money because it charges for each study, whereas with per diem payment the hospital receives no additional money for expensive procedures. Per diem bundling of services into one fee removes the hospital's financial incentive because it loses, rather than profits, by performing expensive studies.

With per diem payment, the insurer continues to be at risk for the number of days a patient stays in the hospital because it must pay for each additional day. However, the hospital is at risk for the number of services performed on any given day because it incurs more costs without additional payment when it provides more services. It is in the insurer's interest to conduct utilization review to reduce the number of hospital days, but the insurer is less concerned about how many services are performed within each day; that fiscal concern has been transferred to the hospital.

▶ Payment per Episode of Hospitalization: Diagnosis-Related Groups

Bill is a 67-year-old man who enters the hospital for acute pulmonary edema. He is treated with furosemide and oxygen in the emergency room, spends 36 hours in the hospital, and is discharged. The cost to the hospital is $4,000. The hospital receives a $5,000 DRG payment from Medicare for heart failure without complications.

Will is an 82-year-old man who enters the hospital for acute pulmonary edema. In spite of aggressive treatment with diuretics and ACE inhibitors,

he remains in heart failure. He requires oxygen, telemetry, daily blood tests, several chest x-rays, electrocardiograms, and an echocardiogram, and is finally discharged on the ninth hospital day. His hospital stay costs $23,000 and the hospital receives $8,000 from Medicare for heart failure with complications.

The DRG method of payment for Medicare patients started in 1983. Rather than pay hospitals on a fee-for-service basis, Medicare pays a lump sum for each hospital admission, with the size of the payment dependent on the patient's diagnoses. The DRG system has gone one step further than per diem payments in bundling services into one payment. While per diem payment lumps together all services performed during 1 day, DRG payment lumps together all services performed during one acute care hospital episode.

With the DRG system, the Medicare program is at risk for the number of admissions, but the hospital is at risk for the length of hospital stay and the resources used during the hospital stay. Medicare has no financial interest in the length of stay, which (except in unusually long "outlier" stays) does not affect Medicare's payment. In contrast, the hospital has a keen interest in the length of stay and in the number of expensive procedures performed; a long, costly hospitalization such as Will's produces a financial loss for the hospital, whereas a short stay yields a profit. Hospitals therefore conduct internal utilization review to reduce the costs incurred by Medicare patients.

▶ Payment per Patient: Capitation

With capitation payment, hospitals are at risk for admissions, length of stay, and resources used; in other words, hospitals bear all the risk and the insurer, usually an HMO, bears no risk. Capitation payment to hospitals is uncommon in the United States.

▶ Payment per Institution: Global Budget

Don Samuels, a member of the Kaiser Health Plan, suffers a sudden overwhelming headache and is hospitalized for 1 week at Kaiser Hospital in Oakland, California, for an acute cerebral hemorrhage. He goes into a coma and dies. No hospital bill is generated as a result of Mr. Samuels' admission, and no capitation payments are made from any insurance plan to the hospital.

Kaiser Health Plan is a large integrated delivery system that in some regions of the United States operates its own hospitals. Kaiser hospitals are paid by the Kaiser Health Plan through a global budget: a fixed payment is made for all hospital services for 1 year. Global budgets are also used in Veterans Health Administration and Department of Defense hospitals in the United States, as well as being a standard payment method in Canada and many European nations. In managed care parlance, one might say that the hospital is entirely at risk because no matter how many patients are admitted and how many expensive services are performed, the hospital must figure out how to stay within its fixed budget. Global budgets represent the most extensive bundling of services: Every service performed on every patient during 1 year is aggregated into one payment.

VALUE-BASED PAYMENT AND PAYMENT REFORM

The health system is witnessing a flurry of new approaches to paying physicians and hospitals. The National Commission on Physician Payment Reform (2013) called for fundamental changes, including the eventual elimination of fee-for-service payment in favor of payment that rewards value (i.e., high quality at reasonable cost) rather than volume. A number of "value-based" payment models are currently in use.

Pay-for-Performance

One of the most basic reforms is paying not just for units of service—whether they be visits, hospital episodes, or hours of work—but for how well physicians and other providers perform in delivering those services. Many public and private payers are supplementing the basic mode of payment with bonus payments to physicians and hospitals that achieve a specified high level of performance on certain measures such as preventive care services, diabetes care, patient experience, and cost reduction (Mendelson et al., 2017; New England Journal of Medicine Catalyst, 2018). In the United States, these payments tend to be small relative to the dominant payment mechanisms of fee-for-service for physicians and per diem or DRGs for hospitals. Pay-for-performance is discussed further in Chapter 13.

Bundled Payments

The term "bundled payment" has taken on a specific meaning under Medicare payment reform. Medicare launched bundled payment programs in 2013 on a voluntary basis and now has more than 25 conditions for which hospitals and physicians can elect to be paid using this method. Under this model, Medicare not only bundles payments into more aggregated units using an episode-based rather than fee-for-service method; the physician and hospital payments are also bundled together into a single payment (Bundled payments, 2018). In 2020, over 1,000 hospitals and 700 physician groups participated in the voluntary Medicare bundled payment program.

An example is bundled payment for a joint replacement. Medicare negotiates with a hospital and the members of its medical staff involved in joint replacements (orthopedic surgeons, anesthesiologists, and others) to agree on a total payment for the joint replacement services, set at a level somewhat below what Medicare estimates it has paid for those services to the same groups of providers under fee-for-service. Bundled payment provides an incentive for the hospital and its medical staff to collaborate to eliminate unnecessary costs, such as by selecting a limited number of joint prostheses and negotiating lower prices with supply vendors for those prostheses, resulting in savings to Medicare and higher earnings for the hospital and physicians. The hospital and physicians share the risk of potentially losing money relative to the traditional payment model if they cannot control the average total cost for joint replacements. Also, bundled payments typically place the hospital and physicians at financial risk for postacute care expenses, such as outpatient physical therapy and a postoperative stay in a skilled nursing facility, since Medicare defines the episode as lasting at least 30 days after the date of surgery, and often 90 days (Ryan, 2018).

Care Coordination Payments

Medicare and some private insurers are paying some primary care practices through a blended model that adds a small capitation payment to the main fee-for-service payment to provide resources and incentives for better management of patients with chronic conditions. For example, a primary care practice caring for

100 patients with diabetes might receive $25 per diabetes patient per month, and use those funds to hire a health coach to help patients control their diabetes.

▶ Accountable Care Organizations

The term "accountable care organization" was introduced in 2006 by Elliott Fisher. Since that time, more than one thousand ACOs have sprung up around the United States, involving both public and private payers (Muhlestein et al., 2018).

In 2019, Northeast Hospital System organized the NewCare ACO to participate in the Medicare ACO program. To form NewCare ACO, Northeast brought together both hospital-owned and independent physician practices, laboratories, imaging centers, and home care agencies in its suburban town. The physician members of NewCare cared for 10,000 Medicare beneficiaries. In the year prior to the ACO's formation, those 10,000 patients cost Medicare an average of $14,000 per patient, a total of $140 million. Based on typical annual health care cost inflation of 5%, Medicare estimated that those same patients would cost $147 million in 2019. Under the ACO contract with Medicare, if NewCare held total Medicare costs for those 10,000 patients in 2019 below $142 million, NewCare would retain half of every dollar saved by Medicare below that $142 million target. Medicare would still pay NewCare constituent providers in the usual way: DRGs for hospitals and fee-for-service for physicians. However, all payments would be tracked against the shared-savings target to determine at the end of the year if NewCare would receive a supplemental payment from Medicare for achieving the threshold cost reductions. To ensure that patients would not suffer from cost-saving measures compromising access and quality, Medicare would not share the savings with NewCare unless NewCare achieved certain quality benchmarks. Medicare expenses in 2019 for NewCare patients wound up to be $140 million and NewCare hit its quality benchmarks. Medicare paid NewCare a $1 million shared saving bonus, which NewCare distributed equally to Northeast Hospital and the physician members of NewCare.

ACO payment models try to make fee-for-service payments to physicians and per diem or episode payments to hospitals function more like a globally budgeted payment model. While retaining the basic disaggregated payments, ACOs create an overall budget target that puts physicians and hospitals at financial risk for overall expenditures. In the case of NewCare, the risk was exclusively "upside" risk, meaning that NewCare could share in savings if it was successful in holding down costs but would not have to pay Medicare back if its Medicare expenditures exceeded the budget target ("downside" risk). Medicare ACO models provide an opportunity for physician and hospital organizations to retain a greater share of the upside risk if they are willing to also assume some downside risk. Similar to bundled payment, the ACO payment model provides an incentive for physicians, hospitals, and other involved providers to collaborate in eliminating wasteful spending. ACO models typically include an element of pay for performance insofar as provider organizations are only eligible for shared savings bonuses if they achieve quality targets.

CONCLUSION

Paying physicians and hospitals by fee-for-service, particularly when physicians and hospitals had considerable control over the fees to be paid, fueled rapid increases in health care costs in the United States. The push for cost containment led to two fundamental changes in how physicians and hospitals are paid:

1. Whereas levels of payment were formerly set largely by providers themselves (reasonable cost reimbursement for hospitals and usual, customary, and reasonable fees for physicians), payment levels are increasingly determined by negotiation between payers and providers or by fee schedules set by payers.
2. Private insurers, Medicare, and Medicaid are gradually replacing fee-for-service payment, which encourages use of more services, with more aggregated payment mechanisms that shift financial risk away from payers toward physicians and hospitals in an effort to control costs.

While fee-for-service encourages expensive over-treatment (Relman, 2007), payments that place physicians and hospitals at risk raise concerns about restricting needed care. Although the perfect payment method that strikes the right balance between economic incentives for overtreatment and undertreatment remains elusive (Casalino, 1992), payers continue to experiment by blending units of payment and reforming payment models to achieve the right recipe for producing "value"–high quality, affordable care.

REFERENCES

Bodenheimer T, Berenson RA, Rudolf P. The primary care-specialty income gap: why it matters. *Ann Intern Med.* 2007;146:301–306.

Bundled payments. NEJM Catalyst, February 28, 2018. https://catalyst.nejm.org/what-are-bundled-payments/.

Casalino LP. Balancing incentives: how should physicians be reimbursed? *JAMA.* 1992;267:403–405.

Hunter K, Ahmadi L, Kendall D. The case against fee-for-service health care. Third Way, September 9, 2021. http://thirdway.imgix.net/pdfs/the-case-against-fee-for-service-health-care.pdf.

Law SA. *Blue Cross: What Went Wrong?* New Haven, CT: Yale University Press; 1974.

Mendelson A, Kondo K, Damberg C, et al. The effects of pay-for-performance programs on health, health care use, and processes of care. *Ann Intern Med.* 2017;166:341–353.

Muhlestein D, Saunders RS, Richards R, McClellan MB. Recent progress in the value journey: growth of ACOs

and value-based payment in 2018. Health Affairs blog, August 14, 2018. www.healthaffairs.org/do/10.1377/hblog20180810.481968/full.

National Commission on Physician Payment Reform, March 2013. http://physicianpaymentcommission.org/.

National Quality Forum. Evaluation of the NQF trial period for risk adjustment for social risk factors. July 18, 2017. www.qualityforum.org/Projects/sz/SES_Trial_Period/Final_Report.aspx.

New England Journal of Medicine Catalyst. What is pay for performance in healthcare? March 1, 2018. https://catalyst.nejm.org/doi/full/10.1056/cat.18.0245. Accessed August 31, 2022.

Phillips RL Jr, Ostrovsky A, Bazemore AW. Adjusting Medicare payment for social risk to better support social needs. Health Affairs Blog, June 1, 2021. https://www.healthaffairs.org/do/10.1377/forefront.20210526.933567/.

Relman A. *Second Opinion: Rescuing America's Health Care.* New York, NY: Public Affairs; 2007.

Robinson JC, Casalino LP. The growth of medical groups paid through capitation in California. *N Engl J Med.* 1995; 333:1684–1687.

Rodwin MA. *Medicine, Money, and Morals: Physicians' Conflicts of Interest.* New York, NY: Oxford University Press; 1993.

Ryan AM. Medicare bundled payment programs for joint replacement. *JAMA.* 2018;320:877–879.

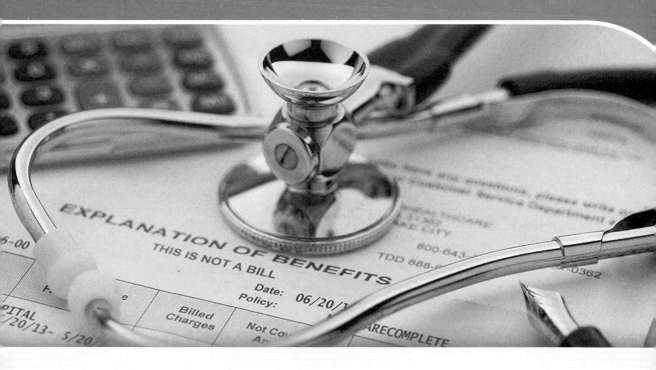

EQUITY AND RESOURCE ALLOCATION

Health Equity

If health care is a right, then it is unfair that some people can pay for care while others cannot. Moreover, as discussed in Chapter 2, regressive methods of financing health services that place a disproportionate burden on lower-income populations are an "unhealthy" way of funding health care. But affordability is only one factor that determines whether people have adequate access to health care. Health care, in turn, is but one element among many that shape people's actual health. This chapter begins by defining the concepts of health equity and health *care* equity, and then reviews factors that influence equity. Because race is such a powerful factor associated with health inequities in the United States, the chapter discusses the concept of race as a social construct and how racism and other forms of oppression produce inequities.

EQUITY: CONCEPTS AND DEFINITIONS

The World Health Organization (WHO) defines *health equity* as "the absence of avoidable, unfair, or remediable differences [in health status] among groups of people, whether those groups are defined socially, economically, demographically or geographically or by other means of stratification (WHO, 2023)." The WHO emphasizes that "everyone should have a fair opportunity to attain their full health potential." *Health care equity* refers more specifically to equitable access to and quality of health care services. Stated another way, health care equity means that everyone is able to receive the health care they need to be as healthy as possible. Equity is not the same as equality. To achieve health equity, a person with greater health care needs

requires not the same level of care as someone with less need, but a greater level of care.

Achieving health care equity is important for advancing the goal of health equity. But health care is not the dominant factor influencing the overall health of a population. Of the four categories of modifiable health determinants, clinical care is generally considered to contribute about 20% (Fig. 5–1). Achieving health equity requires also addressing social and environmental factors—often referred to as the "social determinants of health."

RACE, RACISM, AND HEALTH

Individuals from marginalized racial groups in the United States experience inequities in both health care and health. Black and Latino individuals are much less likely to have a regular source of medical care than White individuals (Jabbarpour et al., 2022). Analyzing a group of quality measures in 2022, Black individuals on average received worse care than White individuals for 45% of these quality measures and Latino and American Indian populations received worse care than the White population for 38% and 43% of the indicators, respectively; quality was better among these populations than among the White population for only 10–17% of the measures. These heath care inequities have persisted over time, with disparities narrowing between 2000 and 2020 for only about 10% of the quality measures (Agency for Healthcare Research and Quality, 2022).

Life expectancy for American Indian men and women in 2020 was 10 years shorter than life expectancy for White men and women. Life expectancy for

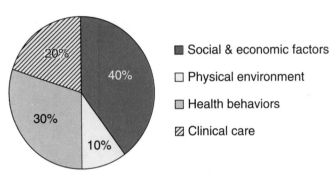

▲ **Figure 5–1.** Determinants of health. The chart shows the relative contribution of modifiable factors that influence health. Genetic susceptibility to illness is not considered a modifiable factor and therefore not included. It is important to recognize the dynamic interplay among the factors displayed in the chart; for example, social and economic factors contribute to behaviors such as smoking and diet. (Source: Remington PL, Catlin BB, Gennuso KP. The County Health Rankings: rationale and methods. *Population Health Metrics* 2015;13.)

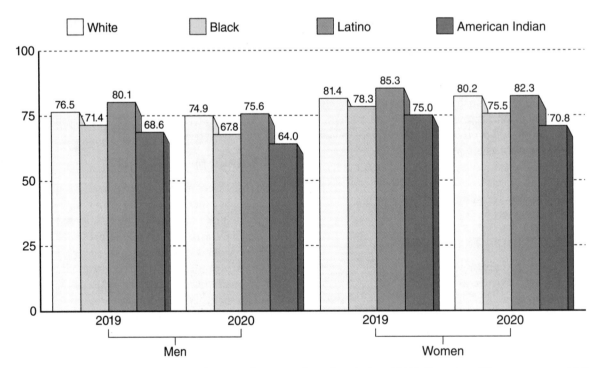

▲ **Figure 5–2.** Life expectancy in years, by race-ethnicity and gender: 2019 and 2020. Data show life expectancy at birth in years. (Source: Aburto et al., 2022; Goldman and Andrasfay, 2022.)

Black men and women was also many years shorter than for their White counterparts (Fig. 5–2). In 2019, the Black infant mortality rate was more than double the rate for White infants, with mortality rates also much higher among Native Hawaiian/Pacific Islander and American Indian infants than among White infants (Fig. 5–3). The maternal mortality rate among Black women is increasing, with the rate among Black women in 2020 more than three times higher than the rate among White women (Hoyert, 2022).

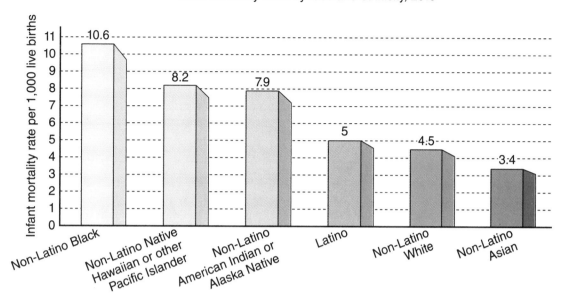

▲ **Figure 5–3.** Infant mortality rates by race and ethnicity, 2019. (Source: Centers for Disease Control Infant Mortality in the United States, 2019: Data from the Period Linked Birth/Infant Death File.)

Race as a Social Construct

To understand the reasons for these stark racial inequities, one must first consider the meaning of race. Historically, the dominant social, political, scientific, and medical cultures in the United States regarded race as a *biologic construct*. An ideology of White supremacy sorted populations based on characteristics such as skin color, regarding those groups defined as "other" than White to be innately inferior. This ideology was used to justify brutal appropriation of land from indigenous populations, enslavement of African people and their descendants, discrimination against immigrants, and other acts of oppression. It abetted a harrowing history of exploitation of people of color by some physicians and researchers, including performance of experimental gynecologic surgery on unanesthetized enslaved Black women in the pre-Civil War era, the unethical syphilis study conducted by the US Public Health Service in Tuskegee in the 1900s which withheld penicillin treatment for Black men infected with syphilis, and coerced gynecologic operations performed on immigrant women at a US detention center in the past decade. White supremacy ideology ascribed

health inequities as being largely due to genetic or other "biologic" deficiencies among the groups experiencing these disparities.

The complete sequencing of the human genome at the turn of the twenty-first century exposed the fallacy of the race-as-innate-biology construct. There is more genetic variation among individuals within a racial group than there is between racial groups. The notion of race as a biologic construct is being replaced by an understanding of race as a *social construct*: a scheme to categorize people based on superficial characteristics, invented to reinforce the exercise of privilege and power by certain groups. The social construct of race is inextricably tied with the concept of racism. Camara Jones defines racism as "a system of structuring opportunity and assigning value based on the social interpretation of how one looks (which is what we call 'race'), that unfairly disadvantages some individuals and communities, unfairly advantages other individuals and communities, and saps the strength of the whole society through the waste of human resources (Jones, 2020)." Jones points out that racism operates at both interpersonal and institutional (or systemic) levels (Jones, 2000).

Interpersonal racism often occurs implicitly—not as intentionally harmful acts of prejudice, but as behaviors emanating from unconscious bias. There is ample evidence that both interpersonal and systemic racism contribute to persistent health care inequities and health inequities in the United States.

Interpersonal Racism and Health Care

James Roto, an airport worker in Florida of Afro-Cuban heritage, is suffering. The pain from his fractured femur is excruciating, and the emergency department physician has given him no pain medication. In the next room, Joe Comfort, a White man, is at ease. He has received 10 mg of morphine for his femur fracture.

Studies of emergency departments in the United States found that Black and Latino patients with extremity fractures were much less likely to receive potent pain medication than non-Latino White patients with similar fractures. This marked difference in treatment was attributable not to insurance status but to race-ethnicity. Even Latinos fluent in English were much less likely than non-Latino White patients to receive pain medication (Todd et al., 1993; Todd et al., 2000). A study conducted several years later provides insights into the implicit bias that may result in these types of inequities. In this study of White medical students and residents, the researchers found that many trainees held biased beliefs that Black patients have an innately different experience of pain (e.g., agreeing with the statement, "Blacks' nerve endings are less sensitive than Whites'"); when shown equivalent scenarios of a patient in pain, the trainees with racial bias rated a Black person as having less pain than a White person and made less appropriate treatment recommendations (Hoffman et al., 2016).

Studies in other settings have found that African American and Latino patients receive poorer interpersonal communication with physicians, including greater physician verbal dominance, less patient-centeredness, and shorter visits, compared with White patients (Johnson et al., 2004; Martin et al., 2013). These disparities are often mitigated when patients from historically marginalized populations are cared for by a clinician of the same race, with patients in racially concordant relationships having higher use of preventive services, patient satisfaction, and ratings of the physician's participatory decision-making style (Saha et al., 2000; Cooper et al., 2003; Alsan et al., 2019). Patients with limited English proficiency cared for by language concordant clinicians tend to have better patient experiences and outcomes such as reductions in patient reports of medication errors (Wilson et al., 2005; Parker et al., 2017).

Interpersonal Racism and Health

The adverse effects of interpersonal racism on health are not limited to those occurring in health care settings. Being subjected to racism in any context may have a toxic effect on an individual's health (Williams & Mohammed, 2013; Bailey et al., 2017; Braveman et al., 2022). A study of women in California who had recently given birth found that Black women were seven times more likely than White women to have experienced chronic worry about racial discrimination, and this worry about discrimination partly explained the higher rate of preterm birth among the Black women (Braveman et al., 2017). Asian Americans in the United States experienced a surge in anti-Asian discrimination during the COVID-19 pandemic; experiences of racial discrimination during the pandemic are associated with poorer mental and physical health among Asian Americans (Lee & Waters, 2021). Experiencing racism damages health through many possible mechanisms, such as chronic stress that adversely affects the immune and cardiovascular systems or produces deleterious epigenetic changes (changes in gene expression provoked by social or environmental stresses).

Systemic and Structural Racism and Health Care

Systemic racism refers to the structures and policies that "reinforce discriminatory beliefs, values, and distribution of resources (Bailey et al., 2017)."

Jeanette Blew and Susanna Redd were both minimum wage, part-time workers at fast food restaurants when the Affordable Care Act was enacted. Because neither had children in the household, they were not at the time eligible for Medicaid coverage. Four years later, Jeanette, who lived in

Minnesota, had health insurance under the state's Medicaid expansion program. Susanna, living in Texas, remained uninsured due to her state's refusal to implement Medicaid expansion.

As of 2023, 10 states had not implemented Medicaid expansion. Texas and southeastern states comprised 7 of the 10 states. These 7 states have relatively high proportions of Black and Latino residents, which is one of the factors contributing to the disproportionately high rates of uninsurance among Black and Latino individuals in the United States overall (see Chapter 3). The federalist model of government in the United States that delegates to states decisions about Medicaid participation may be considered a form of structural racism reinforcing inequitable distribution of health care resources. Similarly, systemic inequities in educational and employment opportunity for people of color mean that fewer of them work in jobs that confer private health insurance benefits—a form of structural racism embedded in a health financing system relying heavily on employment-based private insurance. The disproportionate racial impact of uninsurance and underinsurance is reflected in Black and Latino adults being more likely than White adults to experience debt for a medical or dental bill (Levey, 2022). Another example of a systemic inequity is the Federal government spending much less on the Indian Health Service on a per capita basis than it does on Medicare, despite the high health needs of American Indians.

Medicine in the United States has not escaped the nation's legacy of systemic racism. Many hospitals, including institutions in the North, were for much of the twentieth century either completely segregated or had segregated wards, with inferior facilities and services available to Black, Latino, Asian, and other people of color. The enactment of Medicare and Medicaid catalyzed racial integration by prohibiting segregated hospitals from receiving payments from public insurance programs. Despite these gains, considerable *de facto* hospital segregation continues, with hospitals serving a high proportion of Black patients receiving significantly lower payments per patient day than other hospitals (Himmelstein et al., 2023). Systemic racial segregation in medical education gave rise to the establishment of historically Black medical schools such as the Howard, Morehouse, and Meharry schools of medicine. Until the mid-twentieth century, the American Medical Association effectively barred Black physicians from membership, which in turn often impeded a physician's ability to obtain hospital-admitting privileges. Neighborhoods that have high proportions of Black or Latino residents have far fewer physicians practicing in these communities. Black, Latino, and Asian health professionals are more likely than White physicians to locate their practices in underserved communities (Komaromy et al., 1996; Mertz & Grumbach, 2001; Walker et al., 2012). Black, Latino, and American Indian individuals remain extremely underrepresented among physicians, dentists, and many other health professions relative to their share of the total US population, an issue addressed further in Chapter 9.

Systemic and Structural Racism and Health

William Smith, a Black bus driver working for the New Orleans transportation agency, was considered an essential worker when the first devastating wave of COVID-19 swept through New Orleans. He was required to keep staffing his shifts. He died of COVID-19 acquired from a passenger on his bus.

Lilly Masangkay, a Filipino-American licensed practical nurse working at a nursing home in Saint Louis, also had to keep working during the pandemic. She was infected with COVID-19 during an outbreak among patients at the nursing home, and succumbed to the disease.

Chayton Begay was an elder of the Navajo Nation, living with his extended family in a crowded trailer home at the time the pandemic arrived in Navajo lands. When his daughter caught COVID-19, she had no way to isolate from other family members, resulting in Chayton becoming fatally infected with COVID-19.

Sue Pierce was a White tech worker living with her partner in a condominium in Seattle during the first phase of the pandemic. She started working remotely from home during the initial shut down, and continued to work entirely from home throughout the pandemic. She has never had a case of COVID-19.

During the first year of the pandemic, prior to the availability of vaccines, COVID-19 had an especially crushing impact on Black, Latino, and American Indian populations in the United States. In 2020, life expectancy decreased by 4.6 years for American Indian men, 3.6 years for Black men, and 4.5 years for Latinos, compared with a decrease of 1.6 years for White men. Life expectancy among women decreased by 4.2 years for American Indian women, and about 3 years among Black and Latina women, compared with 1.2 years among White women (Fig. 5–2) (Aburto et al., 2022; Goldman & Andrasfay, 2022). COVID-19 death rates were also much higher among the Pacific Islander population in the United States than among the White population (Feldman & Bassett, 2021). These inequities were not because of any innate greater susceptibility to COVID-19 among these populations. They were largely due to social and environmental factors putting marginalized populations at greater risk of COVID-19 infection, such as working in "essential" occupations (e.g., transportation, health care, food), living in crowded housing, and not having resources to isolate and quarantine.

One prominent form of structural racism in the United States is residential segregation. Concentration of Black residents and other marginalized groups in segregated, under-resourced neighborhoods has been fueled by discriminatory "redlining" of home mortgage lending and by "urban renewal" projects that destroyed many vibrant middle-class neighborhoods in Black communities. COVID-19 mortality is higher among Black residents of highly segregated states than among those residing in states with less residential segregation (Franz et al., 2022). Residential segregation is associated with many other poor health outcomes among Black and other marginalized populations (Williams & Mohammed, 2013; Bailey et al., 2017; Braveman et al., 2022). Closely related to housing segregation is school segregation. Both residential and school segregation are associated with long-lasting adverse health trajectories that begin in childhood (Kim et al., 2022; Wang et al., 2022). Under-resourced neighborhoods often have a paucity of retail establishments selling fresh produce and other healthful foods. Black and Latino households experience twice the level of food insecurity as White households (Coleman-Jensen et al., 2022); among

people with diabetes, food insecurity is associated with poorer control of blood sugar levels.

SOCIOECONOMIC STATUS AND HEALTH

Socioeconomic status can be defined using several metrics (often in combination), including income, wealth (which incorporates financial assets such as the value of a home in addition to income), level of education, and occupation. In many nations, socioeconomic status is referred to as social class. The income gap widened markedly in the United States. The top 10% of earners received 50% of the nation's total income in 2017 compared with 33% in 1965 (Saez, 2019). The top 10% control three-quarters of all the wealth in the United States (Khullar & Chokshi, 2018). Household income for the average family has stagnated (Khullar & Chokshi, 2018). As noted in Chapter 3, lack of health insurance is strongly associated with income, with individuals in households with less than $25,000 in annual income being about three times more likely to be uninsured than individuals in households with greater than $100,000 in income. Individuals with lower educational attainment and lower incomes are much less likely to have a regular source of primary care than those with higher educational and income status, even after accounting for differences in insurance coverage by education and income (Jabbarpour et al., 2022). In 2002, difficulty affording health care was reported by 69% of individuals with household incomes less than $40,000, compared with 49% with incomes of $40,000–89,999 and 21% with incomes of $90,000 or greater (Montero et al., 2022).

People in the United States with incomes above four times the poverty level live on average 7 years longer than those with incomes below the poverty level. Low-income adults are three times more likely to report being in poor or fair health than those with incomes above 400% of the federal poverty level (Fig. 5–4). Middle-aged persons in the highest quintile of wealth had a 5% chance of dying and 15% chance of becoming disabled over the next decade compared with those in the lowest wealth quintile who had a 17% chance of dying and 48% chance of becoming disabled (Khullar & Chokshi, 2018). Among people diagnosed with cancer, 58% of those in the highest income decile survive their cancer for at least 12 years compared with 39% of those in the lowest income decile (Singh & Jemal, 2017).

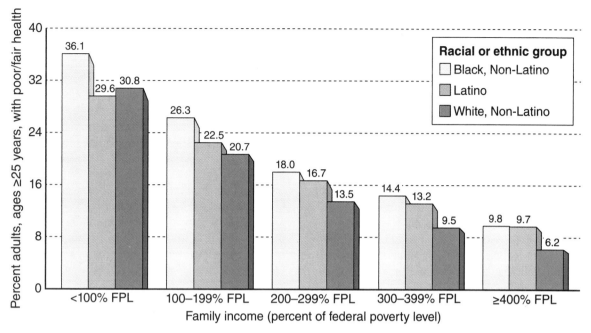

▲ **Figure 5–4.** Percentage of adults in poor or fair health, by income and race-ethnicity. Data are age adjusted. (Source: Braveman P, Egerter P. Overcoming Obstacles to Health. Robert Wood Johnson Foundation, 2008.)

THE INTERSECTIONALITY OF RACE AND SOCIAL CLASS

Race-ethnicity and socioeconomic status are not unrelated. In 2021, median household income was $77,999 for White, $57,981 for Latino, and $48,297 for Black Americans (Semega & Kollar, 2022). Inequities in wealth are even starker, with the median net worth of White households in 2016 being 8.3 times that of Latino households and 10 times that of Black households (Braveman et al., 2018). Both race-ethnicity and socioeconomic status matter for health. Racial-ethnic health inequities are not fully explained by racial-ethnic differences in income or education. At any given income level, Black adults are more likely to be in poor health than their White counterparts. Similar patterns hold when comparing Latino and White adults across income groups (Fig. 5–4). A striking example of the effects of race and class on health inequities may be found in a study of preterm births in California. White and Black women of lower socioeconomic status had similarly high rates of preterm birth. Among White women, the rate of preterm births was progressively lower as socioeconomic status increased.

No such decrease was found for Black women. Rates of preterm births were higher among Black women than White women in all socioeconomic strata other than the lowest one (Braveman et al., 2015).

GENDER IDENTITY AND SEXUAL ORIENTATION

Women's Health

For several months something did not feel right in Nida Moore's chest when she walked uphill near her home. She had difficulty getting time off work to see a physician and worried about the cost of medical care given her high deductible health plan. When she finally saw a physician, he told her that at age 46 she was "too young" to have heart problems, even though Nida's mother had died of a heart attack in her 50s. A few weeks later, Nida woke up with intense chest pain, called 911, and in the emergency department was diagnosed with an acute myocardial infarction. She felt much better after getting a stent placed to remove the blockage in her coronary artery. But now she is experiencing a different kind of heartache. Her daughter is in an abusive relationship and just told Nida that she is 8 weeks pregnant and wants an abortion. Nida and her daughter live in Idaho, a state that has just banned all abortions. Nida tells her daughter she will try to come up with the money to help her travel to another state to get this procedure, but worries she might face legal prosecution or retaliation from her daughter's partner for doing this.

Interpersonal and structural bias results in health care and health inequities for women. In 2017, 26% of adult women in the United States reported delaying or going without care due to cost, compared with 19% of men. The percentage foregoing care was even higher (39%) among low-income women. In addition to problems of affordability, about a quarter of women reported not obtaining care because of not having time (24%) and not being able to take time off work (23%) (Kaiser Family Foundation, 2018). Unlike most high-income nations, the United States has no federally mandated national policy for paid parental leave and the states that have enacted mandatory paid leave provide much shorter duration of leave than the benefit offered in other nations. Paid parental leave is associated with improved health outcomes for mothers and fathers (Nandi et al., 2018; Irish et al., 2021). In addition to these types of structural barriers, many women experience interpersonal bias in health care. In a 2017 survey, nearly 1 in 5 women reported experiencing gender discrimination in a health care setting (SteelFisher et al., 2019). Among patients with pain, women are more likely than men to have clinicians attribute their pain to psychological and emotional rather than somatic causes (Samulowitz et al., 2018). Even though more women than men die of cardiovascular disease each year, many studies show undertesting and undertreatment of women for cardiovascular disease, resulting in higher case fatality rates for women (Bairey Merz, 2014).

For women of reproductive age, access to contraception and abortion is particularly challenging, with barriers in many states becoming more formidable following the 2022 Supreme Court decision in Dobbs vs. Jackson Women's Health Organization overturning the constitutional right to abortion. This decision occurred on a backdrop of preexisting difficulties and inequities many people experience in obtaining high-quality family planning services. The Affordable Care Act reduced financial barriers by requiring health insurance plans to cover "female controlled" contraceptive methods as preventive services exempt from deductibles or copayments. However, contraceptive counseling is often provided with inadequate information and lack of patient-centered communication (Dehlendorf et al., 2014).

Pregnancy termination is one of the most common and safe procedures in the United States, with about 1 in 4 women having an abortion at some point in their lifetime. Two-thirds of abortions occur within 8 weeks of pregnancy (Ranji et al., 2023). About two-thirds of adults in the United States support the Supreme Court's decision in 1973 in Roe vs. Wade that affirmed a constitutional right to abortion, prior to the reversal in the Dobbs decision. But abortion has long been a politically charged issue. Beginning in 1976, annual Congressional action (known as the Hyde Amendment) prohibited use of federal funds to pay for abortion except in cases of rape, incest, or pregnancy endangering the pregnant person's life. The Hyde Amendment applies to programs such as Medicaid, the Indian Health Service, and private insurance for federal employees. Sixteen states cover abortion under their Medicaid programs by only using state funds for these services (Ranji et al., 2023). Because of coverage restrictions, about half of women pay the entire cost of their abortions out of pocket. People seeking abortions are disproportionately in low-income brackets and women of color; coverage restrictions produce class and racial inequities in access to abortion (Salganicoff et al., 2021). The Dobbs decision is accentuating geographic and racial inequities in abortion access, with more than 15 states enacting complete or partial bans on abortion within 6 months of the Supreme Court decision. Post-Dobbs, 33% of women of reproductive age lived more than 60 minutes from the nearest abortion facility, compared with 15% pre-Dobbs, with travel times being longest for American Indian women (Rader et al., 2022). The Dobbs decision drew widespread condemnation from most major physician organizations in the United States. The American Medical Association characterized the Supreme Court's decision as "an egregious allowance of government intrusion into the medical examination room, a direct attack on the practice of medicine and the patient-physician relationship, and a brazen violation of patients' rights to evidence-based reproductive health services (AMA, 2022)."

▶ LGBTQ+ Health

LGBTQ+ refers to lesbian, gay, bisexual, transgender, queer, and related sexual orientations and gender identities marginalized by a dominant culture of heterosexual orientation and traditional definitions of gender. Lesbian, gay, and bisexual refer to sexual orientation, and transgender (and non-binary) to gender identity. The former groups are often referred to as "sexual minorities" and the latter groups as "gender minorities." Common to both groups are experiences of stigma and discrimination; there is often intersectionality among these groups (e.g., transgender individuals with gay, lesbian, or bisexual sexual orientations). Policies promulgated by the medical profession in the United States historically abetted systemic discrimination against the LGBTQ+ community. When the American Psychiatric Association issued its first Diagnostic and Statistical Manual of Mental Disorders (DSM) in 1952, the manual categorized homosexuality as a sociopathic personality disturbance. Laws and regulations discriminating against lesbian and gay people in employment, housing, marriage, and other sectors often cited the DSM categorization as justification (Institute of Medicine, 2011). In 1973, gay rights activists succeeded in convincing the American Psychiatric Association to declassify homosexuality as a mental illness.

Sexual Minority Health

Inequities in insurance coverage between LGB and non-LGB individuals decreased following the enactment of the Affordable Care Act and the Supreme Court's decision in Obergefell vs. Hodges in 2015 legalizing same-sex marriage, which allowed many LGB individuals to gain health insurance under a spouse's employment-based plan. However, LGB individuals remain much more likely than non-LGB individuals to have Medicaid—a type of insurance not accepted by many physicians (Bosworth et al., 2021). LGB individuals are twice as likely as non-LGB individuals to have delayed obtaining medical care or a prescription due to cost (Bosworth et al., 2021). Although prejudice among health professionals against sexual minority patients

appears to have decreased in recent years in tandem with broader societal changes such as legalization of same sex marriage, concerns about potential bias and clinicians' cultural and medical competence in the care of sexual minority patients results in patients not always disclosing their sexual orientation to their clinicians. One study found much higher rates of non-disclosure to health care providers of sexual orientation among bisexual men (39%) and women (33%) than among gay men (10%) and lesbians (13%) (Durso & Meyer, 2013). Among gay men and lesbians in this study, persons of color were much more likely than White individuals to not disclose their sexual orientation.

The explosion of the HIV epidemic in the 1980s decimated the health of gay men. By 1995, 1 in 9 gay men in the United States had been diagnosed with AIDS, and 1 in 15 had died of AIDS (Rosenfeld, 2018). The failures and successes of the US response to AIDS hold myriad lessons for health policy, including the shameful delay in mounting a national public health and clinical care strategy to combat HIV, the role of patient and community activists in groups such as ACTUP to democratize science and health care, and the Federal government's eventual establishment and sustained funding of programs such as the domestic Ryan White program and global PEPFAR program. The advent of highly effective anti-viral medications transformed HIV infection from an invariably fatal disease to a chronic condition compatible with a long life-span for individuals able to access necessary health care. The epidemiology of HIV infection in the United States has shifted over time from one predominantly affecting men who have sex with men to a condition affecting additional populations at risk for infection. In 2019 in the United States, one quarter of people living with HIV were women; 40% were Black people and 24% Latino people (CDC, 2021).

A focus on HIV and sexual health often overshadows other compelling health inequities among LGB individuals. LGB youth have higher rates of depression and suicidality than heterosexual youth; the higher prevalence of mental health conditions is largely attributable to experiences of victimization and discrimination (Institute of Medicine, 2011). LGB youth initiate smoking and substance use at a younger age than their heterosexual counterparts and are more likely than heterosexual individuals to smoke as adults. Lesbians are much less likely than heterosexual women to be up to date on screening for cervical cancer, even though the human papilloma virus, the agent causing most cases of cervical cancer, may be transmitted by intimate contact among women who have sex with women and not only through heterosexual relations (Tracy et al., 2013).

Gender Minority Health

Transgender and other gender minority individuals experience especially harsh stigmatization in the United States. Gender minority individuals have traditionally experienced major barriers to obtaining gender affirming medical and surgical treatment due to discrimination, a paucity of physicians trained to provide gender affirming care, and exclusion of these services from health insurance benefits. Rates of attempted suicide are nine times higher among transgender individuals than among the population at large, with rates particularly high among youth. Family rejection places a gender minority young person at particularly high risk of attempting suicide (Austin et al., 2022).

Health professionals have played a role, along with sexual minority advocates, in beginning to shift cultural norms about diversity of gender expression and the medical appropriateness of gender affirming care (American Medical Association, 2019). Research suggests that gender affirming care results in improved mental health and well-being (White Hughto & Reisner, 2016). Including coverage of medically necessary hormonal and surgical treatment for gender minority patients as a health insurance benefit is more cost-effective than many other commonly covered services, and was estimated to add less than 2 cents per month in 2013 dollars to the cost of health insurance for an insured population (Padula et al., 2016). Over the past decade, the Federal government has acted to expand access to services by including coverage of gender affirming care in programs such as Medicare and interpreting denial of coverage by employment-based health plans as violating the Civil Rights Act. However, beginning in 2021, several states enacted laws banning gender affirming hormonal and/or surgical treatment for minors, with additional states considering similar laws. These measures continue to be highly contentious as they play out in state legislatures and the courts.

RURAL POPULATIONS

About 15% of Americans reside in rural communities. Although residing in a rural area is conceptually very different from marginalized racial-ethnic, gender, and sexual identities, one commonality is systemic inequities in health care and health. The age-adjusted mortality rate in rural communities is 20% higher than the rate in urban communities, with the rural-urban disparity widening between 2000 and 2020 (Curtin & Spencer, 2021). This recent adverse trajectory in health corresponds with a period of economic decline in rural America, with many communities not recovering following the recession of 2008 and experiencing persistently high rates of unemployment. Although a slightly greater proportion of people in rural than urban communities have no health insurance, the biggest barrier to health care access in rural communities is not lack of insurance but the scant supply of health professionals and medical facilities. About two-thirds of federally designated primary care health professional shortage counties are located in rural areas; shortages are even more pronounced for specialist physicians and mental health and dental clinicians. Rural hospitals play a critical role as a hub for health services in sparsely populated areas yet are much more financially distressed than most urban hospitals. Between 2010 and 2020, 135 rural hospitals closed in the United States, resulting in residents in these communities having to travel great distances to access health services (Agency for Healthcare Research and Quality, 2021). Policy strategies to improve access to care in rural communities include educational loan repayment for health professionals practicing in these areas, special payments for critical access rural hospitals, facilitating telehealth and broadband access, and outreach programs to vulnerable populations such as migrant farm workers.

OTHER MARGINALIZED POPULATIONS

Many other groups experience stigma, discrimination, and marginalization, including individuals living with disabilities, people with substance use disorders, unhoused populations, immigrants, and religious minorities. The book *Medical Management of Vulnerable and Underserved Patients* (King & Wheeler, 2016) provides a more thorough presentation of populations experiencing disparities and approaches to promoting health equity.

STRATEGIES TO ADVANCE EQUITY

▶ Strategies for Health Care Organizations

Equity First Paradigm

Too often, health care practitioners and organizations are either largely unaware of the extent of health care and health inequities among the patients they care for, or reactive after a specific inequity comes to their attention. Equity First has been proposed as an approach to center equity in core mission, values, and goals and apply an equity lens at the earliest stages of all activities, moving from disparity resolution to disparity prevention (Collins & Grumbach, 2022). Table 5–1 summarizes the key components of this paradigm.

Identifying and Intervening on Social Needs

With growing recognition of the powerful influence of social drivers of health, many health care providers are implementing processes to more systematically identify patients' social needs. One common approach is routinely screening for these needs using questionnaires that ask about food and housing insecurity, transportation barriers, and related issues. At a minimum, greater awareness of these social needs may inform clinical teams to adjust their care plans to mitigate inequities, such as by accounting for food insecurity when prescribing diabetes medications. A more ambitious goal is to actively help connect patients to community-based and government resources, such as food banks and tenant advocacy organizations. Some studies have demonstrated beneficial health outcomes from screening and linkage programs; Medicare and Medicaid have launched several initiatives in this area. Ongoing research continues to investigate how to feasibly and effectively implement these types of screening and referral programs in routine care settings (DeMarchis et al., 2022).

Diversity, Inclusion, and Anti-Racism

Achieving a more racial-ethnically diverse health workforce is another strategy to reduce health care inequities. As noted above, health professionals underrepresented in health care are more likely than their counterparts to practice in communities with workforce shortages and care for marginalized populations; receiving care from racial-ethnically and linguistically concordant clinicians may improve the quality of care received by communities experiencing inequities. Lack of greater health professions diversity is rooted in systemic injustices in educational opportunity beginning at the earliest years of schooling, with definitive solutions requiring large-scale investment in and revitalization of public schools, school desegregation, and other public policies. However, health care and health education institutions may take action in areas under their direct control. For example, sponsorship of postbaccalaureate pre-medical and pre-dental programs and reform of health profession school admissions policies to place less emphasis on test scores and grade point averages are evidence-based strategies for advancing a diverse, highly skilled health workforce (Grumbach & Mendoza, 2008). Health care settings, from a small private practice to a large health system, also have a responsibility not just to promote diversity, but to foster a climate of inclusion that creates a sense of belonging

Table 5–1. Equity First Paradigm in health care: key components

The Equity First Paradigm is an approach to centering equity in all health care operations.

1. Prioritize and invest in the equity portfolio. Make equity one of the explicit goals for all care improvement initiatives, include individuals with expertise in health equity on improvement project work groups, provide adequate resources for equity improvement, and hold leadership accountable for equity results.
2. Collect and regularly apply data on equity-relevant patient variables. Accurately ascertain and record patient self-reported identities (race-ethnicity, gender, sexual orientation, etc.), and use these data in analyses to identify inequities in care and health and track progress in closing equity gaps.
3. Challenge "business as usual" operating practices that perpetuate structural inequities. Examples include institutionalizing multilingual communication, facilitating digital literacy and digital access, scheduling services in a patient-centered manner such as including evening and weekend hours.
4. Engage and support patients, employees, and community members from marginalized groups as partners in health equity initiatives.

Source: Collins P, Grumbach K. The UCSF Health COVID Equity Work Group: Report of Goals, Accomplishments, and Lessons Learned, March, 2022. https://ucsf.app.box.com/file/953982583370?s=1dyfybbqfrcte6m7mq86wsnqchq4kptc.

among health workers of marginalized identities. Many institutions are incorporating training about racism, homophobia, and other forms of interpersonal and systemic oppression into their core curricula in health professions schools and continuing education programs for health workers.

Anchor Institutions

Hospitals and health systems are among the largest economic forces in communities across the nation. These institutions are often referred to as "anchor institutions" to indicate their position as influential place-based businesses. Growing attention is being paid to how anchor institutions might more intentionally use their economic power to advance social and health equity in their local communities. This approach emphasizes going beyond equity in direct health care services and focusing on how an institution may direct its employment, procurement, and investment practices to better support economic development in nearby under-resourced neighborhoods. Examples include implementing workforce development programs, purchasing goods and services from local businesses owned by people of color, women, veterans, and other priority groups, and earmarking a portion of institutions' large investment portfolios to provide loans for building affordable housing or similar types of social investment (Koh et al., 2020).

▶ Addressing the Political Determinants of Health

To fully achieve health equity requires changes in the social and environmental conditions that are the root cause of disparities. Daniel Dawes uses the term "the political determinants of health" to highlight how the influences upon the social determinants of health lie in the policy and political sphere (Dawes, 2020). Political determinants shape almost all the key issues discussed in this chapter, such as residential and school segregation, access to abortion or gender affirming care, affordable housing and living wages, and state decisions to expand Medicaid. Health professionals have an important role to play as advocates for policies that promote health equity. This may take the form of individual activism, working within professional organizations and other groups to influence their advocacy positions on legislation and regulations, and allyship with community members and organizations with shared interests.

CONCLUSION

Comprehensive health insurance coverage is necessary for equitable access to health care. But it is not sufficient for achieving health equity. Eliminating persistent inequities among racial-ethnic, socioeconomic, and other marginalized groups requires addressing many factors within health care practices and organizations that contribute to inequities, as well as the broader social and political drivers of health. Making headway on the path to equity may benefit from shifting from a deficit-based to asset-based framework, leveraging the resilience and vitality of communities that have found ways to build a culture of health despite facing systemic adversity.

REFERENCES

Aburto JM, Tilstra AM, Floridi G, Dowd JB. Significant impacts of the COVID-19 pandemic on race/ethnic differences in US mortality. *Proc Natl Acad Sci USA.* 2022;119(35):e2205813119.

Agency for Healthcare Research and Quality. 2022 National Healthcare Quality and Disparities Report Appendixes. AHRQ Publication No. 22(23)-0030. October, 2022. www.ahrq.gov/research/findings/nhqrdr/index.html.

Agency for Healthcare Research and Quality. National Healthcare Quality and Disparities Report Chartbook on Rural Healthcare. AHRQ Publication No. 22-0010. November 2021. https://www.ahrq.gov/research/findings/nhqrdr/chartbooks/ruralhealth/index.html.

Alsan M, Garrick O, Graziani G. Does diversity matter for health? Experimental evidence from Oakland. *Am Econ Rev.* 2019;10:4071–4111.

American Medical Association and Health Professionals Advancing LGBTQ Equity. Issue Brief: Health insurance coverage for gender-affirming care of transgender patients. 2019. https://www.ama-assn.org/system/files/2019-03/transgender-coverage-issue-brief.pdf.

American Medical Association. Ruling an egregious allowance of government intrusion into medicine. Press Release, June 24, 2022.

Austin A, Craig SL, D'Souza S, McInroy LB. Suicidality among transgender youth: elucidating the role of interpersonal risk factors. *J Interpers Violence.* 2022;37(5-6):NP2696–NP2718.

Bailey ZD, Krieger N, Agénor M, Graves J, Linos N, Bassett MT. Structural racism and health inequities in the USA: evidence and interventions. *Lancet.* 2017;389(10077):1453–1463.

Bairey Merz CN. Sex. Death and the diagnosis gap. *Circulation.* 2014;130:740–742.

Bosworth A, Turrini G, Pyda S, et al. Health Insurance Coverage and Access to Care for LGBTQ+ Individuals: US Department of Health and Human Services, Issue Brief HP-2021-14, June, 2021. https://aspe.hhs.gov/sites/default/files/2021-07/lgbt-health-ib.pdf.

Braveman P, Acker J, Arkin E, et al. *Wealth Matters for Health Equity.* Princeton, NJ: Robert Wood Johnson Foundation; 2018. https://www.rwjf.org/en/library/research/2018/09/wealth-matters-for-health-equity.html.

Braveman P, Heck K, Egerter S, et al. The role of socioeconomic factors in Black-White disparities in preterm birth. *Am J Public Health.* 2015;105(4):694–702.

Braveman P, Heck K, Egerter S, et al. Worry about racial discrimination: a missing piece of the puzzle of Black-White disparities in preterm birth? *PLoS One.* 2017;12(10):e0186151.

Braveman PA, Arkin E, Proctor D, Kauh T, Holm N. Systemic and structural racism: definitions, examples, health damages, and approaches to dismantling. *Health Aff (Millwood).* 2022;41:171–178.

CDC. Estimated HIV incidence and prevalence in the United States, 2015–2019, HIV Surveillance Supplemental Report 2021;26(1) and US Census Bureau, Quick Facts—United States.

Coleman-Jensen A, Rabbitt MP, Gregory CA, Singh A. *Household Food Security in the United States in 2021.* Washington: U.S. Economic Research Service; 2022. https://www.ers.usda.gov/webdocs/publications/104656/err-309.pdf?v=132.4.

Collins P, Grumbach K. The UCSF Health COVID Equity Work Group. Report of Goals, Accomplishments, and Lessons Learned, March, 2022.

Cooper LA, Roter DL, Johnson RL, Ford DE, Steinwachs DM, Powe NR. Patient-centered communication, ratings of care and concordance of patient and physician race. *Ann Intern Med.* 2003;139:907–915.

Curtin SC, Spencer MR. Trends in death rates in urban and rural areas: United States, 1999–2019. NCHS Data Brief, no 417. Hyattsville, MD: National Center for Health Statistics. 2021. http://dx.doi.org/10.15620/cdc:109049.

Dawes DE. *The Political Determinants of Health.* Baltimore, MD: Johns Hopkins University Press; 2020.

De Marchis EH, Brown E, Aceves B, et al. *State of the Science of Screening in Healthcare Settings.* Social Interventions Research & Evaluation Network; 2022. https://sirenetwork.ucsf.edu/sites/default/files/2022-06/final%20SCREEN%20State-of-Science-Report%5B55%5D.pdf.

Dehlendorf C, Krajewski C, Borrero S. Contraceptive counseling: best practices to ensure quality communication and enable effective contraceptive use. *Clin Obstet Gynecol.* 2014;57:659–673.

Durso LE, Meyer IH. Patterns and predictors of disclosure of sexual orientation to healthcare providers among lesbians, gay men, and bisexuals. *Sex Res Social Policy.* 2013;10(1):35–42.

Feldman JM, Bassett MT. Variation in COVID-19 mortality in the US by race and ethnicity and educational attainment. *JAMA Netw Open.* 2021;4(11):e2135967.

Franz B, Parker B, Milner A, Braddock JH 2nd. The relationship between systemic racism, residential segregation, and racial/ethnic disparities in COVID-19 deaths in the United States. *Ethn Dis.* 2022;32:31–38.

Goldman N, Andrasfay T. Life expectancy loss among Native Americans during the COVID-19 pandemic. *Demogr Res.* 2022;47:233–246.

Grumbach K, Mendoza R. Disparities in human resources: addressing the lack of diversity in the health professions. *Health Aff (Millwood).* 2008;27(2):413–422.

Himmelstein G, Ceasar JN, Himmelstein KE. Hospitals that serve many black patients have lower revenues and profits: structural racism in hospital financing. *J Gen Intern Med.* 2023;38:586–591.

Hoffman KM, Trawalter S, Axt JR, Oliver MN. Racial bias in pain assessment and treatment recommendations, and false beliefs about biological differences between blacks and whites. *Proc Natl Acad Sci USA.* 2016;113(16):4296–4301.

Hoyert DL. Maternal mortality rates in the United States, 2020. NCHS Health E-Stats. 2022. https://dx.doi.org/10.15620/cdc:113967.

Institute of Medicine. *The Health of Lesbian, Gay, Bisexual, and Transgender People: Building a Foundation for Better Understanding.* Washington, DC: National Academies Press; 2011.

Irish AM, White JS, Modrek S, Hamad R. Paid family leave and mental health in the US: a quasi-experimental study of state policies. *Am J Prev Med.* 2021;61:182–191.

Jabbarpour Y, Greiner A, Jetty A, et al. *Relationships Matter: How Usual is Usual Source of (Primary) Care.* Primary Care Collaborative; November, 2022. https://bit.ly/PCCEvidenceReport2022.

Johnson RL, Roter D, Powe NR, Cooper LA. Patient race/ethnicity and quality of patient-physician communication during medical visits. *Am J Public Health.* 2004;94:2084–2090.

Jones CP. Levels of racism: a theoretic framework and a gardener's tale. *Am J Public Health.* 2000;90:1212–1215.

Jones CP. Seeing the water: seven values targets for anti-racism action. Harvard Medical School Primary Care Review, April 25, 2020.

Kaiser Family Foundation. Women's Coverage, Access, and Affordability: Key Findings from the 2017 Kaiser Women's Health Survey. March, 2018.

Khullar D, Chokshi DA. Health, income and poverty: where we are and what could help. Health Affairs Policy Brief, October 4, 2018.

Kim MH, Schwartz GL, White JS, et al. School racial segregation and long-term cardiovascular health among Black adults in the US: a quasi-experimental study. *PLoS Med.* 2022;19(6):e1004031.

King TE, Wheeler MB. *Medical Management of Vulnerable and Underserved Patients.* New York, NY: McGraw-Hill; 2016.

Koh HK, Bantham A, Geller AC, et al. Anchor Institutions: best practices to address social needs and social determinants of health. *Am J Public Health.* 2020;110:309–316.

Komaromy M, Grumbach K, Drake M, et al. The role of black and Hispanic physicians in providing health care for underserved populations. *N Engl J Med.* 1996;334:1305–1310.

Lee S, Waters SF. Asians and Asian Americans' experiences of racial discrimination during the COVID-19 pandemic: impacts on health outcomes and the buffering role of social support. *Stigma Health.* 2021;6:70–78.

Levey NM. Diagnosis: Debt. 100 million people in America are saddled with health care debt. KHN, June, 2022. https://khn.org/news/article/diagnosis-debt-investigation-100-million-americans-hidden-medical-debt/.

Martin KD, Roter DL, Beach MC, Carson KA, Cooper LA. Physician communication behaviors and trust among black and white patients with hypertension. *Med Care.* 2013;51:151–157.

Mertz EA, Grumbach K. Identifying communities with low dentist supply in California. *J Public Health Dent.* 2001;61:172–177.

Montero A, Kearney A, Hamel L, Brodie M. *Americans' Challenges with Health Care Costs.* Kaiser Family Foundation; 2022.

Nandi A, Jahagirdar D, Dimitris MC, et al. The impact of parental and medical leave policies on socioeconomic and health outcomes in OECD countries. *Milbank Q.* 2018;96:434–471.

Padula WV, Heru S, Campbell JD. Societal implications of health insurance coverage for medically necessary services in the US transgender population: a cost-effectiveness analysis. *J Gen Intern Med.* 2016;31:394–401.

Parker MM, Fernández A, Moffet HH, Grant RW, Torreblanca A, Karter AJ. Association of patient-physician language concordance and glycemic control for limited-English proficiency Latinos with type 2 diabetes. *JAMA Intern Med.* 2017;177:380–387.

Rader B, Upadhyay UD, Sehgal NKR, Reis BY, Brownstein JS, Hswen Y. Estimated travel time and spatial access to abortion facilities in the US before and after the *Dobbs v Jackson Women's Health* decision. *JAMA.* 2022;328:2041–2047.

Ranji U, Diep K, Salganicoff A. Key Facts on Abortion in the United States. Jan 20, 2023. https://www.kff.org/womens-health-policy/report/key-facts-on-abortion-in-the-united-states/.

Rosenfeld D. The AIDS epidemic's lasting impact on gay men. British Academy, Feb, 2018. https://www.thebritishacademy.ac.uk/blog/aids-epidemic-lasting-impact-gay-men/.

Saez E. Striking it richer: the evolution of top incomes in the United States. UC Berkeley, 2019. https://eml.berkeley.edu/~saez/saez-UStopincomes-2017.pdf.

Saha S, Taggart SH, Komaromy M, Bindman AB. Do patients choose physicians of their own race? *Health Aff (Millwood).* 2000;19:76–83.

Salganicoff A, Sobel L, Ramaswamy A. *The Hyde Amendment and Coverage for Abortion Services.* Kaiser Family Foundation; 2021.

Samulowitz A, Gremyr I, Eriksson E, Hensing G. "Brave men" and "emotional women": a theory-guided literature review on gender bias in health care and gendered norms towards patients with chronic pain. *Pain Res Manag.* 2018;2018:6358624.

Semega J, Kollar M. Income in the United States: 2021. US Census Report P60-276, September, 2022. https://www.census.gov/library/publications/2022/demo/p60-276.html.

Singh GK, Jemal A. Socioeconomic and racial/ethnic disparities in cancer mortality, incidence, and survival in the United States, 1950–2014. *J Environ Public Health.* 2017;2017:2819372.

SteelFisher GK, Findling MG, Bleich SN, et al. Gender discrimination in the United States: experiences of women. *Health Serv Res.* 2019;54:1442–1453.

Todd KH, Deaton C, D'Adamo AP, Goe L. Ethnicity and analgesic practice. *Ann Emerg Med.* 2000;35:11–16.

Todd KH, Samaroo N, Hoffman JR. Ethnicity as a risk factor for inadequate emergency department analgesia. *JAMA.* 1993;269:1537–1539.

Tracy JK, Schluterman NH, Greenberg DR. Understanding cervical cancer screening among lesbians: a national survey. *BMC Public Health.* 2013;13:442.

Walker KO, Moreno G, Grumbach K. The association among specialty, race, ethnicity, and practice location among California physicians in diverse specialties. *J Natl Med Assoc.* 2012;104(1-2):46–52.

Wang G, Schwartz GL, Kershaw KN, McGowan C, Kim MH, Hamad R. The association of residential racial segregation with health among U.S. children: a nationwide longitudinal study. *SSM Popul Health*. 2022;19:101250.

White Hughto JM, Reisner SL. A systematic review of the effects of hormone therapy on psychological functioning and quality of life in transgender individuals. *Transgender Health*. Dec 2016;21–31.

Williams DR, Mohammed SA. Racism and health I: pathways and scientific evidence. *Am Behav Sci*. 2013;57:1152–1173.

Wilson E, Chen AH, Grumbach K, Wang F, Fernandez A. Effects of limited English proficiency and physician language on health care comprehension. *J Gen Intern Med*. 2005;20:800–806.

World Health Organization. Health Equity. 2023. https://www.who.int/health-topics/health-equity#tab=tab_1.

Medical Ethics and Rationing of Health Care

For those who work in the healing professions, ethical values play a special role. The specific content of medical ethics was first formulated centuries ago, based on the sayings of Hippocrates and others. The refinement of medical ethics has continued up to the present by practicing health caregivers, health professional and religious organizations, and individual ethicists. As medical technology, health care financing, and the organization of health care transform themselves, so must the content of medical ethics change in order to acknowledge and guide new circumstances.

FOUR PRINCIPLES OF MEDICAL ETHICS

Over the years, participants in and observers of medical care have distilled widely shared human beliefs about healing the sick into four major ethical principles: beneficence, nonmaleficence, autonomy, and justice (Beauchamp & Childress, 2023) (Table 6–1).

Beneficence is the obligation of health care providers to help people in need.

Dr. Rolando Bueno is a hard-working family physician practicing in a low-income neighborhood of a large city. He shows concern for his patients, and his knowledge and judgment are respected by his medical and nursing colleagues. On one occasion, he was called before the hospital quality assurance committee when one of his patients unexpectedly died; he agreed that he had made mistakes in his care and incorporated the lessons of the case into his future practice.

Dr. Bueno tries to live up to the ideal of beneficence. He does not always succeed; like all health professionals, he sometimes makes clinical errors. Overall, he treats his patients to the best of his ability. The principle of beneficence in the healing professions is the obligation to care for patients to the best of one's ability.

Nonmaleficence is the duty of health care providers to do no harm.

Mrs. Lucy Knight suffers from insomnia and Parkinson's disease. The insomnia does not bother her but it irritates her husband. Mr. Knight requests his wife's physician to order strong sleeping pills for her, but the physician declines, saying that the combination of sleeping pills and Parkinson's disease places Mrs. Knight at high risk for a serious fall.

The modern array of medical interventions has the capacity to do good or harm or both, thereby enmeshing the principle of nonmaleficence with the principle of beneficence. In the case of Mrs. Knight, the prescribing of sedatives has more potential for harm than for good, particularly because Mrs. Knight does not see her insomnia as a problem.

Autonomy is the right of a person to choose and follow his or her own plan of life and action.

Mr. Winter is a frail 88-year-old found by Dr. James Choice, his family physician, to have colon cancer, which has spread to the liver. The cancer is causing no symptoms. An oncologist gives Mr. Winter the option of transfusions, parenteral nutrition, and surgery, followed by chemotherapy; or watchful waiting with palliative and hospice

Table 6–1. The four principles of medical ethics

Beneficence	The obligation of health care providers to help people in need
Nonmaleficence	The duty of health care providers to do no harm
Autonomy	The right of patients to make choices regarding their health care
Justice	The concept of treating everyone in a fair manner

care when symptoms appear. Mr. Winter is terrified of hospitals and prefers to remain at home. He feels that he might live a comfortable couple of years before the cancer claims his life. After talking it over with Dr. Choice, he chooses the second option.

The principle of autonomy adds another consideration to the interrelated principles of beneficence and nonmaleficence. Would Mr. Winter enjoy a longer life by submitting himself to aggressive cancer therapy that does harm in order to do good? Or, does he sense that the harm may exceed the good? The balance of risks and benefits confronts each physician on a daily basis (Eddy, 1990). But the decision cannot be made solely by a risk–benefit analysis; the patient's preference is a critical addition to the equation.

In medical ethics, autonomy refers to the right of competent adult patients to consent to or refuse treatment. While the clinician has an obligation to respect the patient's wishes, he or she also has a duty to fully inform the patient of the probable consequences of those wishes. For children and adults unable to make medical decisions, a parent, guardian, other family member, or surrogate decision maker named in a legal document becomes the autonomous agent on behalf of the patient.

Justice refers to the ethical concept of treating everyone in a fair manner.

Joe, a White businessman in the suburbs, suffers crushing chest pain and within 5 minutes is taken to a nearby private emergency department, where he receives immediate coronary stenting and state-of-the-art treatment for a heart attack. Five miles away, in a low-income neighborhood, Josephine, a Black woman, experiences severe chest pain,

calls 911, waits 25 minutes for help to arrive, and is brought to a public hospital whose emergency department staff is attending to five other acutely ill patients. Before receiving appropriate attention, she suffers an arrhythmia and dies.

The principle of justice as applied to medical ethics is harder to define than the principles of beneficence, nonmaleficence, and autonomy. In one sense, it is unjust to discipline a physician for a poor patient outcome that she did not cause. In another meaning, justice refers to universal rights: to receive enough to eat, to be afforded shelter, to have access to basic medical care and education, and to be able to speak freely. If these rights are denied, justice has been violated. In yet another version, justice connotes equal opportunity: All people should have an equal chance to realize their human potential. Justice might be linked to the golden rule: Treat others as you would want others to treat you. These notions are central to the concept of health equity discussed in Chapter 5. Viewed through this lens, the differential treatment of Joe and Josephine is an unjust inequity. The structural racism producing delay in care for Josephine violates the ethical principle of justice.

▶ Distributive Justice

The principle of justice includes consideration of the allocation of benefits and burdens in society. This realm of ethical thinking is called *distributive justice*, involving such questions as: Who receives what amount of wealth, of education, or of medical care? Who pays what amount of taxes?

The principle of justice is linked to the idea of fairness. In the arena of distributive justice, no agreement exists on what formula for allocating benefits and costs is fair. Should each person get an equal share? Should those who work harder receive more? Should the proper formula be "to each according to ability to pay," as determined by a free market? Or "to each according to need?" In allocating costs, should each person pay an equal share or should those with greater wealth pay more? Most societies construct a mixture of these allocation formulas. Unemployment benefits consider effort (having had a job) and need (having lost the job). Welfare benefits are primarily based on need. Job promotions may be based on merit. Many goods are distributed according to ability to pay. Primary education in theory (but not always in practice) is founded on the belief that everyone should receive an equal share (Jonsen et al., 2021; Beauchamp & Childress, 2023).

How is the principle of distributive justice formulated for health care? The concept that health care is a privilege, allocated according to ability to pay, has long competed with the idea that health care is a right and should be distributed according to need. In most high-income nations, the allocation of health care according to need has become the dominant political belief, as demonstrated by the passage of universal or near-universal health insurance laws. In the United States, the failure of the 100-year battle to enact national health insurance, and the widely divergent public opinions on the 2010 Affordable Care Act, attest to the ongoing debate between health care as a privilege and health care as a right (see Chapter 16).

If the overwhelming opinion in the developed world holds that health care should be allocated according to need, then all people should have equitable access to a reasonable level of medical care without financial barriers (i.e., people should have a right to health care). In this chapter, we consider that the principle of distributive justice requires all people to receive high-quality medical services based on medical need without regard to ability to pay, race-ethnicity, or other social characteristics.

ETHICAL DILEMMAS, OLD AND NEW

Ethical dilemmas (Lo, 2020) are situations in which a provider of medical care is forced to make a decision that violates one of the four principles of medical ethics in order to adhere to another of the principles. Financial conflicts of interest on the part of physicians (see Chapters 4 and 13), in contrast, pit ethical behavior against individual gain and are not ethical dilemmas.

Anthony, a 22-year-old Jehovah's Witness, is admitted to the intensive care unit for gastrointestinal bleeding. His hematocrit has fallen from 38% to 21%. The medical resident implores Anthony to accept lifesaving transfusions, but he refuses, saying that his religion teaches him that death is preferable to receiving blood products. When the blood pressure reaches 60/20 mm Hg,

the desperate resident decides to give the blood while Anthony is unconscious. The attending physician vetoes the plan, saying that the patient has the right to refuse treatment, even if an avoidable death is the outcome.

In Anthony's case, the ethical dilemma is a conflict between beneficence and autonomy. Which principle has priority depends on the particular situation, and in this case, autonomy supersedes beneficence. If the patient were a child without sufficient knowledge or reasoning capability to make an informed choice, the physician would be obligated to give the transfusions, even if the family disagreed (Jonsen et al., 2021).

Pedro Navarro has lung cancer that has metastasized to his brain. No effective treatment is available, and Mr. Navarro is confused and unable to understand his medical condition. Ms. Navarro demands that her husband undergo craniotomy to remove the tumor. The neurosurgeon refuses, arguing that the operation will do Mr. Navarro no good whatsoever and will cause him additional suffering.

The case of Mr. Navarro pits the principle of autonomy against the principle of nonmaleficence. Mr. Navarro's surrogate decision maker, his wife, wants a particular course of treatment, but the neurosurgeon knows that this treatment will cause Mr. Navarro considerable harm and do him no good. In this case, nonmaleficence triumphs. Whereas patient autonomy allows the right to refuse treatment, it does not include the right to demand a harmful or ineffectual treatment.

In the late twentieth century, a new generation of ethical dilemmas emerged, moving beyond the individual physician–patient relationship to involve the broader society. These social–ethical problems derive from the new reality that money may not be available to pay for a reasonable level of medical services for all people. When money and resources are bountiful, the issue of distributive justice refers to equity in medical care access and health outcomes (see Chapter 5). When money and resources become scarce, the issue of justice takes on a new twist. Should limits be set on treatments given to people with high-cost medical needs, so that other people can receive basic services? If not, might health care consume so many resources that other social needs are sacrificed? If limits should be set, who decides these limits?

Angela and Amy Lakeberg [actual names] were Siamese twins sharing one heart. Without surgery, they would die shortly. With surgery, Amy would die and Angela's chance of survival would be less than 1%. On August 20, 1993, a team of 18 physicians and nurses performed an all-day operation to separate the twins. Amy died. The cost of the treatment was $1 million. The Medicaid program covered $700 to $1,000 per day. On June 9, 1994, Angela died; she had spent her brief life on a respirator in the hospital.

Fiscal reality has spawned two related dilemmas.

1. The first involves a conflict between the duty of the physician to follow the principles of beneficence and nonmaleficence and the growing sentiment that physicians should pay attention to distributive justice. In the case of the Lakeberg twins, the hospital and surgeons adhered to the principle of beneficence: Even a remote chance of aiding one twin was seen as worthwhile.
2. The second category of social–ethical dilemma is the conflict between the individual patient's (and family's) right to autonomy and society's claim to distributive justice. In the Lakeberg case, individual autonomy won out.

Health professionals have a duty to help and not harm their patients. Individuals claim a right to health care and do not want others to restrict that care. Yet the principle of distributive justice (recognizing that resources for health care are limited and should be fairly allocated among the entire population) might lead to denying costly services.

To live in a civilized society, each person must balance the concerns of the individual with the needs of the larger community. The Lakeberg surgery must be seen as a choice. The $1 million spent on the twins might have been spent on immunizing 10,000 children, with greater overall benefit. When health resources are scarce, the principle of justice creates ethical dilemmas that touch many people beyond those involved in an individual therapeutic relationship. The imperatives of cost control have thrust the principle of justice to the forefront of health policy in the debate over rationing.

WHAT IS RATIONING?

Dr. Everett Wall works for a medical group that participates in an Accountable Care Organization (ACO). Betty Ailes came to him with a headache and wanted a magnetic resonance imaging (MRI) scan. After a complete history and physical examination, Dr. Wall prescribed medication and denied the scan. Ms. Ailes wrote to the medical director, complaining that Dr. Wall was rationing services to her.

Perry Hiler arrives at Vacant Hospital with fever and severe cough. His chest x-ray shows an infiltrate near the hilum of the lung consistent with pneumonia or tumor. Since Mr. Hiler has no insurance, the emergency department physician sends him to the county hospital. At the time, Vacant Hospital has 35 empty beds and plenty of staff. When he recovers, Mr. Hiler calls the newspaper to complain. The next day, a headline appears: "Vacant Hospital Rations Care."

Jim Delacour is a 50-year-old man with terminal disease of the heart muscle. He is an ideal candidate for a heart transplant. Because the number of transplant candidates is larger than the supply of donor hearts available, Mr. Delacour is placed on the waiting list. After waiting 6 weeks, he dies.

When the emergency department called, Dr. Marco Intensivo's heart sank. The eight-bed intensive care unit is filled with extremely ill patients, all capable of full recovery. He has worried all day about another patient needing intensive care. Now that call has come: a 55-year-old with a heart attack complicated by unstable arrhythmias. Which one of the nine needy cases will not get intensive care? Dr. Intensivo needs to make a decision, and fast.

The general public and the media often view rationing as a limitation of medical care such that "not all care expected to be beneficial is provided to all patients" (Aaron & Schwartz, 1984). Such a view only partially explains the concept of rationing. More precisely, rationing means a conscious policy of equitably

Table 6–2. Two definitions of rationing

Popular usage of the term "rationing":

A limitation of medical care such that not all care expected to be beneficial is provided to all patients.

Precise usage of the term "rationing":

The limitation of resources, including money, going to medical care such that not all care expected to be beneficial is provided to all patients; and the distribution of these limited resources in a fair manner.

distributing needed resources that are in limited supply (Reagan, 1988) (Table 6–2). Under this definition, only the last two cases presented above can be considered rationing. In the first case, Dr. Wall did not feel that the MRI was a resource needed by Betty Ailes. In the second, Vacant Hospital's refusal to care for Perry Hiler was a decision on the part of a private institution to place its financial well-being above a patient's health; there was no scarcity of resources. In the heart transplant and intensive care unit cases, in contrast, donor hearts and intensive care unit beds were in fact scarce. For Mr. Delacour, the scarcity was nationwide and prolonged; for Dr. Intensivo, the scarcity was within a particular hospital at a particular time. In both cases, decisions had to be made regarding the allocation of those resources.

During World War II, insufficient gasoline was available to both power the military machine and satisfy the demands of automobile owners in the United States. The government rationed gasoline, giving priority to the military, yet allowing each civilian to obtain a limited amount of fuel. In a rural area, there may be a shortage of health care providers; in an overcrowded urban public hospital, there may be an insufficient number of beds; in the transplant arena, donor organs are in short supply. These are cases of commodity scarcity, wherein specific items are in limited supply.

The United States is a nation with an adequate supply of hospital beds and physicians in most communities; commodity scarcity in health care is the exception, though scarcity of primary care resources is a reality. But a different kind of health resource is becoming scarce, and that is money, creating fiscal scarcity.

In summary, rationing in medical care means the limitation of resources, including money, going to health care such that not all care expected to be beneficial is provided to all patients, and the fair distribution of these limited resources.

COMMODITY SCARCITY

Commodity scarcity provides an instructive example of the interaction between ethics and rationing. *Macroallocation* refers to the amount and distribution of resources within an entire society or among large populations, whereas *microallocation* refers to resource constraints at the level of an individual physician or institution.

Macroallocation and Rationing at the System Level: Organ Transplants

Mr. George Elder is a 76-year-old nonsmoking retired business executive with end-stage heart failure. He has good pulmonary and renal function and is not diabetic; thus, he is a good candidate for a heart transplant. His life expectancy without a transplant is 1 month. He has a loving family, with the resources to pay the $300,000 cost of the procedure.

Mr. Matt Younger is a 46-year-old divorced man who is unemployed, having lost his job as an auto worker 3 years ago. He has a history of smoking and alcohol use. He suffers a heart attack, develops intractable heart failure, and will die within 1 month without a heart transplant. He has good pulmonary and renal function and is not diabetic, making him a good candidate for the procedure.

Mr. Elder and Mr. Younger applied for donor hearts on the same day. One donor heart—histocompatible with both patients—has become available. Who should receive it?

In 1967, when Dr. Christiaan Barnard sewed a living heart into the chest of a person suffering end-stage cardiac disease, modern medicine entered the age of transplantation. In 2021, about 25,000 kidney, 9,000 liver, and 4,000 heart transplants were performed in the United States. Transplants are truly lifesaving in most cases. Mean survival after transplant in 2020 was over 22 years for kidney, 21 years for liver, and 15 years for heart.

Transplantation of organs is both a medical miracle and an ethical watershed. A central ethical issue is: Who should receive organs that are in short supply?

The number of persons on the national waiting list for organ transplants rose from 16,000 in 1988 to 106,000 in 2021. The number of organs that could be harvested each year falls short of the number needed. On average in 2021, 17 patients in the United States died each day awaiting organs.

Transplantation presents a classic case of commodity scarcity: there is insufficient supply to meet demand. In the early 1980s, the major heart transplant center at Stanford University excluded people with "a history of alcoholism, job instability, antisocial behavior, or psychiatric illness," and required transplant recipients to enjoy "a stable, rewarding family and/or vocational environment." Stanford's recipients had a better than 50% chance of surviving 5 years, signifying that acceptance or rejection from the program was a matter of life and death. The US Department of Health and Human Services was concerned about Stanford's discriminatory selection criteria. Moreover, the $100,000 cost restricted heart transplants to those with insurance coverage or ability to pay out of pocket. Both the social and economic criteria for access to this lifesaving surgery raised serious issues of distributive justice and health equity.

Following the passage of the National Organ Transplantation Act of 1984, the federal government designated the United Network for Organ Sharing (UNOS) as a national system for matching donated organs and potential recipients (www. unos.org). According to the Task Force on Organ Transplantation (1986), organ allocation should be governed by medical criteria, with the major factors being urgency of need and probability of success. The Task Force recommended that if two or more patients are equally good candidates for an organ according to the medical criteria, length of time on the waiting list is the fairest way to make the final selection. However, Black people are four times more likely than White people to have kidney failure but are less likely to get transplants (Stolberg, 2023). Also, haunting the ethics of the prioritization process is ability to pay. In 2020, the average kidney transplant cost $440,000 and heart transplant $1,665,000. Persons needing a transplant are often rejected if they lack health insurance coverage (Aleccia, 2018).

▶ Microallocation and Rationing at the Institutional Level

Ms. Wilson is a 71-year-old woman with pneumonia caused by COVID-19. Ms. Wilson is admitted to the ICU in her rural town, requiring a respirator. By the eighth hospital day, she is no better. On that day, Louis Ford, a previously healthy 27-year-old, is brought to the hospital, also with COVID pneumonia, in immediate need of a respirator. None of the six patients in the ICU can be removed from respirators without dying; of the six, Ms. Wilson has the poorest prognosis. She has no family. No other respirators exist within a 50-mile radius. Should Ms. Wilson be removed from the respirator in favor of Mr. Ford?

Whereas macroallocation decisions may be based on a set of rules governing rationing, as for organ transplant, microallocation choices typically operate in a less formal way, bringing ethical dilemmas into stark focus and placing issues of resource allocation squarely in the lap of the practicing physician. The microallocation choice involving Ms. Wilson incorporates all four ethical principles, which must be weighed and acted on within minutes: (1) Beneficence: For whom? This ideal cannot be realized for both patients. (2) Nonmaleficence: If Ms. Wilson is removed from the respirator, harm is done to her, but the price of not harming her is great for Mr. Ford. (3) Autonomy: Withdrawal of therapy requires the consent of the patient or family, which is impossible in Ms. Wilson's case. (4) Justice: Should resources be distributed on a first-come first-served basis or according to need?

These are tragic decisions. Many physicians would remove Ms. Wilson from the respirator and make all efforts to save Mr. Ford. The main consideration would be medical effectiveness: Ms. Wilson's chance of living is slim, while Mr. Ford could be cured and live for many decades.

Less stark but similar decisions face physicians on a daily basis. On a busy day, which patients get more of the physician's time? In a public hospital caring for low-income people, with an MRI waiting list, when should a physician call the radiologist and argue for an urgent scan, thereby pushing other people down on the waiting list? Situations involving microallocation demonstrate why in daily practice health care professionals are often forced to balance the interests of one patient against those of another and the interests of the larger group.

FISCAL SCARCITY AND RESOURCE ALLOCATION

During the 1980s, advances in medicine combined with the rapid rise in health care costs led to the belief that medical care rationing was upon us. However, great differences separate the case of organ transplants from that of medical care as a whole.

1. Medical care in general is not a scarce resource; in most population centers, facilities and personnel are abundant.
2. Whereas a nationwide structure is in place to decide who will receive a transplant, no such structure exists for medical care as a whole.

Dr. Ernest, who works for a multispecialty group practice, wants to do her part to keep medical costs down. She prescribes low-cost amoxicillin at 60 cents per capsule rather than ciprofloxacin at $12 for each dose. She teaches back pain patients home exercises at no cost rather than sending them to physical therapy visits at $125 per session. At the end of each year, she enjoys calculating how many thousands of dollars she has saved compared with one of her colleagues, who ignores costs in making medical decisions.

While Dr. Ernest can be praised for attempting to reduce costs without sacrificing quality, her cost savings probably did not reap benefits for other patients. There is no US national structure within which to effect a trade-off between savings in one area and benefits in another. According to analyst Joshua Wiener (1992),

In countries that have a socially determined health budget, cuts in one area can be justified on the grounds that the money will be spent on other, higher-priority services... In the United States, it is difficult to refuse additional resources for patients, because there is no certainty that the funds will be put to better use elsewhere.

Persuading physicians to save money on one patient in order to improve services for someone else is as illogical as telling a child to eat all the food on the plate because children in countries with famines are starving (Cassel, 1985).

For health care providers like Dr. Ernest to make their cost savings socially useful, two things are needed: a closed system of health care funding, whether governmental or private, and a decision-making structure with responsibility to allocate budgets to health care interventions in a fair manner.

For the purposes of the following discussion, let us assume that the United States is in a position of fiscal scarcity and that a mechanism exists to fairly allocate medical care resources from one individual or population group to another. Which ethical conflicts arise between beneficence, nonmaleficence, and autonomy on the one hand and justice (equitable distribution of resources) on the other?

THE RELATIONSHIP OF RATIONING TO COST CONTROL

Assume that Limittown, USA, has a fixed budget of $400 million for medical care in 2020. Limittown has three imaging centers, each with an MRI scanner that is used only 4 hours each weekday. None of the medical facilities perform bone marrow transplantation, a procedure that can prolong the lives of some leukemia patients. In 2020, Limittown spent $10 million to pay for bone marrow transplants at a university hospital 50 miles away.

Limittown's health commissioner projects that 2022 medical care expenditures will be $5 million over budget; she must implement cost savings. She considers two choices: (1) Two of the three MRI scanners could be closed, allowing the remaining scanner's cost per procedure to be drastically reduced or (2) Limittown could stop paying for bone marrow transplantation for leukemia patients.

Is rationing the same as cost containment? While the limitation of money going to medical care is cost containment, not all cost containment reduces beneficial care to patients. In the case of Limittown, both options for saving $5 million can be considered cost containment, but only denial of coverage for bone

Table 6–3. Rationing and cost control

Not all cost control is rationing.
Painless cost control is not rationing, because no limitation is placed on medical care expected to be beneficial.
Painful cost control may require rationing because limits are placed on medical care expected to be beneficial.

marrow transplants requires rationing. Consolidating MRI scanning at a single facility would allow the same number of scans to be performed, but at a lower cost. Rationing is associated with painful cost control (reducing effective medical care), but cost containment (see Chapter 11) can be either painful or painless (Table 6–3). The reality that 25% of total US health spending goes to unnecessary care and administrative waste (Shrank et al., 2019) means that the United States does not need to ration effective medical services. No rationing of beneficial services should take place until all wasteful practices are curtailed; painless cost control should precede painful cost control.

▶ Care Provided to Profoundly Ill People

Lula Rogers is an 84-year-old diabetic woman; multiple strokes have rendered her unable to move, swallow, understand, or speak. She has been in a nursing home for 3 years, Ms. Rogers' son wishes to remove her feeding tube, but her physician and the nursing staff disagree. Ms. Rogers lives for 3 more years, costing $400,000.

Were Lula Rogers' caregivers right to prolong her life? Or were they prolonging Ms. Rogers' suffering and denying her a peaceful death? Should cost be a factor in such decisions, or should such matters of life and death be governed by autonomy, beneficence, and non-maleficence alone?

Patients in hospice programs have lower end-of-life costs than those not in hospice programs (Obermeyer et al., 2014), and have better quality care compared with those not in hospice (Kumar et al., 2017). Thus, reduced expenditures can go hand in hand with better care.

RATIONING BY COST-EFFECTIVENESS

Eliminating administrative waste, medical waste, and unwanted interventions for the profoundly and incurably ill before rationing needed services best realizes the principles of beneficence and justice. However, if rationing of truly beneficial services were needed, the issues become more difficult and cost-effectiveness comes into play (see Chapter 11). If intervention A increases person-years of reasonable-quality life more than intervention B, intervention A is more medically effective. The cost of the two interventions is not considered. Cost-effectiveness adds dollars to the equation: If intervention A increases person-years of reasonable-quality life per dollar spent more than intervention B, it is more cost-effective. If money were not scarce, medical effectiveness (maximizing benefit and minimizing harm) would be the ideal standard upon which to ration care. But if rationing is needed, then costs cannot be ignored (Garber & Sox, 2010).

Yet the ethical aspects pose challenges. In 1991, Dr. David Eddy (1991a) published a compelling article entitled "The individual vs society: Is there a conflict?" Dr. Eddy posed the case of Mrs. Smith, a woman with widely metastatic breast cancer, and noted that screening mammography was eight times as cost-effective as intensive treatment for metastatic breast cancer. If medical care must be rationed, it seems logical to spend funds on mammography rather than intensive treatment of metastatic disease because the former intervention is more cost-effective. Dr. Eddy (1991a) did not confine his analysis to cost-effectiveness, however, but moved on to the ethical issues.

Each of us can be in two positions when we make judgments about the value of different health care activities. We are in one position when we are healthy…. Call this the "first position." We are in a different position when we actually have a disease (the "second position")…. Imagine that you are a 50-year-old woman employed by Mrs. Smith's corporation…. [The company] is considering two options: (1) cover screening for breast cancer … or (2) cover [treatment of metastatic cancer]…. Now imagine you are in the first position … as long as you do not yet have the disease (the first position), option 1 will always deliver greater benefit at lower cost than option 2…. Now, let us switch you to the second position. Imagine that you already have breast cancer and have just been told that it has metastasized.... The value to you of the screening option has plummeted because you already have breast cancer and can no longer benefit from screening....

Maximizing care for individual patients attempts to maximize care for individuals when they are in the second position. Maximizing care for society expands the scope of concern to include individuals when they are in the first position. As this example illustrates, the program that delivers the most benefit for the least cost for society (option 1) is not necessarily best for the individual patient (option 2), and vice versa. But as this example also illustrates, individual patients and society are not distinct entities. Rather, they represent the different positions that each of us will be in at various times in our lives.

Health professionals generally care for patients in Dr. Eddy's second position—when they are sick. But if the cost of treating those in the second position reduces resources available to prevent illness for the far larger number of people in the first position, the individual principles of beneficence and autonomy are superseding the societal principle of justice. One could even say that choosing for individuals in the second position violates beneficence for those in the first position. On the other hand, if all resources go to those in the first position (e.g., to cost-effective screening rather than expensive treatment for those with life-threatening disease), injustice is committed in the other direction by ignoring the costly needs of the very ill.

Clearly, no ideal method of rationing medical care exists. All efforts should be made to control costs painlessly before resorting to the painful limitation of effective medical care. But if rationing is inevitable, a balance must be struck among many legitimate needs: the concerns of healthy people for illness prevention, the imperative for acutely sick people to obtain diagnosis and treatment, and the obligation to provide care and comfort to those with untreatable chronic illness.

For rationing to be ethical, there must be vigilance to guard against discrimination that violates the principle

of justice, as discussed in Chapter 5. As revealed by the organ transplantation example, bias may insinuate itself into rationing guidelines and aggravate inequity. Patients from marginalized communities may have justified apprehension about rationing reinforcing longstanding bias in health care.

A BASIC LEVEL OF GUARANTEED MEDICAL BENEFITS

Don Rich is a bank executive with a strong family history of heart disease who receives his care through a New York City ACO. He begins having occasional episodes of chest pain. An exercise treadmill test does not show evidence of coronary artery disease. Yet Mr. Rich asks his cardiologist to perform a coronary angiogram. He is told that the ACO has finite resources for such procedures and limits their use to patients with abnormal treadmill tests. Mr. Rich flies to Texas, consults with a cardiologist there, and receives a coronary angiogram at his own expense.

Most people in the United States believe that health care should be a right. But how much health care? If every person has a right to all beneficial health care, the nation may be unable to pay the bill or may be forced to limit other rights such as education or environmental protection. One approach to this problem is to limit the health care right to a basic package of services. In the case of Don Rich's ACO, angiography after a negative stress test is not within the basic package. Any services beyond the basics can be purchased by individuals who choose to spend their own money. This solution creates an ethical problem. If a service that does produce medical benefit is not included in the basic package or is denied by an insurance company medical director, that service becomes available only to those who can afford it. Where should society draw the line between a basic level of care that should be equally available to all, and "more than basic" services that may be purchased according to individual ability and willingness to pay (Eddy, 1991b)? Unless the basic package covers all beneficial health services, the principle of distributive justice, that all people equally receive a reasonable level of medical services without regard to ability to pay, will be compromised.

THE ETHICS OF HEALTH CARE FINANCING

The principle of distributive justice holds that young and healthy people should pay more in health costs than they use in health services so that older and less healthy people can receive health services at a reasonable cost. Even from the perspective of one's own long-term self-interest, it makes sense to pay more for health care while young and healthy, and to benefit when advanced age creates a greater risk of becoming sick.

A much-discussed issue involves individuals whose behavior, particularly smoking, eating unhealthy diets, and drinking alcohol in excess, is seen as contributing to their ill health.

Jim Butts, a heavy smoker, develops emphysema and has multiple hospitalizations for respiratory failure, including many days on the respirator. Randy Schipp, a former shipyard worker, develops work-related asbestosis and has multiple hospitalizations for respiratory failure, including many days on the respirator. Should Jim pay more for health insurance than Randy?

Gene eats a healthy diet, exercises regularly, but has a strong family history of heart disease; he suffers a heart attack at age 44. Mac eats fast food, does not exercise, and has a heart attack at age 44. Should Mac pay more for health care coverage than Gene?

One view holds that individuals who fall sick as a result of high-risk behavior such as smoking, substance abuse including use of alcohol, and consumption of unhealthy foods are entirely responsible for their behavior and should pay higher health insurance premiums. Opponents of this idea see it as "blaming the victim" and argue that high-risk behaviors have a complex causation that may involve genetic, social, and environmental factors. The food industry spends billions of dollars each year on television advertising, most for products with poor nutritional value. Low-income people often cannot afford healthy foods. The tobacco industry heavily advertises to the Black and LGBTQ communities. To the extent that the causes of high-risk behaviors are multifactorial, it would be unfair to charge individuals more for health insurance based on these behaviors.

WHO ALLOCATES HEALTH CARE RESOURCES?

The predicament of limited resources has been likened to a herd of cattle grazing on a common pasture. The total grazing area may be regarded as the entirety of economic resources in the United States. A smaller pasture, the *medical commons*, comprises that portion of the grazing area dedicated to health care. The herd represents the nation's physicians and other providers, using the resources of the commons in the process of caring for patients. Physicians, guided by medicine's moral imperative to "do everything possible for the patient," continually attempt to extend the borders of the medical commons. But communities outside the medical commons have legitimate claims to societal resources and view the herd as encroaching on resources needed for other social goods (Grumbach & Bodenheimer, 1990).

Who decides the magnitude of the medical commons, that is, the resources devoted to health care? Physicians and other health care providers, whose interventions on behalf of their patients add up to the totality of medical resources used? The sum of individual consumer choices operating through a free market? Health insurance plans, watching over their particular piece of the commons? Or government, using the political process to set budgetary limits on the entire health care system?

Traditionally, physicians and patients have had a great deal to say about the size of the medical commons. In the United States, the medical commons has been an open range. The quantity and price of medical visits, hospital days, diagnostic studies, and pharmaceuticals determine the total costs of medical care. This is not the case in other nations, where government health care budgets constitute a "fence" around the medical commons, setting a clear limit on the quantity of resources available. Some advocates of fence-building in the United States have considered parceling the medical commons into numerous subpastures, each representing an integrated health system working within the constraints of fixed, prepaid budgets. Not all pastures would be equal in size, and the fences might have holes, allowing patients to purchase additional services outside the organized systems of care.

Ethical considerations play a role in both open and closed medical care systems. In the United States open range, the principles of beneficence and autonomy have the upper hand, tending toward an expanding, though not equitable, system. Fenced-in systems, in contrast, balance the more expansive principles of beneficence and autonomy with the demands of distributive justice to fairly allocate resources within the medical commons.

If the United States moves toward a more fenced-in medical commons, decisions will be needed about who gets what. Do all 90-year-old people with multiple organ failure receive kidney dialysis that may extend their lives only a few months? Which patients should be eligible for effective but phenomenally expensive treatments, such as $1 million chimeric antigen receptor T-cell (CAR-T) therapy for cancer? Do individual physicians, interacting with their patients, have the final say in making these decisions? Should societal bodies such as government, commissions of interested parties, or professional associations set the rules?

Microallocation issues come down to daily clinical decisions about which individual patients will receive what types of care (Lo, 2020). Physicians and other caregivers may well recoil from the prospect of "bedside rationing," believing that allocative decision making unduly compromises their commitment to the principles of beneficence and autonomy. Yet if health care professionals abstain from making allocative decisions, then medicine will be granting these decisions to insurance company and governmental officials.

If health care professionals are to maintain their dedication to individual patients while at the same time responsibly managing resources, they need rules to assist them. At the population level, society should decide which general treatments are to be collectively paid for. At the individual level, rules are needed to guide decisions about the prioritization of resources for specific patients. Rules at both the population and individual level must center equity and ensure that rules do not perpetuate systemic harm of marginalized populations. Organ transplantation provides a model: do everything possible to procure organs for your transplant patients, but also accept the rules of the system that attempt to allocate organs in a fair manner (Benjamin et al., 1994). The modern health care professional is caught in a global ethical dilemma. On the one hand, patients and their families expect the best that modern technology can offer, paid for through private or public insurance. The imperatives of beneficence, nonmaleficence, and autonomy rule the bedside. On the other hand, grave injustices take place on a daily basis. An underinsured young person with a curable illness is unable to pay for care, while a well-insured, bedridden individual who experiences a stroke causing brain hemorrhage incurs vast medical bills during the last weeks of her ebbing life. Should not the physician at the stroke patient's bedside be concerned about both patients? However this dilemma is resolved, the principle of justice will relentlessly peek at the physician from under the bed.

REFERENCES

Aaron HJ, Schwartz WB. *The Painful Prescription*. Washington, DC: The Brookings Institution; 1984.

Aleccia J. No cash, no heart. Transplant centers require proof of payment. Kaiser Health News, December 5, 2018.

Beauchamp TL, Childress JF. *Principles of Biomedical Ethics*. 8th ed. New York, NY: Oxford University Press; 2023.

Benjamin M, Cohen C, Grochowski E. What transplantation can teach us about health care reform. *N Engl J Med*. 1994;330:858–860.

Cassel CK. Doctors and allocation decisions: a new role in the new Medicare. *J Health Polit Policy Law*. 1985;10:549–564.

Eddy DM. Comparing benefits and harms: the balance sheet. *JAMA*. 1990;263:2493.

Eddy DM. Clinical decision making: from theory to practice. The individual vs society: is there a conflict? *JAMA*. 1991a;265:1446–1450.

Eddy DM. What care is "essential?" What services are "basic?" *JAMA*. 1991b;265:782, 786–788.

Garber AM, Sox HC. The role of costs in comparative effectiveness research. *Health Aff (Millwood)*. 2010;29:1805–1811.

Grumbach K, Bodenheimer T. Reins or fences: a physician's view of cost containment. *Health Aff (Millwood)*. 1990;9:120–126.

Jonsen AR, Siegler M, Winslade WJ. *Clinical Ethics: A Practical Approach to Ethical Decisions in Clinical Medicine*. 9th ed. New York, NY: McGraw-Hill; 2021.

Kumar P, Wright AA, Hatfield LA, Temel JS, Keating NL. Family perspectives on hospital care experiences of patients with cancer. *J Clin Oncology*. 2017;35:432–439.

Lo B. *Resolving Ethical Dilemmas. A Guide for Clinicians*. 6th ed. Wolters Kluwer; 2020.

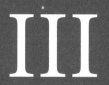

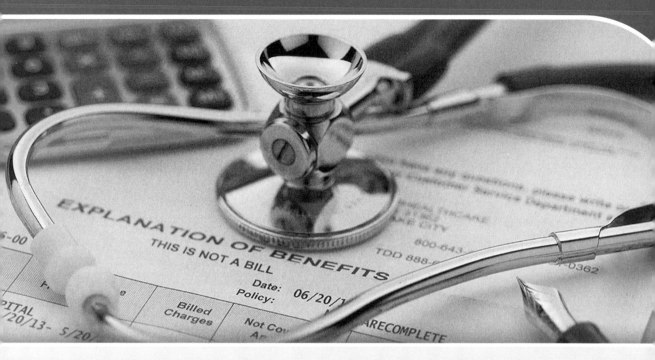

THE ORGANIZATION OF HEALTH CARE

How Health Care Is Organized—I: Primary, Secondary, and Tertiary Care

In 1989, Frank Hope developed Acquired Immune Deficiency Syndrome (AIDS) and was in and out of the hospital with debilitating infections. Yet he remained hopeful that a scientific breakthrough would give him a chance. By 1995, with the discovery of life-saving protease inhibitors, his wish had come true. Many years later he continues to enjoy life and has a non-detectable viral level on his regular blood tests. In Frank's mind, these types of scientific discoveries attest to the wonders of the US health care system.

Frank's grandson attends a day care program. Ruby, a 3-year-old girl in the program, was recently hospitalized for a severe asthma attack complicated by pneumococcal pneumonia. She spent 2 weeks in a pediatric intensive care unit, including several days on a respirator. Ruby's mother works full time as a bus driver while raising three children. She has comprehensive private health insurance through her job but has difficulty finding a physician's office that offers convenient appointment times. She takes Ruby to an evening-hours urgent care center when Ruby has wheezing but never sees the same physician twice. Ruby never received all her pneumococcal vaccinations or a prescription of a steroid inhaler to prevent a severe asthma attack. Ruby's mother blames herself for her child's hospitalization.

People in the United States rightfully take pride in the technologic accomplishments of their health care system. Innovations in biomedical science have almost eradicated such scourges as polio, and measles, and transformed HIV infection from an invariably fatal illness to a manageable chronic disease. Yet for all its successes, the health care system also has its failures. In cases such as Ruby's, the failure to prevent a severe asthma flare-up is not related to financial barriers, but rather reflects organizational problems, particularly in the delivery of primary care services.

The organizational task facing all health care systems is one of "assuring that the right patient receives the right service at the right time and in the right place" (Rodwin, 1984). An additional criterion could be "… and by the right caregiver." The fragmented care Ruby received for her asthma is an example of this challenge. While Ruby received an abundance of care, she did not receive critical services that might have prevented a need for more intensive and costlier care. Who is responsible for planning and ensuring that every child receives the right services at the right time? What is the proper balance between intensive care units that provide life-saving services to critically ill patients and primary care services geared toward less dramatic medical and preventive needs?

In this chapter and the following one, the organization of the health care system will be the main focus. While a debate persists on how to improve financial access to care, less emphasis is given to the question "access to what?" This chapter views organizational systems through a wide-angle lens, examining such broad concepts as the relationship between primary, secondary, and tertiary levels of care, and the influence of the biomedical paradigm and medical professionalism in shaping US health care delivery. In Chapter 8, a zoom lens will be used to focus on specific organizational models that have appeared (often only to disappear) in this country.

MODELS OF ORGANIZING CARE

▶ Primary, Secondary, and Tertiary Care

One concept is essential in understanding the topography of any health care system: the organization of care into primary, secondary, and tertiary levels. In the Lord Dawson Report, an influential British study written in 1920, Dawson (1975) proposed that each of the three levels of care should correspond with certain unique patient needs.

1. Primary care involves common health problems (e.g., sore throats, diabetes, arthritis, depression, or hypertension) and preventive measures (e.g., vaccinations or mammograms) that account for 80% to 90% of visits to a physician or other caregiver.
2. Secondary care involves problems that require more specialized clinical expertise such as hospital care for a patient with acute renal failure.
3. Tertiary care, which lies at the apex of the organizational pyramid, involves the management of rare disorders such as pituitary tumors and congenital malformations.

Two contrasting approaches can be used to organize a health care system around these levels of care: (1) the carefully structured Dawson model of regionalized health care and (2) a more free-flowing model.

1. One approach uses the Dawson model as a scaffold for a highly structured system. This model is based on the concept of regionalization: the organization and coordination of all health resources and services within a defined area (Bodenheimer, 1969). In a regionalized system, different types of personnel and facilities are assigned to distinct tiers in the primary, secondary, and tertiary levels, and the flow of patients across levels occurs in an orderly, regulated fashion. This model emphasizes the primary

care base and a population-oriented framework for health planning.
2. An alternative model allows for more fluid roles for caregivers, and more free-flowing movement of patients across all levels of care. This model tends to place a higher value on services at the tertiary care apex than at the primary care base.

Although most health care systems embody elements of both models, some gravitate closer to one polarity or the other. The traditional British National Health Service (NHS) and some large integrated delivery systems in the United States resemble the regionalized approach, while US health care as a whole follows the more dispersed format.

▶ The Regionalized Model: The Traditional British National Health Service

Basil, a 60-year-old man living in a London suburb, is registered with Dr. Prime, a general practitioner in his neighborhood. Basil goes to Dr. Prime for most of his health problems, including hay fever, back spasms, and hypertension. One day, he experiences numbness and weakness in his face and arm. By the time Dr. Prime examines him later that day, the symptoms have resolved. Suspecting that Basil has had a transient ischemic attack, Dr. Prime prescribes aspirin, orders a brain CT scan, and refers him to the neurologist at the local hospital, where a carotid artery sonogram reveals high-grade carotid stenosis. Dr. Prime and the neurologist agree that Basil should make an appointment at a London teaching hospital with a vascular surgeon specializing in head and neck surgery. The surgeon recommends that Basil undergo carotid endarterectomy on an elective basis to prevent a major stroke. Basil returns to Dr. Prime to discuss this recommendation and inquires whether the operation could be performed at a local hospital closer to home. Dr. Prime informs him that only a handful of London hospitals are equipped to perform this type of specialized operation. Basil schedules his operation in London and several months later has an uncomplicated carotid endarterectomy. Following the operation, he returns to Dr. Prime for his ongoing care.

The British NHS traditionally typified a relatively regimented primary–secondary–tertiary care structure (Fig. 7–1).

1. For physician services, the primary care level is virtually the exclusive domain of general practitioners (commonly referred to as GPs), who practice in small- to medium-sized groups and whose main responsibility is ambulatory care. About half of all physicians in the United Kingdom are GPs.

2. The secondary tier of care is occupied by physicians in such specialties as internal medicine, pediatrics, neurology, psychiatry, obstetrics and gynecology, and general surgery. These physicians are located at hospital-based clinics and serve as consultants for outpatient referrals from GPs, in turn routing most patients back to GPs for ongoing care needs. Secondary-level physicians also provide care to hospitalized patients.

3. Tertiary care subspecialists such as cardiac surgeons, immunologists, and pediatric hematologists are located at a few tertiary care medical centers.

Hospital planning followed the same regionalized logic as physician services. District hospitals were local facilities equipped for basic inpatient services. Regional tertiary care medical centers handled highly specialized inpatient care needs.

Planning of physician and hospital resources within the traditional NHS occurred with a population focus. GP groups provided care to a base population of 5,000 to 50,000 persons, depending on the number of GPs in the practice. District hospitals had a catchment area population of 50,000 to 500,000, while tertiary care hospitals served as referral centers for a population of 500,000 to 5 million (Fry, 1980).

While this regionalized structure has recently become more fluid (Chapter 15), patient flow still moves in a stepwise fashion across the different tiers. Except in emergency situations, all patients are first seen by a GP, who may then steer patients toward more specialized levels of care through a formal process of referral. Patients may not directly refer themselves to a specialist.

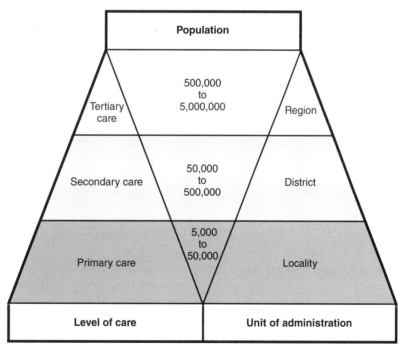

▲ **Figure 7–1.** Organization of services under the traditional National Health Service model in the United Kingdom. Care is organized into distinct levels corresponding to specific functions, roles, administrative units, and population bases.

While nonphysician health professionals, such as nurses, play an integral role in staffing hospitals at the secondary and tertiary care levels, especially noteworthy is the NHS' multidisciplinary approach to primary care. GPs work in close collaboration with practice nurses (similar to nurse practitioners in the United States), home health visitors, public health nurses, and midwives (who attend most deliveries in the United Kingdom). Such teamwork, along with accountability for a defined population of enrolled patients and universal health care coverage, helps to avert such problems as missed childhood vaccinations. Public health nurses visit all homes in the first weeks after a birth to provide education and assist with scheduling of initial GP appointments. A national vaccination tracking system notifies parents about each scheduled vaccination and alerts GPs and public health nurses if a child has not appeared at the appointed time. As a result, more than 90% of British preschool children receive a full series of immunizations.

A number of other nations, ranging from industrialized countries in Scandinavia to developing nations in Latin America, have adopted a similar approach to organizing health services. In low-income nations, the primary care tier relies more on community health educators and other types of public health personnel than on physicians.

▶ The Dispersed Model: Traditional US Health Care Organization

Polly Seymour, a 55-year-old woman with private health insurance who lives in the United States, sees several different physicians for a variety of problems: a dermatologist for eczema, a gastroenterologist for recurrent heartburn, and an orthopedist for tendinitis in her shoulder. She may ask her gastroenterologist to treat a few general medical problems, such as borderline diabetes. On occasion, she has gone to the nearby hospital emergency department for treatment of urinary tract infections. One day, Polly feels a lump in her breast and consults a gynecologist. She is referred to a surgeon for biopsy, which indicates cancer. After discussing treatment options with Polly, the surgeon performs a lumpectomy and refers her to an oncologist and radiation therapy specialist for further therapy. She receives all these treatments at a local hospital, a short distance from her home.

The US health care system has had a far less structured approach to levels of care than the British NHS. In contrast to the stepwise flow of patient referrals in the United Kingdom, insured patients in the United States, such as Polly Seymour, have traditionally been able to refer themselves and enter the system directly at any level. While many patients in the United Kingdom have a primary care physician (PCP) to initially evaluate all their problems, many people in the United States have become accustomed to taking their symptoms directly to the specialist of their choice.

For many decades, PCPs in the United States assumed a number of secondary care functions by providing substantial amounts of inpatient care. Only recently has the United States moved toward the European model that removes inpatient care from the domain of some PCPs and assigns this work to "hospitalists"—physicians who exclusively practice within the hospital (Wachter & Goldman, 1996; Goroll & Hunt, 2015).

The total supply of PCPs amounts to 31% of all physicians in the United States (Robert Graham Center, 2021). Traditionally, 50% of physicians in the United Kingdom have been GPs, though the number of GPs per capita has fallen slightly since 2009 (Palmer, 2019). Many nurse practitioners and physician assistants in the United States work in primary care settings, and in 2019 constituted 37% of the primary care practitioner workforce (Robert Graham Center, 2021).

US hospitals are not constrained by secondary and tertiary care boundaries. Instead of a pyramidal system featuring a large number of general community hospitals at the base and a limited number of tertiary care referral centers at the apex, hospitals in the United States each aspire to offer the latest in specialized care. In most urban areas, for example, several hospitals compete with each other to perform open heart surgery, organ transplants, radiation therapy, and high-risk obstetric procedures. The resulting structure resembles a diamond more than a pyramid, with a small number of hospitals (mostly rural) that lack specialized units at the base, a small number of elite university medical centers providing super-specialized referral services at the apex, and the bulk of hospitals providing a wide range of secondary and tertiary services in the middle.

Which Model Is Right?

Critics of the US health care system find fault with its "top-heavy" specialist and tertiary care orientation and lack of organizational coherence. Analyses of health care in the United States over many decades abound with such descriptions as "a nonsystem with millions of independent, uncoordinated, separately motivated moving parts," "fragmentation, chaos, and disarray," and "uncontrolled growth and pluralism verging on anarchy" (Somers, 1972; Halvorson & Isham, 2003). The high cost of health care has been attributed in part to this organizational disarray. Quality of care may also suffer. For example, when many hospitals each perform small numbers of surgical procedures such as coronary artery bypass grafts, mortality rates are higher than when such procedures are regionalized in a few high-volume centers (Gonzalez et al., 2014).

Defenders of the dispersed model reply that pluralism is a virtue, promoting flexibility and convenience in the availability of facilities and personnel. In this view, the emphasis on specialization and technology is compatible with values and expectations in the United States, with patients placing a high premium on autonomy in selecting caregivers of their choice for a particular health care need. Similarly, the desire for the latest in-hospital technology available at a convenient distance from home competes with plans to regionalize tertiary care services at a limited number of hospitals.

Balancing the Different Levels of Care

Dr. Billie Ruben completed her residency training in internal medicine at a major university medical center. Like most of her fellow residents, she went on to pursue subspecialty training, in her case gastroenterology. Dr. Ruben chose this career after caring for a young woman who developed irreversible liver failure from autoimmune hepatitis. After a nerve-racking, touch-and-go effort to secure a donor liver, transplantation was performed and the patient made a complete recovery.

Upon completion of her training, Dr. Ruben joins a growing subspecialty practice at Atlantic Heights

Hospital, a successful private hospital in the city. Even though the metropolitan area of 2 million people already has two liver transplant units, Atlantic Heights just opened a third such unit, feeling that its reputation for excellence depends on delivering services at the cutting edge of biomedical innovation. In her first 6 months at the hospital, Dr. Ruben participates in the care of only two patients requiring liver transplantation. Most of her patients seek care for chronic, often ill-defined digestive problems. As Dr. Ruben begins seeing these patients on a regular basis, she starts to give preventive care and treat nongastrointestinal problems such as hypertension and diabetes. At times she wishes she had experienced more general medicine during her training.

Advocates of a stronger role for primary care in the United States believe that it is too important to be considered an afterthought in health planning. In this view, overemphasis on the tertiary care apex of the pyramid creates a system in which health care resources are not well matched to the prevalence and incidence of health problems in a community. In an article entitled "The Ecology of Medical Care" published more than 5 decades ago, Kerr White recorded the monthly prevalence of illness for a general population of 1,000 adults (White et al., 1961). In this group, 750 experienced one or more illnesses or injuries during the month. Of these patients, 250 visited a physician at least once during the month, nine were admitted to a hospital, and only one was referred to a university medical center. Dr. White voiced concern that the training of health care professionals at tertiary care–oriented academic medical centers gave trainees like Dr. Billie Ruben an unrepresentative view of the health care needs of the community. Updating Kerr White's findings, Larry Green found precisely the same patterns 4 decades later (Fig. 7–2) (Green et al., 2001).

The ecological framework uses a population-based approach: For a defined population in the community, what is the incidence and prevalence of disease and health care needs and patterns of care seeking? This framework confirms the adage that "common disorders commonly occur and rare ones rarely happen" (Fry, 1980). The dominant pathology in an unselected population consists of minor ailments, chronic conditions

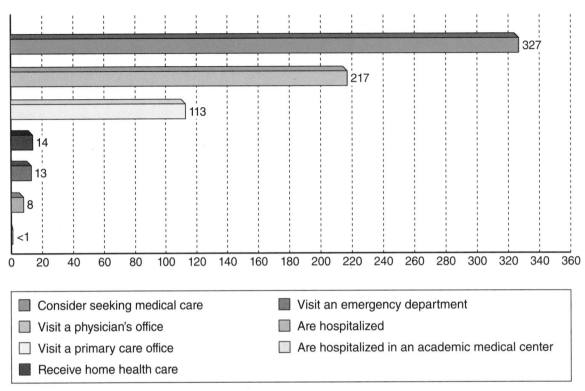

▲ Figure 7–2. Monthly prevalence of illness in a community of 1000 persons, and the use of various sources of health care. Each bar represents a subgroup of the community of 1000 persons.

such as hypertension and arthritis, and an array of behavioral conditions ranging from children with attention deficit and hyperactivity disorder to adults with depression and substance use disorders to older adults with cognitive decline. The incidence of new cancers is relatively rare, and only a handful of patients manifest complex syndromes such as multiple sclerosis. This is very different from the pattern of disease viewed from the reference point of an emergency department or intensive care unit, where distinct subsets of patients are encountered.

The ecological framework does not imply that most health care resources should be devoted to primary care. The minority of patients with severe conditions requiring secondary or tertiary care will command a much larger share of health care resources per capita than the majority of people with less dramatic health care needs. Treating a patient with liver failure costs a great deal more than treating a patient for hypertension. Even in the United Kingdom, where GPs provide the majority of ambulatory care, expenditures on their services account for about 10% of the overall NHS budget. In the United States, primary care receives a scant 5% of all health care spending (National Academies of Sciences, Engineering, and Medicine, 2021). Thus, the pyramidal shape shown in Fig. 7–1 better represents the distribution of health care problems in a community than the apportionment of health care expenditures. While almost all industrialized nations devote a dominant share of health care resources to secondary and tertiary care, the ecologic view reminds us that most people have health care needs at the primary care level.

The Functions and Value of Primary Care

Dr. O. Titus Wells has cared for all four of Bruce and Wendy Smith's children. As a family physician whose practice includes obstetrics, Dr. Wells attended the births of all but one of the children. The Smiths' 18-month-old daughter Ginny has had many ear infections. Even though this is a common problem, Dr. Wells finds that it presents a real medical challenge. Sometimes examination of Ginny's ears indicates a raging infection and at other times shows the presence of middle ear fluid, which may or may not represent a bona fide bacterial infection. He tries to reserve antibiotics for clear-cut cases of severe bacterial otitis. He feels it is important that he be the one to examine Ginny's ears because her eardrums never look entirely normal and he knows what degree of change is suspicious for a genuinely new infection.

When Ginny is 2 years old, Dr. Wells recommends to the Smiths that she see an otolaryngologist and audiologist to check for hearing loss and language impairment. The audiograms show modest diminution of hearing in one ear. The otolaryngologist informs the Smiths that ear tubes are an option. At Ginny's return visit with Dr. Wells, he discusses the pros and cons of tube placement with the Smiths. He also uses the visit as an opportunity to encourage Mrs. Smith to quit smoking, mentioning that research has shown that exposure to tobacco smoke may predispose children to ear infections.

Barbara Starfield, a foremost scholar in the field of primary care, conceptualized the key tasks of primary care as (1) first contact care, (2) continuity, (3) comprehensiveness, and (4) coordination. Dr. Wells' care of the Smith family illustrates these essential features of primary care. He is the *first-contact* physician performing the initial evaluation when Ginny or other family members develop symptoms of illness. *Continuity* refers to sustaining a patient–caregiver relationship over time. Dr. Wells' familiarity with Ginny's condition helps him to better discern an acute infection. *Comprehensiveness* consists of the ability to manage a wide range of health care needs, in contrast with specialty care, which focuses on a particular organ system or procedural service. Dr. Wells' comprehensive, family-oriented care makes him aware that Mrs. Smith's smoking cessation program is an important part of his treatment plan for Ginny. *Coordination* builds upon longitudinality. Through referral and follow-up, the primary care

clinician integrates services delivered by other caregivers. These tasks performed by Dr. Wells meet the standard definition of primary care: "Primary care is the provision of integrated, accessible health care services by clinicians who are accountable for addressing a large majority of personal health care needs, developing sustained partnerships with patients, and practicing in the context of family and community" (Institute of Medicine, 1996).

A functional approach helps characterize which health care professionals truly fill the primary care niche. Among physicians in the United States, family physicians, general internists, and general pediatricians typically provide first contact, longitudinal, comprehensive, coordinated care. Emergency medicine physicians provide first contact care that may be relatively comprehensive for acute problems, but they do not provide continuity of care or coordinate care for patients on an ongoing basis. Some obstetrician-gynecologists provide first contact and longitudinal care, but usually only for reproductive health conditions. Similarly, a patient with kidney failure or cancer may have a strong continuity of care relationship with a nephrologist or an oncologist, but these medical subspecialists rarely assume responsibility for comprehensive care of clinical problems outside of their specialty area or coordinate most ancillary and referral services.

Studies have found that the core elements of good primary care advance the "triple aim" of health system improvement: better patient experiences, better patient outcomes, and lower costs (Starfield, 1998; Bodenheimer & Grumbach, 2007; Friedberg et al., 2010). For example, continuity of care is associated with greater patient satisfaction, higher use of preventive services, reductions in hospitalizations, and lower costs (Saultz & Albedaiwi, 2004; Saultz & Lochner, 2005). Care that is comprehensive, provided by family physicians, is associated with a 10% to 15% reduction in Medicare expenditures per beneficiary (Bazemore et al., 2015). Persons whose care meets a primary care–oriented model have better perceived access to care, are more likely to receive recommended preventive services, are more likely to adhere to treatment, and are more satisfied with their care (Bindman et al., 1996; Stewart et al., 1997; Safran et al., 1998). International comparisons have indicated that nations with a greater primary care orientation tend to have more satisfied patients and better performance on health indicators such as infant mortality, life expectancy, and total health expenditures (Starfield et al., 2005). Similar observations have been made comparing regions in the United States (Starfield et al., 2005). In an analysis of quality and cost of care across states for Medicare beneficiaries, Baicker and Chandra (2004) found that states with more PCPs per capita had lower per capita Medicare costs and higher quality. States with more specialists per capita had lower quality and higher per capita Medicare expenditures. An analysis by county showed that greater PCP supply was associated an increase in life expectancy and lower cardiovascular, cancer, and respiratory mortality from 2005 to 2015 (Basu et al., 2019).

▶ Care Coordination Versus "Gatekeeping"

Polly Seymour, described earlier in the chapter, feels terrible. Every time she eats, she feels nauseated and vomits frequently. She has lost 8 lb, and her oncologist is worried that her breast cancer has spread. She undergoes blood tests, an abdominal CT scan, and a bone scan, all of which are normal. She returns to her gastroenterologist, who tells her to stop the ibuprofen she has been taking for tendinitis. Her problem persists, and the gastroenterologist performs an endoscopy, which shows mild gastric irritation. A month has passed, $7,000 has been spent, and Polly continues to vomit.

Polly's friend Martha recommends a nurse practitioner, Sara Steward, who has been caring for Martha for many years and who spends more time talking with patients than do many physicians. Ms. Steward takes a complete history, which reveals that Polly is taking tamoxifen for her breast cancer and that she began to take aspirin after stopping the ibuprofen. Ms. Steward explains that either of these medications can cause vomiting and suggests that they be stopped for a week. Polly returns in a week, her nausea and vomiting resolved. Ms. Steward then consults with Polly's oncologist, and together they decide to restart the tamoxifen but not the aspirin. Polly becomes nauseated again, but eventually begins to feel well and gains weight

while taking a reduced dose of tamoxifen. In the future, Ms. Steward handles Polly's medical problems, referring her to specialty physicians when needed, and making sure that the advice of one consultant does not interfere with the therapy of another specialist.

A concept that incorporates many of the elements of primary care is that of the primary care clinician as gatekeeper who manages referrals to specialists. Gatekeeping took on pejorative connotations in the heyday of managed care, when, as described in Chapter 4, some types of financial arrangements with PCPs provided incentives for them to "shut the gate" in order to limit specialist referrals, diagnostic tests, and other services (Grumbach et al., 1998). A more accurate designation of the role of the PCP in helping patients navigate the complexities of the health care system is that of care coordinator (Bodenheimer et al., 1999). Stories such as Polly's demonstrate the importance of having a generalist care coordinator who can advocate on behalf of his or her patients and work in partnership with patients to integrate an array of services involving multiple providers to avoid duplication of services, enhance patient safety, and care for the whole person.

▶ The Patient-Centered Medical Home

Dr. Funk is counting the days until he can retire from his solo practice of general internal medicine. He feels overwhelmed most days. The next available appointment in his office is in 10 weeks, and patients call every day frustrated about lack of access. A health plan just sent him a quality report card indicating that many diabetic patients in his practice have not achieved the targeted levels of control of their blood sugar, blood pressure, and lipids. Dr. Funk is also behind in keeping his patients up to date on their mammograms and colorectal cancer screening. Many days he has trouble finding information in the thick paper medical records about when his patients last received their preventive care services or diabetic tests. He never has time to take his daughter to her soccer games. He was hoping to recruit a new residency graduate to take over his practice, but most young internists in his region are pursuing highly paid careers in subspecialties.

Dr. Avantgard has always embraced innovation. When she read a book about new primary care practice models, she proposed to her three physician and two nurse practitioner partners that their primary care practice become a Patient Centered Medical Home. Dr. Avantgard starts by revamping the scheduling system to a "same-day" appointment system, where 50% of appointment slots are left unbooked until the day prior so that patients can call and be guaranteed a same day or next day appointment. Despite her partners' concerns about being overrun with patient appointments, the new scheduling system results in the same number of patients being seen each day, but with happier patients who are delighted to be able to get prompt access to care. The practice uses its new electronic health record system to develop registries of all the patients in the practice due for preventive and chronic care services. Dr. Avantgard and her associates train their medical assistants to use the EHR, along with standing orders, to proactively order mammograms and blood lipid tests when due and to administer vaccinations and screen for depression during patient intake at medical visits. Now that many of the routine preventive and chronic care tasks are being capably handled by other staff, Dr. Avantgard and her clinician colleagues have more time during office visits to focus on the problems patients wish to discuss. With quality indicators and patient satisfaction scores for the practice rising to the top decile of scores for practitioners in the region, Dr. Avantgard plans to start negotiations with several health plans to add a monthly care coordination payment to the current fee-for-service payments, so that the practice can be compensated for the hours spent on coordinating care outside of office visits. Ultimately, she hopes to join one of the new programs changing the payment model for one of the largest insurers from fee-for-service to capitation (see Chapter 4).

By the turn of the twenty-first century, primary care in the United States had reached a critical juncture, with alarms warning an impending collapse of primary care (American College of Physicians, 2006; Bodenheimer, 2006). The primary care report of the National Academies of Sciences, Engineering, and Medicine (2021) proclaimed that "primary care is slowly dying." Primary care clinicians like Dr. Funk struggled to meet patient demands for accessible, comprehensive, well-coordinated care. Many gaps in quality existed, and care often fell short of being patient-centered. PCPs were demoralized by paltry compensation for primary care relative to specialty care that contributed to understaffing. Outmoded practice models were ill-equipped to meet the demands of modern-day primary care, not to mention an ever-widening gap between PCP take-home pay and the escalating earnings of specialists. In the face of these challenges, decreasing numbers of US medical school graduates selected careers in primary care and many policy analysts concluded that the nation faced a major shortage of PCPs (Bodenheimer, 2022).

In response to this crisis, the four major professional organizations representing the nation's PCPs—the American Academy of Family Physicians, American College of Physicians, American Academy of Pediatrics, and American Osteopathic Association—came together in 2007 and issued a report on a common vision for reform of primary care. The *Patient-Centered Medical Home* has served as a rallying point for building a broad movement to revitalize primary care in the United States (National Academies of Sciences, Engineering, and Medicine, 2021). A more inclusive group with consumer advocates and representatives from nursing and other professions in addition to physicians updated the medical home concept in 2018 in the *Shared Principles of Primary Care* (Epperly et al., 2019).

The term "medical home" dates back to 1967, when it was first used by the American Academy of Pediatrics to describe the notion of a primary care practice that would coordinate care for children with complex needs. Contemporary frameworks begin by reaffirming Starfield's fundamental functions of primary care and build on those principles by calling for greater attention to patient-centeredness, such as the type of same-day scheduling methods adopted by Dr. Avantgard; implementation of innovative practice models, such as Dr. Avantgard's development of team-care models that reengineer workflows and tasks; and changes in physician payment, such as blending fee-for-service with partial capitation and quality incentives.

Table 7–1. "Old" and "new" model primary care: some elements of transforming a practice into a patient-centered medical home

Traditional Model	Patient-Centered Medical Home
My patients are those who make appointments to see me	Our patients are those who are registered in our medical home
Care is determined by today's problem and time available today	Care is determined by a proactive plan to meet health needs, with or without visits
Care varies by scheduled time and memory or skill of the doctor	Care is standardized according to evidence-based guidelines
I know I deliver high-quality care because I'm well trained	We measure our quality and make rapid changes to improve it
Patients are responsible for coordinating their own care	A prepared team of professionals works with all patients to coordinate care
It's up to the patients to tell us what happened to them	We track tests and consultations, and follow-up after ED and hospital care
Clinic operations center on meeting the doctor's needs	An interdisciplinary team works at the top of our licenses to serve patients

Source: Adapted with permission from F. Daniel Duffy, MD, MACP, Senior Associate Dean for Academics, University of Oklahoma School of Community Medicine.

A perspective on the patient-centered medical home is shown in Table 7–1.

The Affordable Care Act set in motion several programs to support patient-centered medical home reforms, such as the Medicare Comprehensive Primary Care Initiative (Peikes et al., 2018). Organizations such as the National Committee on Quality Assurance (NCQA) created a checklist of requirements for grading practices applying to be recognized as patient-centered medical homes. Evaluation of the first wave of patient-centered medical home reforms has demonstrated mixed results in quality of care improvement and health care cost reduction (Peikes et al., 2018; Bodenheimer, 2022). Groups facilitating comprehensive reengineering of primary care practices issued roadmaps to transformation, such as the Building Blocks of High-Performing Primary Care (Bodenheimer et al., 2014) and the Change Concepts of the Safety Net Medical Home Initiative (Wagner et al., 2012).

FORCES DRIVING THE ORGANIZATION OF HEALTH CARE IN THE UNITED STATES

The Biomedical Model

The growth of the dispersed mode of health care delivery in the United States was shaped by several forces. One factor was the preeminence of the biomedical model among medical educators. An influential national study, the Flexner report of 1906, led to consolidation of medical training in academically oriented medical schools (Starr, 1982). These academic centers embraced the biomedical paradigm that was the legacy of such renowned nineteenth-century European microbiologists as Pasteur and Koch. The antimicrobial model engendered the faith that every illness has a discrete, ultimately knowable cause and that "magic bullets" can be crafted to eradicate these sources of disease. Physicians were trained to master pathophysiologic changes within a particular organ system, leading to the development of specialization (Luce & Byyny, 1979).

Advocates of a larger role for generalism and primary care in US health care have not so much rejected the concepts of scientific medicine and professional specialism as they have attempted to broaden the interpretation of these terms. They have called for a more integrated scientific approach to understanding health and illness that incorporates information about the individual's psychosocial experiences and family, cultural, and environmental context as well as physiologic and anatomic constitution (Engel, 1977). The attempt to more rigorously define the scientific and clinical basis of generalism contributed to the emergence of family medicine in 1969 as a specialty discipline in its own right, and the 1-year general practice internship was replaced by a 3-year residency program and specialty board certification.

Financial Incentives

A second and related factor influencing the structure of health care was the financial incentive for physician specialization and hospital expansion, which played out in a number of ways.

1. Insurance benefits first offered by Blue Cross covered hospital costs but not physician visits and other outpatient services.

2. As physician services came to be covered later under Blue Shield and other plans, a growing differential in payment between generalist and specialist physicians developed. New technologic and other procedures often required considerable physician time when first introduced, and higher fees were justified for these procedures. But as the procedures became routine, fees remained high, while the time and effort required to perform them declined (Starr, 1982); this resulted in an increasing disparity in income between PCPs and specialists (Bodenheimer et al., 2007; Urwin and Emanuel, 2019). In the mid-1980s, the average PCP's income was 75% of the average specialist's income; by 2006, PCP income had dropped to only 50% of specialists' income (Council of Graduate Medical Education, 2010). In 2020, orthopedists and cardiologists earned more than twice as much as family physicians. As Fig. 7–3 shows, the percentage of graduating medical students planning to enter careers in primary care has tracked the PCP-specialist income gap closely, with the proportion of students entering primary care decreasing as the earnings of PCPs relative to specialists declines.

3. Federal involvement in health care financing further fueled the expansion of hospital care and specialization. The Hill–Burton Hospital Construction Act of 1946 allocated billions of dollars between 1946 and 1971 for expansion of hospital capacity rather than development of ambulatory services (Starr, 1982). The enactment of Medicare and Medicaid in 1965 perpetuated the private insurance tradition of higher payment for procedurally oriented specialists than for generalists. Medicare further encouraged specialization through its policy of extra payments to hospitals to cover costs associated with residency training. Linking Medicare teaching payments to the hospital sector added yet another bias against community-based primary care training.

The growth of hospitals and medical specialization was intertwined. As medical practice became more

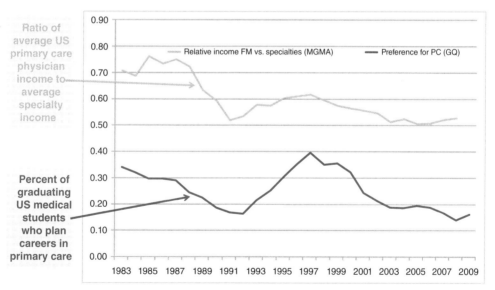

▲ **Figure 7–3.** Proportion of US medical students entering primary care strongly tracks relative incomes of primary care physicians. The figure shows trends over time in the average income of primary care physicians relative to specialist physicians in the United States, and in the percentage of graduating medical students in the United States planning on entering careers in primary care. In 1990, when the average primary care physician income was about half that of specialists, fewer than 20% of graduating students planned to enter primary care fields. By 1997, when primary care physician incomes had risen to more than 60% that of specialists, the proportion of graduating students entering primary care had increased in a parallel direction with 40% of graduates planning to enter primary care fields in 1997. Both relative incomes and intentions to enter primary care decreased after 1997. (Council on Graduate Medical Education, 2010).

specialized and dependent on technology, the site of care increasingly shifted from the patient's home or physician's office to the hospital. The emphasis on acute hospital care had an effect on the nursing profession comparable to that on physicians. World War I was a watershed period in the transition of nursing from a community-based to a hospital-based orientation. During the war, US military hospitals overseas were much heralded for their success in treating acute war injuries. At the war's conclusion, the nation rallied behind a policy of boosting the civilian hospital sector. According to Rosemary Stevens (1989),

> Before the war, public-health nursing was the elite area; nurses had been instrumental in the campaigns against tuberculosis and for infant welfare. In contrast, the war emphasized the supremacy and glamour of hospitals ... nurses, like physicians, were trained—and ready—to perform in an increasingly specialized, acute-care medical environment rather than to expand their interests in social medicine and public health.

▶ Professionalism

The final factor accounting for the organizational evolution of US health care delivery was the nature of control over health planning. The United States is unique in its laxity of public regulation of health care resources. In most industrialized nations, governments wield considerable control over health planning through measures such as regulation of hospital capacity and technology, allocation of the number of residency training positions in generalist and specialist fields, and coordination of public health with medical care. In the United States, the government has provided much of the financing for health care, but without an attendant degree of administrative control. The Hill–Burton program, for example, did not make grants for hospital construction contingent upon any rigorous community-wide plan for regionalized hospital services. Medicare funding for physician training did not stipulate any particular distribution of residency positions according to specialty.

With government controls kept largely at bay, the professional "sovereignty" of physicians emerged as the preeminent authority in health care (Starr, 1982).

Their professional status vested physicians with special authority to guide the development of the US health care system. As described in Chapter 2, third-party payment for physician services was established with physician control of the initial Blue Shield insurance plans. Physician judgment about the need for technology and greater inpatient capacity drove the expansion of hospital facilities.

What was the nature of the profession that so heavily influenced the development of the US health care organization? It was a profession that, because of the primacy of the biomedical paradigm and the nature of financial incentives, was weighted toward hospital and specialty care. Small wonder that US health care has emphasized its tertiary care apex over its primary care base. In Chapter 17, we discuss the shifting power relationships in health care that are challenging the professional dominance of physicians.

CONCLUSION

> Jeff leaves a town forum at the local medical center feeling confused. It featured two speakers, one of whom criticized the medical center as being out of touch with the community's needs, and the other of whom defended the center's contributions to society. Jeff found the first speaker convincing about the need to pay more attention to primary care, prevention, and public health. He had never had a regular primary care physician, and the idea of having a family physician appealed to him. He was equally impressed by the second speaker, whose account of how research at the medical center had led to life-saving treatment of children with a hereditary blood disorder was very moving, and whose description of the hospital's plan for a new imaging center was spellbinding. Jeff felt that if he ever became seriously ill, he would certainly want all the specialized services the medical center had to offer.

The professional model and the biomedical paradigm are responsible for many of the successes of the US health care system. The biomedical model has instilled respect for the scientific method and curtailed medical quackery. Professionalism has directed physicians to serve as agents acting in their patients' best interests and has made the practice of medicine more than just another business. Expansion of hospital facilities has meant that people with health insurance have had convenient access to tertiary care services and new technology and the expertise and availability of a wide variety of specialists. In many circumstances, the system is well organized to deliver the "right care." For a patient in cardiogenic shock, the right place to be is an intensive care unit; for a patient with a detached retina, an ophthalmologist's office is the right place to be.

However, there is widespread concern that despite the benefits of biomedical science and medical professionalism, the US health care system is precariously off balance. A model of excellence focused on specialization, technology, and curative medicine has led to relative inattention to basic primary care services that care for the whole person, including disease prevention and supportive care for patients with chronic and incurable ailments. The value placed on autonomy for health care professionals and institutions has contributed to fragmentation of care. A system that prizes specialists who focus on organ systems has bred apprehension that health care has lost sight of the whole person and the whole community. The net result is a system structured to perform miraculous feats for individuals who are ill, but at great expense and often without satisfactorily attending to the full spectrum of health care needs of the entire population. During the 2009 debate in Congress leading up to the passage of the Affordable Care Act, one of the harshest critiques of the status quo in US health care came not from a Congressional Democrat, but from Senator Orrin Hatch, at the time the senior Republican Senator from Utah. At a hearing on health reform, Senator Hatch said, "The US is first in providing rescue care, but this care has little or no impact on the general population. We must put more focus on primary care and preventive medicine" (Grundy et al., 2010).

REFERENCES

American College of Physicians. The Impending Collapse of Primary Care Medicine and its Implications for the State of the Nation's Health Care. January 30, 2006.

Baicker K, Chandra A. Medicare spending, the physician workforce, and beneficiaries' quality of care. *Health Aff (Millwood)*. 2004:W4-184–W4-197.

Basu S, Berkowitz SA, Phillips RL, Bitton A, Landon BE, Phillips RS. Association of primary care physician supply with population mortality in the United States, 2005–2015. *JAMA Intern Med*. 2019;179:506–514.

Bazemore A, Petterson S, Peterson LE, Phillips RL Jr. More comprehensive care among family physicians is associated with lower costs and fewer hospitalizations. *Ann Fam Med*. 2015;13:206–213.

Bindman AB, Grumbach K, Osmond D, Vranizan K, Stewart AL. Primary care and receipt of preventive services. *J Gen Intern Med*. 1996;11:269–276.

Bodenheimer T, Berenson RA, Rudolf P. The primary care-specialty income gap: why it matters. *Ann Intern Med*. 2007;146:301–306.

Bodenheimer T, Ghorob A, Willard-Grace R, Grumbach K. The 10 building blocks of high-performing primary care. *Ann Fam Med*. 2014;12:166–171.

Bodenheimer T, Grumbach K. *Improving Primary Care. Strategies and Tools for a Better Practice*. New York, NY: McGraw-Hill; 2007.

Bodenheimer T, Lo B, Casalino L. Primary care physicians should be coordinators, not gatekeepers. *JAMA*. 1999;281(21):2045–2049.

Bodenheimer T. Primary care–Will it survive? *N Engl J Med*. 2006;355:861–864.

Bodenheimer T. Regional medical programs: no road to regionalization. *Med Care Rev*. 1969;26:1125–1166.

Bodenheimer T. Revitalizing primary care. *Ann Fam Med*. 2022;20:464–468, 469–478.

Council on Graduate Medical Education. Twentieth report: advancing primary care, December 2010. Available at www.hrsa.gov/advisorycommittees/bhpradvisory/cogme/Reports/twentiethreport.pdf.

Dawson W. Interim report on the future provision of medical and allied services. In: Saward EW, ed. *The Regionalization of Personal Health Services*. London, England: Prodist; 1975.

Engel GL. The need for a new medical model: a challenge for biomedicine. *Science*. 1977;196:129–136.

Epperly T, Bechtel C, Sweeney R, et al. The shared principles of primary care: a multistakeholder initiative to find a common voice. *Fam Med*. 2019;52:179–184.

Friedberg MW, Hussey PS, Schneider EC. Primary care: a critical review of the evidence on quality and costs of health care. *Health Aff (Millwood)*. 2010;29:766–772.

Fry J. Primary care. In: Fry J, ed. *Primary Care*. London, England: William Heinemann; 1980.

Gonzalez AA, Dimick JB, Birkmeyer JD, Ghaferi AA. Understanding the volume-outcome effect in cardiovascular surgery: the role of failure to rescue. *JAMA Surg*. 2014;149:119–123.

Goroll AH, Hunt DP. Bridging the hospitalist-primary care divide through collaborative care. *N Engl J Med*. 2015;372:308–309.

Green LA, Fryer GE Jr, Yawn BP, Lanier D, Dovey SM. The ecology of medical care revisited. *N Engl J Med.* 2001;344:2021–2025.

Grumbach K, Osmond D, Vranizan K, Jaffe D, Bindman AB. Primary care physicians' experience of financial incentives in managed care systems. *N Engl J Med.* 1998;339:1516–1521.

Grundy P, Hagan KR, Hansen JC, Grumbach K. The multistakeholder movement for primary care renewal and reform. *Health Affairs.* 2010;29:791–798.

Halvorson GC, Isham GJ. *Epidemic of Care.* San Francisco, CA: Jossey-Bass; 2003.

Institute of Medicine. *Primary Care: America's Health in a New Era.* Washington, DC: National Academies Press; 1996. Available at www.ncbi.nlm.nih.gov/pubmed/25121221.

Luce JM, Byyny RL. The evolution of medical specialism. *Perspect Biol Med.* 1979;22:377–389.

National Academies of Sciences, Engineering, and Medicine. *Implementing High-Quality Primary Care: Rebuilding the Foundation of Health Care.* Washington, DC: The National Academies Press; 2021. https://doi.org/10.17226/25983.

Palmer B. Is the number of GPs falling across the UK? Nuffield Trust blog post, May 8, 2019.

Peikes D, Dale S, Ghosh A, et al. The comprehensive primary care initiative: effects on spending, quality, patients, and physicians. *Health Aff (Millwood).* 2018;37:890–899.

Robert Graham Center. Primary Care in the United States. A Chartbook of Facts and Statistics. 2021.

Rodwin VG. *The Health Planning Predicament.* Berkeley, CA: University of California Press; 1984.

Safran DG, Taira DA, Rogers WH, Kosinski M, Ware JE, Tarlov AR. Linking primary care performance to outcomes of care. *J Fam Pract.* 1998;47:213–220.

Saultz JW, Albedaiwi W. Interpersonal continuity of care and patient satisfaction: a critical review. *Ann Fam Med.* 2004;2:445–451.

Saultz JW, Lochner J. Interpersonal continuity of care and care outcomes: a critical review. *Ann Fam Med.* 2005;3:159–166.

Somers AR. Who's in charge here? Alice searches for a king in Mediland. *N Engl J Med.* 1972;287:849–855.

Starfield B, Shi L, Macinko J. Contribution of primary care to health systems and health. *Milbank Q.* 2005;83:457–502.

Starfield B. *Primary Care.* New York, NY: Oxford University Press; 1998.

Starr P. *The Social Transformation of American Medicine.* New York, NY: Basic Books; 1982.

Stevens R. *In Sickness and in Wealth: American Hospitals in the Twentieth Century.* New York, NY: Basic Books; 1989.

Stewart AL, Grumbach K, Osmond DH, Vranizan K, Komaromy M, Bindman AB. Primary care and patient perceptions of access to care. *J Fam Pract.* 1997;44:177–185.

Urwin JW, Emanuel EJ. The relative value scale update committee: time for an update. *JAMA.* 2019;322:1137–1138.

Wachter RM, Goldman L. The emerging role of "hospitalists" in the American health care system. *N Engl J Med.* 1996;335:514–517.

Wagner EH, Coleman K, Reid RJ, Phillips K, Abrams MK, Sugarman JR. The changes involved in patient-centered medical home transformation. *Prim Care.* 2012;39:241–259.

White KL, Williams TF, Greenberg BG. The ecology of medical care. *N Engl J Med.* 1961;265:885–892.

How Health Care Is Organized—II: Health Care Delivery Systems

The last chapter explored general principles of health care organization, including levels of care, regionalization, and patient flow through the system. This chapter looks at actual structures of medical practice.

The traditional dispersed model of the US medical practice has been referred to as a "cottage industry" of independent private physicians working as solo practitioners or in small groups. By 2020, a major change was evident, with small organizations either banding together to form large enterprises or being swallowed up by health care giants. The dispersed model is evolving into a consolidated model of health care delivery.

THE TRADITIONAL STRUCTURE OF MEDICAL CARE

Physicians and Hospitals

Dr. Harvey Commoner finished his residency in general surgery in 1976. For the next 30 years, he and another surgeon practiced medicine together in a middle-class suburb near St. Peter's Hospital, a nonprofit church-affiliated institution. Dr. Commoner received most of his cases from family physicians and internists on the St. Peter's medical staff. By 1996, the number of surgeons operating at St. Peter's had grown. Because Dr. Commoner was not getting enough cases, he and his partner joined the medical staff of Top Dollar Hospital, a for-profit facility 3 miles away, and University Hospital downtown. On an average morning, Dr. Commoner drove to all three hospitals to perform operations or to do postoperative rounds on his patients. The afternoon was spent seeing patients in his office. He was on call every other night and weekend.

Dr. Commoner was active on the St. Peter's medical staff executive committee, where he frequently proposed that the hospital purchase new radiology and operating room equipment needed to keep up with advances in surgery. Because the hospital received more than 1 million dollars each year for providing care to Dr. Commoner's patients, and because Dr. Commoner had the option of admitting his patients to Top Dollar or University, the St. Peter's administration usually purchased the items that Dr. Commoner recommended. The Top Dollar Hospital administrator did likewise.

During the period when Dr. Commoner was practicing, most medical care was delivered by fee-for-service private physicians in solo or small group practices. Most hospitals were private nonprofit institutions, sometimes affiliated with a religious organization, occasionally with a medical school, often run by an independent board of trustees composed of prominent people in the community. Most physicians in traditional fee-for-service practice were not employees of any hospital, but joined one or several hospital medical staffs, thereby gaining the privilege of admitting patients to the hospital and at times acquiring the responsibility to assist the hospital through work on medical staff committees or by caring for emergency department patients who have no physician.

For many years, physicians were the dominant power in the hospital because physicians admit the patients, and hospitals without patients have no income. Because physicians were free to admit their patients to more than one hospital, the implicit threat to take their patients elsewhere gave them influence. Physicians used informal referral networks, often involving other physicians on the same hospital medical staff. In metropolitan areas with a high ratio of physician specialists to population, referrals could become a critical economic issue. Most surgeons obtained their cases by referral from primary care physicians (PCPs) or medical specialists; surgeons like Dr. Commoner, who were not readily available when called, soon found their case load drying up.

THE SEEDS OF NEW MEDICAL CARE STRUCTURES

The dispersed structure of fee-for-service private practice was not always the dominant model in the United States. When modern medical care took root in the first half of the twentieth century, a variety of structures blossomed. Among these were multispecialty group practices, community health centers, and prepaid group practices. Some of these flourished but then wilted, while others became the seeds from which the emerging health care system of the twenty-first century is germinating.

Multispecialty Group Practice

In 1905, Dr. Geraldine Giemsa joined the department of pathology at the Mayo Clinic. The clinic, led by the brothers William and Charles Mayo, was becoming a nationally renowned referral center for surgery and was recruiting pathologists, microbiologists, and other specialized diagnosticians to support the work of the clinic's surgeons. Dr. Giemsa received a salary and became an employee of the group practice. With time, she became a senior partner and part owner of the Mayo Clinic.

Together with their father, the Mayo brothers, general practitioners skilled at surgical techniques, formed a group practice in the small town of Rochester, MN, in the 1890s. As the brothers' reputation for excellence grew, the practice added surgeons and physicians in laboratory-oriented specialties. By 1929, the Mayo Clinic had more than 375 physicians and 900 support staff and eventually opened its own hospitals (Starr, 1982). Although the clinic paid its physician staff by salary, the clinic itself billed patients, and later insurance plans, on a fee-for-service basis. The Mayo Clinic was the inspiration for other group practices that developed in the United States, such as the Menninger Clinic in Topeka, KS, and the Palo Alto Medical Foundation in California. These clinics were owned and administered by physicians in various specialties—hence the common use of the term *multispecialty group practice* to describe this organizational model. The multispecialty group practices brought a large number of physicians together under one roof to deliver care. By formally integrating physicians into a single clinic structure, group practice attempted to promote a collaborative style of care in which colleagues shared responsibility for the care of patients.

In 1932, the Committee on the Costs of Medical Care recommended that the delivery of care be organized around large group practices (Starr, 1982). The eight private practice physicians on the committee dissented from the recommendations, roundly criticizing the sections on group practice (Committee on the Costs of Medical Care, 1932).

Several multispecialty group practices flourished during the period between the world wars, and to this day remain among the most highly regarded systems of care in the United States. Yet multispecialty group practice did not become the dominant organizational structure, in part due to resistance by professional societies. In addition, as hospitals assumed a central role in medical care, group practice lost some of its unique attractions. Hospitals could provide the ancillary services physicians needed for the increasingly specialized and technology-dependent work of medicine. Hospitals also served as an organizational focus for the informal referral networks that developed among private physicians in independent practice.

Community Health Centers

A far-reaching alternative to private medical practice is the community health center, emphasizing primary and preventive care and striving to take responsibility for the health status of the community served by the health center. An early twentieth-century example of such an institution was the Greater Community

Association at Creston, Iowa. In describing the association, Kepford (1919) wrote:

> We have a hospital that makes no attempt to pattern after the great city institutions, but is organized to meet the needs of a rural neighborhood. The Greater Community Association has been taught to regard the hospital as a repair shop, necessary only where preventive medicine has failed.

The association brought together civic, religious, education, and health care groups in a coordinated system centered on the community hospital serving a six-county area with 100,000 residents. The plan placed its greatest emphasis on preventive care and public health measures administered by public health nurses.

> In 1928, Sherry Kidd joined the Frontier Nursing Service in Appalachia as a nurse midwife. For $5 per year, families could enroll in the service and receive pregnancy-related care. Sherry was responsible for all enrolled families within a 100-mile radius. She referred patients with complications to an obstetrician in Lexington, KY, the service's physician consultant.

Another pioneering model, the Frontier Nursing Service was established by Mary Breckinridge, an English-trained midwife, in 1925 (Dye, 1983). Breckinridge designed the service to meet the needs of a low-income rural area in Kentucky that lacked basic medical and obstetric care and suffered from high rates of maternal and infant mortality. The Frontier Nursing Service shared many features of the Creston model: regionalized services planned on a geographic basis to serve rural populations with an emphasis on primary care and health education. Like the Creston system, the service relied on nurses to provide primary care, with physicians reserved for secondary medical services.

These rural programs had their urban counterparts in health centers that focused on maternal and child health services during the early 1900s (Stoeckle & Candib, 1969; Rothman, 1978). The clinics primarily served populations in low-income districts in large cities, often consisting of large immigrant populations. As in the rural systems, public health nurses played a central role in health education, nutrition, and sanitation. Both the urban and rural models of community health centers waned during the middle years of the

twentieth century. Public health nursing declined in prestige as hospitals became the center of activity for nursing education and practice (Stevens, 1989). A team model of nurses working in collaboration with physicians withered under a system of hierarchical professional roles.

The community health center model was revived in 1965 by the federal Office of Economic Opportunity's "War on Poverty." The program's goals included the combining of comprehensive medical care and public health to improve the health status of defined low-income communities, the building of multidisciplinary teams to provide health services, and participation in the governance of the health centers by community members.

> Dr. Franklin Jefferson was professor of hematology at a prestigious medical school. His distinguished career was based on laboratory research, teaching, and subspecialty medical practice, with a focus on sickle cell anemia. Dr. Jefferson felt that his work was serving his community, but that he would like to do more. In 1965, with the advent of the federal neighborhood health center program, he left his laboratory in the hands of a well-trained assistant and began to talk with community leaders in the low-income neighborhood that surrounded the medical school. After a year, the trust that developed between Dr. Jefferson and members of the neighborhood bore fruit in a decision to approach the medical school dean about a joint medical school–community application for funds to create a neighborhood health center. Two years later, the center opened its doors, with Dr. Jefferson as its first medical director.

In 2021, over 1,400 community health centers at 14,000 sites were serving over 30 million people, most uninsured or covered by Medicaid (National Association of Community Health Centers, 2022). Many of the centers train community members as outreach workers, who became members of health care teams that include public health nurses, physicians, mental health workers, and health educators. Some health centers strive to meld clinical services with public health activities in programs of community-oriented primary care. For example, the rural health center in Mound Bayou, Mississippi helped organize a cooperative farm to improve nutrition in the county, dig wells to supply safe drinking water, and train community residents to become health care professionals (Geiger, 2016). By improving the ambulatory care of low-income patients, the centers were able to reduce hospitalization and emergency department visits by their patients. Community health centers have also had some success in improving community health status, particularly by reducing infant and neonatal mortality rates among African Americans (Geiger, 1984).

▶ Prepaid Group Practice and Health Maintenance Organizations

One alternative to small office-based, fee-for-service practice became the major challenge to that traditional model: prepaid group practice.

In 1929, the Ross–Loos Clinic began to provide medical services for employees of the Los Angeles Department of Water and Power on a prepaid basis. By 1935, the clinic had enrolled 37,000 employees and their dependents, who each paid $2 per month for a specified list of services. Also in 1929, an idealistic physician, Dr. Michael Shadid, organized a medical cooperative in Elk City, OK, run by the patients of the cooperative. In the late 1940s, more than a hundred rural health cooperatives were founded, many in Texas, but they faded away, partly from the stiff opposition of organized medicine. In the 1950s, another version of the consumer-managed prepaid group practice sprang up in Appalachia, where the United Mine Workers established union-run group practice clinics, each receiving a budget from the union-controlled medical care fund. A few years later in Seattle, Group Health Cooperative of Puget Sound acquired its own hospital, began to grow, and by the mid-1970s had 200,000 subscribers, a fifth of the Seattle-area population. In 1947, the Health Insurance Plan of New York opened its doors, operating 22 group practices; within 10 years, its enrollment approached 500,000 (Starr, 1982).

Rather than preserving a separation between insurance plans and the providers of care, these prepaid group practice models meld the financing and delivery of care into a single organizational structure. Patients could pay in advance to directly purchase health services from a particular system of care. In addition to the prepayment component, care is delivered by a large group of practitioners working under a common administrative structure—the "group practice" aspect of prepaid group practice.

The most successful of the prepaid group practices that emerged in the 1930s and 1940s was Kaiser Permanente. In 1938, a surgeon named Sidney Garfield began providing prepaid medical services for industrialist Henry J. Kaiser's employees working at the Grand Coulee Dam in Washington State. Rather than receiving a salary from Kaiser, Garfield was prepaid a fixed sum per employee, a precursor to modern capitation payment. Kaiser transported this concept to 200,000 workers in his shipyards and steel mills on the West Coast during World War II (Garfield, 1970; Starr, 1982). In this way, company-sponsored medical care in a remote area gave birth to today's largest alternative to fee-for-service practice. Kaiser opened its doors to the general public after World War II. In 2022, Kaiser was present in eight states plus Washington, DC, with 12.6 million patients enrolled.

Prepaid group practices were renamed "health maintenance organizations" in the 1970s, with the term health maintenance designed to suggest that these systems would place more emphasis on preventive care than had the traditional medical model. We will return later in the chapter to discuss how health maintenance organizations (HMOs) have taken on a new meaning separate from the prepaid group practice model. But first, we will use the Kaiser Permanente organization to introduce the key concepts of vertical and horizontal integration.

VERTICAL AND HORIZONTAL INTEGRATION

▶ Kaiser Permanente

Maria Fuentes was a professor at the University of California. She and her family belonged to the Kaiser Health Plan, and the university paid most of her family's premium. Professor Fuentes had once fractured her clavicle, for which she went to the urgent care clinic at Kaiser Hospital in Oakland; otherwise, she had not used Kaiser's facilities. Professor Fuentes' wife suffered from rheumatoid arthritis; her regular physician was a salaried rheumatologist at the Permanente Medical Clinic, the group practice in which Kaiser physicians work. One of the Fuentes' sons, Juanito, had been in an automobile accident a year earlier near a town 90 miles away from home. He had been taken to a local emergency department and released; Kaiser had paid the bill because no Kaiser facility was available in the town. Three days after returning home, Juanito developed a severe headache and became drowsy; he was taken to the urgent care clinic, received a CT scan, and was found to have a subdural hematoma (when blood collects between the skull and the surface of the brain). He was immediately transported to Kaiser's regional neurosurgery center in Redwood City, CA, where he underwent surgery to evacuate the hematoma.

Dr. Roberta Short had mixed feelings about working at Kaiser. She liked the salary and the paucity of administrative tasks. She particularly liked working in the same building with other specialists, providing the opportunity for discussions on diagnostic and therapeutic problems. However, she was not happy about the large number of patients she was scheduled to see. Overall, Dr. Short felt that the Kaiser system worked well but perhaps needed more physicians to care for enrolled patients.

Kaiser Permanente is a large integrated health system consisting of three interlocking administrative units: Kaiser Foundation Health Plan, which performs the functions of health insurer, Kaiser Foundation Hospitals, and Permanente Medical Groups, the physician organizations that provide medical services to Kaiser members under a capitated contract with the Health Plan.

This organizational model has come to be known as vertical integration. Vertical integration refers to consolidating under one organizational roof and common ownership all levels of care, from primary to tertiary care, and the facilities and staff necessary to provide this full spectrum of care (Fig. 8–1). Most Kaiser Permanente units own their hospitals and clinics, hire the nurses, pharmacists, and other personnel staffing these facilities, and contract with a single large group practice (Permanente) to exclusively serve patients covered by the Kaiser health plan. The Kaiser Permanente health system differs from traditional fee-for-service models in how it pays physicians (salary) and hospitals

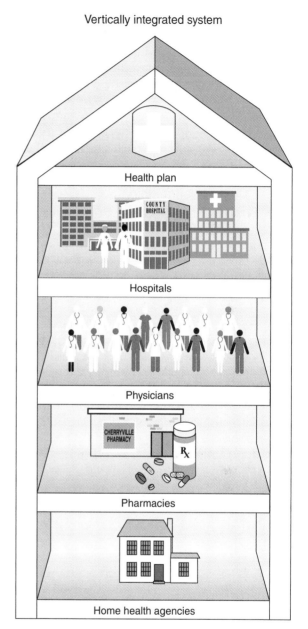

Vertically integrated system

Health plan

Hospitals

Physicians

Pharmacies

Home health agencies

▲ **Figure 8–1.** Vertical integration consolidates health services under one organizational roof.

(global budget). The prepaid group practice structure contrasts with solo, independent private practice.

Kaiser Permanente is also horizontally integrated. Horizontal integration refers to consolidation of health care units providing the same type of services.

Kaiser hospitals in a region operate under common ownership and management rather than as autonomous facilities. Horizontal integration of hospitals has allowed Kaiser to regionalize tertiary care services at a select number of specialized centers. For example, Northern California Kaiser has centralized neurosurgical care at only two hospitals, in contrast to dispersed models in which competing independent hospitals often duplicate many of the same specialized services. Similarly, the Permanente Medical Group represents horizontal integration of physicians and other health professionals. This approach has given Kaiser Permanente considerable control of its internal workforce policy, resulting in the Permanente Medical Group having a greater proportion of PCPs than the overall US workforce and incorporating nurse practitioners and physician assistants into the primary care team. Many observers consider this ability to coherently plan and regionalize services to a defined population to be a strength of vertically and horizontally integrated systems. Structural integration also may facilitate functional integration in patient care, such as by having a shared electronic medical record used throughout the organization. The prepaid nature of enrollment in the Kaiser plan permits Kaiser to orient its care more toward a population health model.

Other Models of Integrated Health Systems

Ollie Gopoly, CEO of California Health, smiled as he reviewed the hospital system's year-end financial report. Fifteen years ago, Ollie was CEO of an independent hospital that was rapidly going from profitable to running in the red as Kaiser gained ever-increasing market share in the region. Ollie realized that the only way to compete was to become more horizontally organized. His first step was to orchestrate a merger with two other local hospitals. Over the ensuing years, the hospital partnership acquired six other hospitals in the region, created a new hospital corporation, California Health, that named Ollie as CEO, and implemented an integrated model with a shared electronic medical record. California Health was now second only to Kaiser in the volume of hospital care in the region. Because of its size, it was able to negotiate higher payment rates with health insurance plans and discounts on the supplies and equipment it purchased. This year's financial performance had generated a substantial positive margin that would allow Ollie to take the next step in his strategic plan: acquiring physician practices.

The greatest growth in integrated models in the past two decades has come not from organizations replicating the Kaiser Permanente model but through consolidation of hospitals into large horizontal systems. Hospitals across the nation have engaged in a process of mergers and acquisitions to create regional systems. Examples of nonprofit systems are Sutter Health in California, Carilion Health System in Virginia, Carolinas Health Care System (now known as Atrium Health), and Banner Health in Arizona. Several for-profit horizontal hospital systems such as Tenet and HCA have a national scope. This consolidation was motivated in part by a desire to achieve the functional benefits and economies of scale of horizontal integration. Another powerful motivator was achieving a stronger bargaining position in the health care marketplace.

The first stage of horizontal consolidation of hospitals into regional health systems has been followed by a second stage of becoming more vertically integrated, principally by purchasing physician practices and converting physicians from independent small business owners to employees of the hospital or of a hospital-sponsored medical group. A tipping point has occurred in the twenty-first century, with the health care cottage industry giving way to larger organizations for delivering care. In 2002, 70% of physicians owned their own practices, dropping to 49% working in physician-owned practices in 2020; 40% of physicians worked in practices with hospital ownership or were hospital employees in 2020 (Kocher & Sahni, 2011; Kane, 2021) (Fig. 8–2). Even as a growing share of physicians are employees of larger systems, one-third of physicians still work in small practices of 4 or fewer physicians (Kane, 2021). In 2020, only one-third of physicians younger than age 40 worked in physician-owned practices (Fig. 8–2). Several of these regional delivery systems, such as Sutter Health and Banner Health, have added the final element of vertical integration—operating their own health insurance plan.

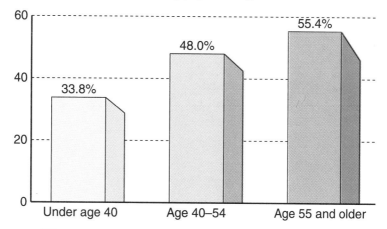

▲ **Figure 8–2.** Percentage of Physicians Working in Physician-Owned Practices by Physician Age, 2020. (Source: Kane CK. Recent Changes in Physician Practice Arrangements. American Medical Association, 2021.) https://www.ama-assn.org/system/files/2021-05/2020-prp-physician-practice-arrangements.pdf.

However, unlike Kaiser Permanente, none of these regional systems relies exclusively on its own health plan; they also contract with other private plans for the majority of their privately insured patients.

VIRTUAL INTEGRATION

We have contrasted the traditional dispersed model of US health care with the growing integration that is occurring. Despite the accelerating consolidation of hospitals and physicians into larger systems, many health care stakeholders remain interested in a third way that brings some of the functional benefits of integration while retaining some of the independence of traditional practice. An example is how a group of physicians in California organized themselves many years ago to create an alternative to the Kaiser Permanente model.

▷ Network Models

In 1954, the medical society in San Joaquin County, CA, fretted about the possibility of Kaiser moving into the county. Patients might go to the lower cost Kaiser, and physicians' incomes would fall. An idea was born: to compete with Kaiser, the San Joaquin Foundation for Medical Care was set up as a network of physicians in independent private practice to contract as a group with employers for a monthly payment per enrollee; the Foundation would then pay the physicians on a discounted fee-for-service basis and conduct utilization review to discourage overtreatment (Starr, 1982). It was hoped that the plan would reduce the costs to employers, who would choose the Foundation rather than Kaiser. This "network model" of horizontal integration spread widely in California as Independent Practice Associations (IPAs) brought together doctors in their private offices to gain more favorable contracts with insurance companies. In the three-tiered payment model described in Chapter 4, insurers pay the IPA which in turn pays its physicians.

This approach of weaving together autonomous physician practices in an IPA in turn engendered a network HMO model of loose vertical integration that became the alternative to the tightly integrated prepaid group practice model. Like the prepaid group practice HMO model, the network HMO model differs from traditional insurance in that the insurance plan only pays for services provided by those physicians and hospitals that participate in the HMO plan—often referred to as a "narrow network" of providers. However, unlike the prepaid group practice model, these providers are not owned or employed by a single organized health delivery system. As shown in Fig. 8–3, the network HMO

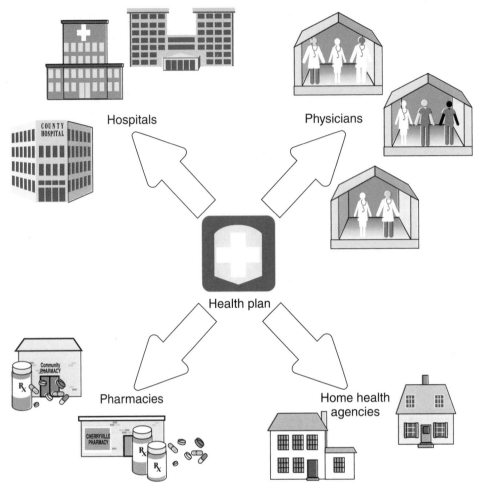

Hospitals

Physicians

Health plan

Pharmacies

Home health agencies

▲ **Figure 8–3.** Virtual integration involves contractual links between HMOs and physician groups, hospitals, and other provider units.

model consists of contractual links between HMO health insurance plans and individual physicians, IPAs, multispecialty medical groups, hospitals, and other provider units, rather than the "everything-under-one-roof" model of vertical integration. Differing from the "monogamous" arrangement between the Kaiser health plan, Kaiser hospitals, and Permanente medical group, network models feature hospitals and physicians having contractual relationships with many different insurance plans. Observers have dubbed the network model of organization "virtual integration," signifying an integration of services based on contractual

relationships rather than unitary ownership (Robinson & Casalino, 1996).

Preferred Provider Organization (PPO) network plans are looser than HMO networks. In response to the reluctance of many patients to be locked into a narrow network of physicians and hospitals in HMO plans, PPO plans have a "preferred" network of physicians and hospitals but allow patients to use physicians and hospitals that are not in the network, with the stipulation that patients pay a higher share of the cost out of pocket when they use non-network physicians and hospitals. Physicians joining the PPO network agree to accept discounted fees from the health plan with the hope that being listed as a "preferred" provider will attract more patients to their practice. Unlike HMO plans, PPO plans use fee for service payment and have not traditionally required patients to select a PCP for their medical home, although some PPOs are now starting to formally link all subscribers to a PCP. PPO enrollment was 166 million in 2018, compared with HMO enrollment of 95 million (MCOL, 2020).

Both network model HMOs and PPOs are considered forms of "managed care." But do these types of managed care truly represent more integrated forms of care delivery? PPOs do not change how care is organized and are simply a minor variation of fee-for-service insurance products. Network HMOs drive a modest degree of change in care organization; they establish a tighter relationship between patients and primary care clinicians and often use capitated payment that emphasizes population health-oriented care. Network HMOs that contract with IPAs rather than directly with individual physicians may also encourage "virtual group practice." Although IPAs initially did little more than to act as brokers between physicians and HMOs, over time IPAs have taken on a larger portion of financial risk for care (see Chapter 4), become more active in attempting to control costs, and assumed responsibility for authorizing utilization of services, profiling physicians' practice patterns, and facilitating quality improvement efforts.

Accountable Care Organizations

As described in Chapter 4, Accountable Care Organizations (ACOs) were developed as a strategy to modify fee-for-service payment to encourage a more integrated, population health approach. In this sense, ACOs can be viewed as another form of virtual integration. Under an ACO model, provider organizations contract with a payer "to manage the full continuum of care and be accountable for the overall costs and quality of care for a defined population" (Rittenhouse et al., 2009). The Affordable Care Act authorized Medicare to initiate an ACO program—the Medicare Shared Savings Program—beginning in 2012 (Gold, 2015). Private insurance plans and large employers have also adopted ACO payment models. In 2018, 53% of ACO contracts were private, 37% Medicare, and

10% Medicaid. In 2021, about 950 ACOs were covering almost 30 million people, a slight decrease from 2018 (Muhlestein et al., 2021). ACOs may include tight structures such as vertically integrated delivery systems or looser federations of independent hospitals and physician networks.

Vertical and Horizontal Integration on the Rise

The various permutations of horizontal and vertical integration are shown in Table 8–1. Health care in the United States is steadily consolidating into the vertically and horizontally integrated systems listed at the bottom half of Table 8–1. One study, using a definition of an integrated health system as one that "included at least one acute care hospital and at least one group of physicians who provided comprehensive care and were connected with each other and the hospital through common ownership or joint management," found that in 2018, half of all physicians and nearly three-quarters of all hospitals were affiliated with an integrated system (Furukawa et al., 2020). The share of physicians affiliated with integrated systems jumped considerably in a very short time, from 40% in 2016 to 51% in 2018. This rapid rise of structurally integrated systems raises a critical question: are patients receiving better care from integrated rather than more dispersed models? The final portion of this chapter addresses this question.

COMPARING STRUCTURALLY AND VIRTUALLY INTEGRATED MODELS

From Medical Homes to Medical Neighborhoods

In Chapter 7, we introduced the concept of medical homes. Much of the current chapter can be described as the attempt to create well-functioning medical neighborhoods (Fisher, 2008). The primary care medical home resides in the medical neighborhood which also includes the secondary, tertiary, community, and related services needed by different patients at different times to meet their comprehensive health care needs. High-performing health care requires both excellent medical homes and excellent medical neighborhoods (Rittenhouse et al., 2009; Huang & Rosenthal, 2014). The distinguishing feature of a hospitable medical

Table 8–1. Varieties of health system integration

	Physicians	Hospitals	Insurance Plan	Organizational Model	Examples
Horizontally loosely integrated medical group	✓	–	–	Independent practice association	Hill Physicians Medical Group
Horizontally tightly integrated medical group	✓	–	–	Integrated multispecialty medical group	Allina Health System Physicians, CHRISTUS Physician Group
Horizontally integrated hospital system	+/–	✓	+/–	Regional or national hospital system	Sutter Health, Tenet Health[*]
Vertically and horizontally tightly integrated delivery system	✓	✓	+/–	Regional health system	Atrium Health, Baylor Scott & White Health, University of Pittsburgh Medical Center
Vertically and horizontally loosely integrated system	✓	✓	✓	HMO Network model	Anthem Blue Cross HMO's provider network
Vertically and horizontally tightly integrated system	✓	✓	✓	Prepaid group practice model HMO	Kaiser Permanente

✓, essential component.
–, not a component.
+/–, optional component; usually a subsidiary element if present.
[*]Over time, horizontally integrated systems added vertical integration; i.e., after several hospitals merged into hospital systems, the hospital systems began to add physician groups either by owning them or contracting with them, thereby becoming a health system rather than only a hospital system.

neighborhood is care that is functionally integrated, but not necessarily structurally integrated. According to one definition, "Integrated health care starts with good primary care and refers to the delivery of comprehensive health care services that are well coordinated with good communication among providers; includes informed and involved patients; and leads to high-quality, cost-effective care. At the center of integrated health care delivery is a high-performing primary care provider who can serve as a medical home for patients" (Aetna Foundation, 2010).

Organizations that are structurally integrated have the potential to provide care that is functionally integrated. These organizations have assets such as multispecialty groups, a unified electronic medical record, interdisciplinary health care teams, and a quality improvement infrastructure equipped to promote care coordination and the free flow of information among all providers involved in a patient's care. One of the ongoing challenges in the United States is whether virtually integrated health systems can achieve the degree of functional integration needed to deliver more effective and efficient care and overcome what we cited

in Chapter 7 as the "fragmentation, chaos, and disarray" that has long plagued the US health system.

▶ Evidence on the Relative Performance of Integrated Models

Does greater organizational integration result in a more functionally integrated medical neighborhood and better patient care? Some research has documented higher quality performance among larger medical groups relative to smaller or less well-organized groups (Weeks et al., 2010; Solberg et al., 2022). Integrated medical groups perform better than IPAs in delivering up-to-date preventive care such as mammograms and Pap tests (Mehrotra et al., 2006). Patients are more satisfied with integrated HMOs such as Kaiser than with network-model HMOs. Compared with physicians in IPAs or those not affiliated with any network, physicians in prepaid group practices report greater adoption of tools for chronic illness care (Rittenhouse et al., 2004). However, many studies show mixed results, often with tradeoffs between benefits and drawbacks of care from more integrated systems. For example, patients in one large study rated comprehensive care highest in prepaid group practice model HMOs, somewhat lower among physicians in IPAs, and lowest among physicians in independent practices not participating in IPAs, whereas ratings of continuity of care were exactly the opposite, being highest among the independent practice physicians (Safran et al., 1994). This same study found that low-income patients had worse outcomes in HMO settings and non-low-income patients fared better in HMOs (Ware et al., 1996). A more recent national study found that patients did not experience care as being more functionally integrated when cared for in more structurally integrated practices than in smaller, more independent practices (Kerrissey et al., 2017).

The dispersed model appears to have one important strength from the patient perspective, which is the satisfaction that comes from receiving care from a small practice where patients have a sense that clinicians and staff know them personally. Patient satisfaction is higher when care is received in small offices rather than larger clinic structures (Rubin et al., 1993). People value having a familiar receptionist at the end of the line when they call about a child with a fever rather than experiencing the frustration of navigating impersonal clinic switchboard operators and voicemail systems—what has been described as the "chain store" persona of some large delivery systems (Mechanic, 1976). Patients whose regular source of care is a small primary care practice with one to two physicians are less likely than patients cared for by larger practices to have preventable hospital admissions, such as admissions for poorly controlled asthma and heart failure, suggesting that the personal touch of a small office may confer meaningful advantages in access and quality to avert deterioration of chronic conditions (Casalino et al., 2014).

Many of the studies described above precede the recent surge of consolidation occurring in health care and the emergence of hospital-dominated, vertically integrated systems. Accumulating research on these systems fails to show any consistent advantage for quality of care (Berenson, 2017; Post et al., 2018). As one analyst concluded, "consolidation is not coordination" (Greaney, 2018). Unlike the more cost-effective care provided by the prepaid group practice form of vertically integrated systems, the integrated systems

resulting from hospital and physician group mergers and acquisitions are increasing health care expenses due to oligopolistic pricing power (Baker et al., 2014; Greaney, 2018; Curto et al., 2022).

THE EXPLOSION OF VIRTUAL CARE

US health care is entering the new era of virtual care. For centuries, health care has been delivered by face-to-face visits between patients and providers of care. Care at a distance, with telephones, video visits, e-mail patient portals, was slowly gaining in popularity during the beginning of the twenty-first century. These modalities exploded with the COVID-19 pandemic of 2020. The new virtual care model has two overlapping components—telehealth and digital care. Telehealth brings together patients and providers at a distance, using scheduled phone and video encounters plus patient portals for electronic communication. Examples include a video physical therapy appointment, a scheduled phone appointment for diabetes care management, or the electronic forwarding of lab results to patients. Digital care reaches patients via software applications (apps) on computers or smart phones. Through apps, patients can access their health data, manage medication dosing, and receive lifestyle coaching. Digital apps can also integrate with other devices, for example, remote monitoring of blood sugar in patients with diabetes using glucose sensors on a patient's skin which electronically transmit results to the care provider. While telehealth is widely recognized as improving patients' access to good quality care, digital apps have rarely been evaluated (Gordon et al., 2020; Li et al., 2021).

CONCLUSION

The process of horizontal and vertical integration described here in fact consolidates the health care system into fewer and larger organizations, as elaborated in Chapter 17. Will the rapid organizational changes occurring in health care in the United States result in a higher-quality, more affordable health system? Will patients be cared for at the proper level of care—primary, secondary, and tertiary? Will a sufficient number of primary care clinicians—generalist physicians, physician assistants, and nurse practitioners—be available so that everyone in the United States can have a regular source of primary care that allows for continuity and coordination of care? What is an ideal health delivery system? Different people would have different answers. One vision is a system in which people choose their own primary care clinicians in modest-sized, decentralized, prepaid group practices that would be linked to community hospitals, including specialists' offices providing secondary care, with shared electronic medical records and other tools to promote functional care integration. Complex cases could be referred to the academic tertiary care center in the region. In the primary care practices, teams of health caregivers would endeavor to provide medical care to those people seeking attention and would also have the resources to address the health status of the entire population served by the practice.

REFERENCES

Aetna Foundation. Program Areas: Specifics, 2010.

Baker LC, Bundorf MK, Kessler DP. Vertical integration: hospital ownership of physician practices is associated with higher prices and spending. *Health Affairs*. 2014;33(5):756–763.

Berenson RA. A physician's perspective on vertical integration. *Health Affairs*. 2017;36:1585–1590.

Casalino LP, Pesko MF, Ryan AM, et al. Small primary care physician practices have low rates of preventable hospital admissions. *Health Aff (Millwood)*. 2014;33:1680–1688.

Committee on the Costs of Medical Care. Editorial. *JAMA*. 1932;99:1950.

Curto V, Sinaiko AD, Rosenthal MB. Price effects of vertical integration and joint contracting between physicians and hospitals in Massachusetts. *Health Aff (Millwood)*. 2022;41:741–750.

Dye NS. Mary Breckinridge, the Frontier Nursing Service and the introduction of nurse-midwifery in the United States. *Bull Hist Med*. 1983;57:485–507.

Fisher ES. Building a medical neighborhood for the medical home. *N Engl J Med*. 2008;359:1202–1205.

Furukawa MF, Kimmey L, Jones DJ, Machta RM, Guo J, Rich EC. Consolidation of providers into health systems increased substantially, 2016-18. *Health Aff (Millwood)*. 2020;39:1321–1325.

Garfield SR. The delivery of medical care. *Sci Am*. 1970;222:15–23.

Geiger HJ. The first community health center in Mississippi: communities empowering themselves. *Am J Pub Health*. 2016;106:1738–1740.

Geiger HJ. Community health centers: health care as an instrument of social change. In: Sidel VW, Sidel R, eds. *Reforming Medicine*. New York, NY: Pantheon Books; 1984.

Gold J. Accountable Care Organizations, explained. Kaiser Health News, September 14, 2015.

Gordon WJ, Landman A, Zhang H, Bates DW. Beyond validation: getting health apps into clinical practice. *Digit Med*. 2020;3:14.

Greaney TL. The new health care merger wave: does the "vertical, good" maxim apply? *J Law Med Ethics*. 2018;46:918–926.

Huang X, Rosenthal MB. Transforming specialty practice—the patient-centered medical neighborhood. *N Engl J Med*. 2014;370:1376–1379.

Kane CK. Recent Changes in Physician Practice Arrangements. American Medical Association, 2021.

Kepford AE. The Greater Community Association at Creston, Iowa. *Mod Hosp*. 1919;12:342.

Kerrissey MJ, Clark JR, Friedberg MW, et al. Medical group structural integration may not ensure that care is integrated, from the patient's perspective. *Health Aff (Millwood)*. 2017 May 1;36(5):885–892.

Kocher R, Sahni NR. Hospitals race to employ physicians—the logic behind a money-losing proposition. *N Engl J Med*. 2011;364:1790–1793.

Li C, Borycki EM, Kushniruk AW. Connecting the world of healthcare virtually: a scoping review on virtual care delivery. *Healthcare*. 2021;9:1325.

MCOL. The facts of managed care. January 10, 2020. https://mcolblog.com/kcblog/2020/1/10/the-facts-of-managed-care.html.

Mechanic D. *The Growth of Bureaucratic Medicine*. New York, NY: John Wiley & Sons; 1976.

Mehrotra A, Epstein AM, Rosenthal MB. Do integrated medical groups provide higher-quality medical care than individual practice associations? *Ann Intern Med*. 2006;145:826–833.

Muhlestein D, Bleser WK, Saunders RS, McClellan MB. All-payer spread of ACOs and value-based payment models in 2021. *Health Affairs Forefront*. June 17, 2021.

National Association of Community Health Centers. America's Health Centers, 2022 Shapshot. August 2022. https://www.nachc.org/research-and-data/americas-health-centers-2022-snapshot/.

Post B, Buchmueller T, Ryan AM. Vertical integration of hospitals and physicians: economic theory and empirical evidence on spending and quality. *Med Care Res Rev*. 2018;75:399–433.

Rittenhouse DR, Grumbach K, O'Neil EH, Dower C, Bindman A. Physician organization and care management in California: from cottage to Kaiser. *Health Aff (Millwood)*. 2004;23:51–62.

Rittenhouse DR, Shortell SM, Fisher ES. Primary care and accountable care—two essential elements of delivery-system reform. *N Engl J Med*. 2009;361:2301–2303.

Robinson JC, Casalino LP. Vertical integration and organizational networks in health care. *Health Aff (Millwood)*. 1996;15:7–22.

Rothman SM. *Woman's Proper Place: A History of Changing Ideals and Practices*. New York, NY: Basic Books; 1978.

Rubin HR, Gandek B, Rogers WH, Kosinski M, McHorney CA, Ware JE Jr. Patients' ratings of outpatient visits in different practice settings. *JAMA*. 1993;270:835–840.

Safran DG, Tarlov AR, Rogers WH. Primary care performance in fee-for-service and prepaid health care systems: results from the medical outcomes study. *JAMA*. 1994;271:1579–1586.

Solberg LI, Carlin CS, Peterson KA, Eder M. Diabetes care quality: do large medical groups perform better? *Am J Manag Care*. 2022 Mar;28:101–107.

Starr P. *The Social Transformation of American Medicine*. New York, NY: Basic Books; 1982.

Stevens R. *In Sickness and in Wealth: American Hospitals in the Twentieth Century*. New York, NY: Basic Books; 1989.

Stoeckle JD, Candib LM. The neighborhood health center: reform ideas of yesterday and today. *N Engl J Med*. 1969;280:1385–1391.

Ware JE Jr, Bayliss MS, Rogers WH, Kosinski M, Tarlov AR. Differences in 4-year health outcomes for elderly and poor, chronically ill patients treated in HMO and fee-for-service systems. *JAMA*. 1996;276:1039–1047.

Weeks WB, Gottlieb DJ, Nyweide DE, et al. Higher health care quality and bigger savings found at large multispecialty medical groups. *Health Aff (Millwood)*. 2010;29:991–997.

The Health Care Workforce and the Education of Health Professionals

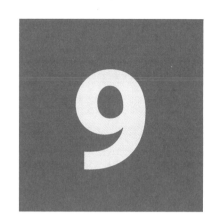

A health care system is only as good as the people working in it. The most valuable resource in health care is not the latest technology or state-of-the-art facility, but the health workers who are the heart of the system.

In this chapter, we discuss the nation's four largest health professions—nurses (including nurse practitioners), physicians, pharmacists and pharmacy technicians, and social workers—as well as physician assistants and medical assistants (Table 9–1). How many of these health care professionals are working in the United States, and where do they practice? Do we have the right number? Too many? Too few? Is the growing racial-ethnic diversity of the nation's population mirrored in the racial-ethnic composition of the health professions? To answer these questions, we begin by providing an overview of each of these professions. In the latter portion of the chapter, we discuss several cross-cutting issues pertinent to all these professions.

As shown in Tables 9–1 and 9–3, an intricate array of entities accredit educational programs and license and certify practitioners across these occupations.

NURSES

Marilyn has worked for 20 years as a registered nurse on hospital medical–surgical wards. She finds it gratifying to care for patients, but lately the work seems more difficult. The pressure to get patients in and out of the hospital as soon as possible has meant that more patients occupying hospital beds are severely ill and require a tremendous amount of nursing care—pressures that intensified during the COVID pandemic when wards were overflowing with critically ill patients and Marilyn had to work additional shifts when many staff were out on sick leave. Marilyn decides that it is time for a change. She takes a job as a visiting nurse with a home health care agency. She likes the pace of her new job and finds the greater clinical independence refreshing after her years of dealing with rigid hospital regimentation of nurses and physicians.

Registered nurses (RNs) represent the single largest health profession, with more than 3,000,000 RNs licensed in the United States. Hospitals employ 60% of nurses, 18% work in ambulatory care or other community-based settings, and 6% in long-term care (US Bureau of Labor Statistics [BLS], 2021). In addition to RNs, there are more than 650,000 Licensed Practical Nurses or Licensed Vocational Nurses in the United States (LPN/LVN; Table 9–2); these two terms are used by different states but are equivalent. Unlike RNs, LPN/LVNs most often work in long-term care facilities (35%), followed by hospitals (15%), home health care services (14%), and physician offices (12%).

Nursing as a profession became formalized in the United States around the time of the Civil War, when prominent people such as Clara Barton, Harriet Tubman, Walt Whitman, and Louisa May Alcott, among others, not only served as nurses to wounded soldiers but wrote and spoke about the importance of nursing as a profession. The first nursing school opened in the Women's Hospital of Philadelphia in 1872. Despite resistance from some physicians, by 1900, 400 schools of nursing had been established at US hospitals. Nurses such as Lillian Wald promoted

Table 9–1. Accreditation, licensure, and certification in the United States: Definition of terms

Accreditation: A determination that an educational institution or program has met minimum standards of quality, as defined by an external non-governmental entity which awards accreditation through a process emphasizing self- and peer-review. Graduation from an accredited educational program is a requirement for becoming a licensed practitioner in that profession.
Example: Accreditation Council for Pharmacy Education

Licensure: A process legally sanctioning an individual to practice and bill for services in a designated profession, typically managed by licensing boards administered by state governments.
Example: State Boards of Nursing or Medicine

Certification: A process administered by non-governmental entities to define standards of training and competence and award credentials for professional categories beyond basic professional licensure.
Example: Physician specialty certification by the American Board of Pediatrics, Family Nurse Practitioner certification by the American Academy of Nurse Practitioners Certification Board

Table 9–2. Number of active practitioners in selected health professions in the United States, 2021

	# Jobs (2021)
Registered nurses	3,130,600
Physicians	940,000
Medical assistants	743,500
Social workers	708,100
Licensed Practical/Vocational Nurse	657,200
Pharmacy techs	447,000
Dental assistants	358,000
Pharmacists	323,500
Nurse practitioners	246,700
Physical therapists	238,800
Dental hygienists	214,000
Psychologists	181,600
Dentists	146,200
Physician assistants	139,100

Source: Bureau of Labor Statistics, Department of Labor, Occupational Outlook Handbook, 2021. https://www.bls.gov/ooh/. Physician data from Association of American Medical Colleges (AAMC). Physician specialty data report. 2020. https://www.aamc.org/about-us/mission-areas/health-care/workforce-studies/data/number-people-active-physician-specialty-2019.

models of care that addressed social determinants of health and placed nursing in the community—what Wald called "Public Health Nursing" (Egenes, 2017).

Historically, most RNs received their education in vocational programs administered by hospitals awarding diplomas of nursing. Over time, nursing education shifted into academic institutions. Of RNs active in 2017, 7% were trained in diploma programs, 28% in associate degree programs, 45% in baccalaureate degree programs, and 17% in master's degree programs (National Council of State Boards of Nursing, 2017). Many nursing leaders have called for RN education to move completely to baccalaureate-level programs because of evidence of better patient outcomes (Yakusheva, 2014). LPN/LVN education usually consists of a 1-year technical program.

▶ **Nurse Practitioners**

Marilyn has been working as a home care nurse for 2 years. She has taken on growing responsibility as a case manager for many home care patients. She decides that she would like to become the primary clinician for these types of patients. She applies to a nurse practitioner training program. After completing her 2 years of nurse practitioner education, she finds a job as a primary care clinician at a geriatric clinic.

A growing number of registered nurses in the United States have obtained advanced practice degrees in addition to their basic nursing training. Advanced practice nurses include clinical nurse specialists, nurse anesthetists, clinical nurse midwives, and nurse practitioners. Nurse practitioners (NPs) represent the largest single group of advanced practice nurses, numbering 246,700. Sixty percent of NPs work in ambulatory offices and 23% work in hospitals (BLS, 2021). An estimated 70% of NPs deliver primary care, and more than 80% participate in Medicaid (American Association of Nurse Practitioners [AANP], 2022).

The first nurse practitioner program was launched in 1965, with early programs focused on increasing pediatric primary care clinicians in underserved areas (Pulcini & Wagner, 2002). Additional programs were established in the 1970s with federal funding as part of a national effort to boost the number of primary care clinicians. Enrollment in nurse practitioner programs

Table 9–3. Educational pathways, accreditation, licensure, and certification

Profession	Most Common Educational Pathways	Degree	Licensing Exams and Certifications
Registered nurses	2–3-year associate programs 4-year baccalaureate program	Registered Nurse (RN) (associates degree) Associate of Nursing (ASN) Bachelors of Nursing (BSN)	National Council of State Boards of Nursing NCLEX-RN exam for licensure Optional specialized certifications
Licensed practical or vocational nurses	1-year program in technical or community college	Licensed Practical Nurse (LPN) Licensed Vocational Nurse (LVN)	National Council of State Boards of Nursing NCLEX-PN exam for licensure Optional specialized certifications
Nurse practitioners	2-year master's level program, typically after a BSN degree	Master of Science in Nursing (MSN)	American Association of Nurse Practitioners (AANP) or American Nurses Credentialing Center (ANCC) exams for licensure Additional specialty certifying boards
Physicians	4-year medical school 3–6-year residency program, depending on specialty	Medical degree (MD) Doctor of osteopathy (DO)	US Medical Licensing Examination for licensure (MD) National Board of Osteopathoc Medical Examiners for licensure (DO) American Board of Medical Specialties and its 24 independent specialty boards for specialty certification after completing residency training
Physician assistants	2–3-year Master's level program	Physician Assistant (PA)	National Commission on Certification of Physician Assistants exam for licensure
Medical assistants	~1-year program Some programs offer 2-year program with associates degree	Not usually a degree program	No formal licensure or certifying exam required but several organizations offer certification: American Association of Medical Assistants American Medical Technologists National Center for Competency Training National Healthcareer Association
Social workers	4-year program for Bachelor's in Social Work 2-year program for Master's in Social Work plus 1–2 years supervised training for clinical social work	Bachelor of Social Work (BSW) Master of Social Work (MSW)	Association of Social Work Boards exam for licensure Additional certifications for advanced practice
Pharmacists	4-year training period Optional 2-year residency to focus on specialty	Doctor of Pharmacy (PharmD)	North American Pharmacist Licensure Exam for licensure Multistate Pharmacy Jurisprudence Exam or state-specific test is also required by most states for licensure
Pharmacy technicians	On the job training or a 1 year certificate program	Not usually a degree program	No licensure required Pharmacy Technician Certification Board exam

Source: Bureau of Labor Statistics, Department of Labor, Occupational Outlook Handbook, 2021. https://www.bls.gov/ooh/.

exploded in the twenty-first century, as the number of nurse practitioner training programs grew from 282 to 424 between 2000 and 2016 (Auerbach et al., 2018).

Licensing and related regulations for nurse practitioners are less uniform across states than those for physicians and registered nurses. State boards of nursing vary in the scope of practice they allow nurse practitioners. Twenty-six states allow nurse practitioners to practice with complete independence from physicians, while other states require physician supervision (AANP, 2018). As a result, nurse practitioners both substitute for physicians and complement physicians in health care teams, often playing a leading role in chronic care management and health promotion. Nurse practitioners working in primary care settings typically perform approximately 80% of the types of tasks performed by physicians. Research suggests that nurse practitioners can generally deliver care of equivalent quality to that delivered by primary care physicians for those tasks (Stanik-Hutt et al., 2013).

Nursing recently added a higher level of training, qualifying graduates for a Doctor of Nursing Practice (DNP) degree. DNP programs require a baccalaureate nursing degree for admission and consist of 3 to 4 years of advanced education compared with the 2 years for NP degrees.

▷ Medical Assistants

Rosalie worked through high school as a receptionist in a local doctor's office. She knew many of the families that came in for care and they knew they could come to her with questions. When she graduated from high school, Rosalie took the advice of a friend at the office and signed up for a program to become a medical assistant.

There were 743,000 medical assistants in 2021. Although medical assistants do not have nursing degrees, their tasks typically complement those performed by RNs and LVNs. Most medical assistants (58%) work in physician offices and 15% work in hospitals (BLS, 2021). The occupation of medical assistant dates to World War II, when a large number of nurses were called on to work in military hospitals and physicians trained other office staff to provide support for medical visits. While some medical assistants are trained on the job, an increasing number are trained through vocational programs of about 1 year in length. There is a national certification program, but to date, most medical assistants do not take part in it. Medical assistants are one of the most racially-ethnically diverse health care occupations (Chapman et al., 2010), and often conceptualize their roles as cultural liaisons (Taché & Hill-Sakurai, 2010). Medical assistants are playing expanded roles in health care teams, such as identifying and reaching out to patients overdue for preventive care or supporting patients with poorly controlled chronic conditions in making plans to become active or take medications regularly. There

is growing evidence that medical assistants in these expanded roles improve quality and increase patients' adherence to treatment (Willard-Grace et al., 2015; Thom et al., 2015a, 2015b).

PHYSICIANS

As a fourth-year medical student preparing to apply for residency training, Susan needed to make a decision about her choice of a specialty. She had particularly enjoyed her medical school experiences in pediatrics. She could complete a pediatrics residency in 3 years to become a general pediatrician, but that was one of the lowest paying specialties and Susan worried about being able to pay off the $175,000 in educational debt she had accumulated. Dermatology, emergency medicine, and ophthalmology residencies required only one more year of training relative to pediatrics, and those specialties paid considerably more than pediatrics and allowed for a more controllable lifestyle.

There are approximately 940,000 active physicians in the United States (AAMC, 2020). More than half of physicians work in ambulatory care offices and 25% work in hospitals. One-third of physicians work in primary care fields and two-thirds in nonprimary care fields (Bazemore et al., 2019).

At the time the University of Pennsylvania opened the first medical school in the colonies in 1765 few regulations governed entry into a medical career; physicians were as likely to have completed informal apprenticeships as to have graduated from medical school (Starr, 1982).

A key event in the creation of a twentieth-century medical profession was the publication of the Flexner Report in 1910. Flexner's report indicted conventional medical education as conducted by most proprietary, nonuniversity medical schools. Flexner held up as a standard the example of Johns Hopkins, which emphasized clinical and laboratory science. More than 30 medical schools closed in the decades following the Flexner Report, and academic standards at the surviving allopathic schools became much more stringent (Starr, 1982). The one alternative medical tradition in the United States that earned the imprimatur of physician licensing boards was osteopathy (Starr, 1982). State licensing boards grant physicians

Doctor of Osteopathy (DO) degrees equivalent scope of practice with MDs. In 2021, nearly 21,000 people graduated from allopathic medical schools and 7,400 from osteopathic medical schools (KFF, 2021).

At least 1 year of formal education after medical school is required for licensure in all states, and most physicians complete additional training to become certified in a particular specialty. Traditionally, the first year of postdoctoral training was referred to as an "internship," with subsequent years referred to as "residency." Now, almost all physicians in the United States complete a full residency training experience of at least 3 years.

PHYSICIAN ASSISTANTS

Arnold was a medic with the US Army for 10 years. As he prepared to leave the armed forces, several senior mentors suggested he look into Physician Assistant training.

An estimated 139,000 physician assistants (PAs) work in the United States (BLS, 2021). PAs work in diverse settings, including private physician offices, community clinics, and hospitals. Only 25% of PAs practice in primary care, with many working in emergency departments and surgical specialties (National Commission on Certification of Physician Assistants, 2020).

The PA profession originated in the United States in 1965 to fill the niche of a broadly skilled clinician who could be trained without the many years of medical school and residency education required to produce a physician, and who would work in close collaboration with physicians to augment the medical workforce. The first wave of PAs included many veterans who had acquired clinical skills working as medical corpsmen in the Vietnam War. PA training programs served as an efficient means to allow these veterans to "retool" their skills for civilian practice. Currently, the 300 accredited PA training programs in the United States award a master's degree program. Several PA programs have established postgraduate training programs, typically 1 year in duration and focused on subspecialty training (Hooker & Cawley, 2021).

PAs are usually licensed by the same state boards that license physicians, with the requirement that PAs work under the delegated authority of a physician. In practical terms, "delegated authority" means that PAs

are permitted to perform many of the tasks performed by physicians as long as the tasks are completed under physician supervision. As with nurse practitioners, scope of practice laws vary widely by state. Between 1998 and 2017, 38 states expanded the scope of practice of physician assistants. As with nurse practitioners, clinical outcomes and patient satisfaction for PAs are comparable to physicians for services within a PA scope of practice (Valentin et al., 2021).

PHARMACISTS & PHARMACY TECHNICIANS

Rex Hall has worked for 5 years as a pharmacist at a chain drug store. He is not sure that his skills as a pharmacist are being fully utilized in his current job. Too much of his time is taken up answering calls from physicians and patients who are ordering prescription refills, counting out pills, filling pill bottles, and determining which medications are covered by which health plan. He sees a job posting for a new pharmacist position at a local hospital. The job description states that the pharmacist will review drug use in the hospital and develop strategies to work with physicians, nurses, and other staff to minimize drug errors and inappropriate prescribing practices. Rex decides to apply for the job.

Of the 323,500 pharmacists in 2021, 43% work in pharmacies and drug stores, 27% in hospitals, and the remainder in grocery stores with pharmacies or clinics. There were also 447,000 pharmacy tech positions (BLS, 2021). Over the past decades, drug store chains have largely displaced the independently owned pharmacy. As they have consolidated, they have increasingly reduced the number of pharmacist positions and increased the number of pharmacy techs.

Pharmacy technicians have worked alongside pharmacists since the eighteenth century under a variety of names. Increases in prescription volume and payment through insurance and computerized systems have contributed to greater demand for pharmacy technicians (Wheeler et al., 2020).

Although historically most pharmacists were educated in baccalaureate degree programs, in 2004 all programs were required to extend the training period by 1 to 2 years and award Doctor of Pharmacy degrees. Pharmacy technicians may receive on the job training or be trained in vocational programs; an increasing number of states require pharmacy technicians to pass a national certification test and to graduate from accredited programs.

Pharmacists play a growing role in direct patient care to improve medication management, including reducing the risk of medication interactions, reducing fall risk due to medications in older adults and actively managing chronic conditions (Johnson, 2008). A systematic review found that adding pharmacists in direct care roles on clinical teams was associated with better quality of care, such as control of diabetes and hypertension (Chisholm-Burns et al., 2010). Pharmacists in some, but not all, states can provide influenza vaccines and smoking cessation medication. In 2019 alone, over 100 pieces of legislation across 34 states could impact pharmacist scope of practice (Pollack et al., 2020).

SOCIAL WORKERS

Almost half of the 708,000 social workers in 2021 were dedicated to health care, many in the fields of mental health and substance abuse. Tasks carried out by social workers include connecting patients to in-home services; helping patients to get health insurance, medical equipment, and other community services; investigating possible neglect or abuse; psychotherapy; and counseling on substance use disorders (BLS, 2021).

Social work arose at the dawn of the 20th Century as a response to concerns about government inaction to growing social needs resulting from urbanization and poverty. In addition to providing direct aid, mutual aid and charitable societies, the precursors of social work, attempted to address the environmental causes of poverty through public health reforms, prohibition of child labor, and establishment of pension programs and social insurance (Simmons University, 2023).

The minimum educational requirement to become a social worker is a bachelor's degree, but most social work positions in the health care field require a master's degree. Licensed clinical social workers (LCSWs) must have at least a master's degree plus 2 years of supervised practical experience in the field. LCSWs may be generalists or specialize in the management of geriatric patients, children, or persons with developmental disabilities, mental health, and substance use diagnoses. LCSWs have gained greater prominence in primary care as a result of the national movement toward behavioral health integrated into primary care

(Block, 2018). Behavioral health professionals, generally LCSWs or psychologists, colocated within primary care teams.

FINANCING HEALTH PROFESSIONS TRAINING AND THE BURDEN OF GROWING EDUCATIONAL DEBT

Unlike most other high-income nations, where health profession schools are government-supported and charge no or nominal tuition, students in the United States pay high and increasing tuition and fees, including for publicly operated state universities. As a result, newly entering health care professionals are shouldering a much heavier financial debt from their education than their predecessors. Median educational debt of medical students increased by 53%, controlling for inflation, over a 10-year period—1998–2008 (King & Scott, 2009) and by 2021 reached $200,000 (AAMC, 2021). The average debt for a pharmacy education almost doubled from $82,000 for pharmacists graduating in 2001–2010 to $143,000 in 2011–2019 (American Association of Colleges of Pharmacy [AACP], 2019). Average educational debt for RNs is considerably lower, at about $20,000. This high financial burden deters promising candidates from entering the health care professions, particularly individuals from lower-income and underrepresented racial-ethnic groups. Half of US medical students come from families in the highest 20% of household income; only 5% come from families in the lowest 20% of income (AAMC, 2018). High educational debt also disincentivizes providing lower-income primary care or accepting positions in underserved areas, thus worsening health inequities (Chisholm-Burns et al., 2019).

The Federal Government plays a minor role in directly financing health professions training with one major exception: funding of residency training for physicians, spending close to $20 million annually for residency training through educational payments to hospitals paid by Medicare, Medicaid, and the Veterans Administration. However, unlike the case in other nations in which taxpayer funding of medical education is tightly linked with public regulation of the physician workforce, public funding of residency education in the United States comes with few strings attached. Hospitals receiving training funds can decide which specialties, and how many slots in each specialty, they wish to sponsor for residency training. As a result, the shortage of primary care physicians in the United States is reinforced by a financing system providing public funding without public accountability, with hospitals preferentially choosing to invest their funds in the training of specialists (Iglehart, 2015).

DIVERSITY OF THE HEALTH WORKFORCE

▷ Women in the Health Professions

Dr. Jenny Wong works as a general internist for the Suburbia Medical Group. As one of only two women in a group of 11 primary care physicians, she is in demand, particularly among female patients. Dr. Wong senses that her patients expect her to spend more time with them to explain diagnoses and treatments and discuss their overall well-being. In seeking to meet those needs, Dr. Wong continually finds herself falling behind in her schedule. Today Dr. Wong is feeling especially stressed. She is scheduled to meet at lunchtime with the director of Suburbia Medical Group to discuss plans for her impending parental leave. She knows he will not take kindly to her intention of taking 4 months off after the birth of her child.

Historically, most physicians and pharmacists in the United States have been men, and most nurses women. For physicians and pharmacists, this demographic pattern is in the midst of a dramatic change, with a rapidly growing share of women (Fig. 9–1). The trends are even more dramatic when examining the makeup of current students: women constituted 56% of entering medical students in 2019 (AAMC, 2021) and 65% of pharmacy students in 2020 (AACP, 2023). In contrast, only 13% of registered nurses were men, up slightly from 5% in 1996 (BLS, 2022).

Female health care professionals on average are more likely to work on a part-time basis. Female physicians attract more female patients and tend to spend more time with their patients than do male physicians (Ganguli et al., 2020). Studies have shown that female physicians deliver more preventive services than male physicians, especially for their female patients, and their patients have fewer preventable hospitalizations (Dahrouge et al., 2016). Female physicians are more likely to discuss lifestyle and social concerns, to

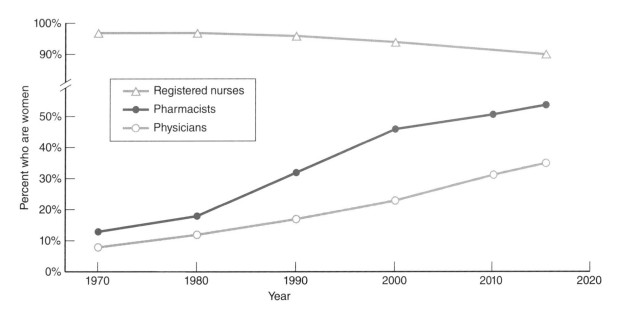

▲ Figure 9–1. Women as a percentage of physicians, nurses, and pharmacists in the United States. (Source: US Bureau of Health Workforce. Sex, Race and Ethnic Diversity of U.S. Health Occupations (2011–2015). August 2017. https://bhw.hrsa.gov/sites/default/files/bhw/nchwa/diversityushealthoccupations.pdf.)

provide more information and explanations, and to involve patients in medical decision-making than male physicians (Roter et al., 2002).

Gender inequity exists in health professional pay. Female physicians and nurses earn less than their male counterparts, even after adjusting for specialty, hours worked, and other factors (Muench et al., 2015; Lo Sasso et al., 2020).

▶ Racial-ethnic Groups Underrepresented in the Health Professions

Cynthia is the first person in her family to go to college and the first to become a health professional. A large contingent of her extended family celebrates her graduation from her family nurse practitioner training program. Although hospitals in the city where Cynthia trained had several open positions for nurse practitioners, she has decided to take a job at a migrant farm worker clinic in a rural community near where she grew up.

The United States is a nation of growing racial and ethnic diversity. People identifying as Black, Latino, or American Indian account for one-third of the population, yet individuals from these groups are profoundly underrepresented in most health professions. One indicator for assessing representation is the diversity index, which measures the percentage of practitioners in a given racial-ethnic group relative to their percentage of the overall US working age population. A diversity index less than 1.0 means that a group is underrepresented in that profession. Diversity indices for health professions requiring at least a college degree are less than 1.0 for Black, Latino, and American Indian groups for all these professions (Fig. 9–2).

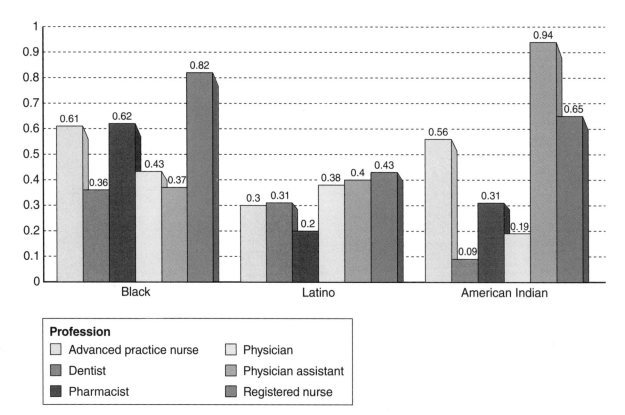

▲ **Figure 9–2.** Diversity index by professional and race-ethnicity, 2019. (Source: Salsberg E, Richwine C, Westergaard S, et al. Estimation and comparison of current and future racial/ethnic representation in the US health care workforce. *JAMA Netw Open.* 2021;4(3):e213789.)

The highest diversity indices are 0.94 for American Indian Physician Assistants and Black Registered Nurses, with diversity indices falling far below this level for most health professions and racial-ethnic groups (e.g., 0.19 for American Indian physicians, 0.20 for Latino pharmacists, and 0.37 for Black Physician Assistants). Diversity indices are greater than 1.0 for the White population for all these professions (Salsberg et al., 2021).

The lack of greater racial and ethnic diversity in the health professions has profound implications for health equity. As discussed in Chapter 5, marginalized racial-ethnic communities experience poorer health and access to health care compared with communities populated primarily by White residents. Black, Latino, American Indian, and Asian health care professionals are more likely than their White counterparts to practice in underserved communities and serve the uninsured and those covered by Medicaid (Walker et al., 2012). Research has found salutary effects of racial-ethnically concordant relationships between Black and Latino patients and health care professionals on the use of preventive services, patient satisfaction, and ratings of the physician's participatory decision-making style. Studies of patients with limited English proficiency have found that access to language concordant clinicians is associated with better patient experiences and outcomes such as reductions in patient reports of medication errors (US Department of Health and Human Services [US DHHS], 2006).

Efforts to increase the diversity of health professions training programs have had mixed success. Underrepresented racial-ethnic groups as a proportion of students in baccalaureate nursing programs increased from 12% in 1991 to 19% in 2020 (American Association of Colleges of Nursing, 2020) and similar gains have occurred for advanced practice nursing programs (Salsberg et al., 2021). Pharmacy schools have had a modest increase in enrollment from underrepresented racial-ethnic groups, from 11% of students in 1990 to 15% in 2017 (AACP, 2017). Gains in medical school diversity have not been sustained over recent decades, with periods of increases offset by years of decline in enrollment of underrepresented groups, coinciding with waves of anti-affirmative action laws and court decisions that curtailed the ability of university admissions committees to give consideration to applicants' race-ethnicity (Grumbach & Mendoza, 2008).

Internationally Educated Professionals in the US Health Workforce

The United States has long relied on health professionals educated in countries outside the United States, particularly for the physician workforce. About one-quarter of licensed physicians in the United States graduated from an international medical school, compared with 7% of RNs.

Internationally educated nurses are eligible to apply for state licensure as an RN if they graduated from an internationally accredited RN school, hold an active license in their country, and pass the US RN licensing exam and an English proficiency test. If they are not a US citizen, they must then apply for a visa to be authorized to work in the United States, which may take many years to obtain. The United States at one time had special visa programs for RNs tied to employment at hospitals in underserved communities, but Congress allowed that program to expire in 2009.

For physicians, graduates of international medical schools must complete at least 1 year of residency training in the United States to be eligible to practice in the United States. They must first certify their medical school education and pass the US national medical licensing examination to be eligible for a residency position. About half of international medical graduates are US citizens who trained abroad, usually due to the limited capacity of US medical schools. International medical graduates who are not US citizens must obtain a temporary educational visa for the duration of their residency, and then apply for a work visa if they wish to remain in the United States to practice medicine. Unlike nursing, the United States has maintained a special employment visa program for physicians linked to a period of service in a US community with a physician shortage. International medical graduates are more likely than US medical school graduates to work in primary care and accept patients with public insurance (Katakam, 2019).

Controversy exists about the reliance on international graduates to meet US health workforce needs. Critics argue that the United States fosters a "brain drain," depleting low- and middle-income nations of vital human resources (Karan et al., 2016), with others responding that emigration to seek better life opportunities is a human right. The World Health Organization and the US Alliance for Ethical International Recruitment Practices have developed standards to make health workforce migration practices more ethical; greater alignment of these principles into US policy would help to improve ethical practices (Chen, 2013).

"RIGHT-SIZING" THE HEALTH CARE WORKFORCE: SUPPLY, DEMAND, AND NEED

The supply of most types of health workers has been growing faster than overall population growth over past decades (Figs. 9–3 to 9–5). Between 1975 and 2020, the number of active registered nurses per capita in the United States nearly doubled, the number of physicians per capita grew by approximately 75%, and the number of pharmacists per capita increased by approximately 50%. Increases in the supply of PAs and NPs have been even more dramatic (Auerbach et al., 2018). For physicians, virtually all the growth in supply

is accounted for by increasing numbers of nonprimary care specialists. Interestingly, although supply steadily increased during these years, health workforce analysts have alternated between sounding alarms about shortages and surpluses of physicians and nurses. For example, in the 1980s and 1990s, several commissions warned of a surplus of physicians in the United States (Pew Health Professions Commission, 1995; Council on Graduate Medical Education [CGME], 1996). By the early years of the twenty-first century, some policy analysts were declaring a physician shortage (CGME, 2005). Similarly, concerns about an oversupply of nurses in the mid-1990s were soon supplanted by declarations of a nursing shortage (Buerhaus et al., 2000), with many analysts concluding the shortage had ended by 2010 (Staiger et al., 2012).

Why did perceptions turned from surplus to shortage when supply was continuing to steadily increase over these decades? The supply of health care professionals is only one part of the equation for determining

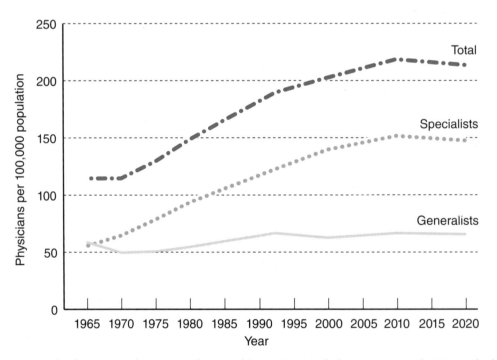

▲ **Figure 9–3.** Supply of practicing physicians in the United States. Note: Includes patient care physicians who have completed training and excludes physicians employed by the federal government. (Source: Council on Graduate Medical Education [COGME]. Patient Care Physician Supply and Requirements: Testing COGME Recommendations. US Department of Health and Human Services; 1996 [HRSA-P-DM 95–3].)

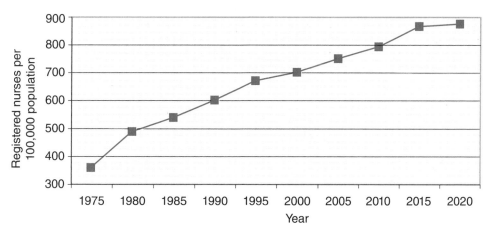

▲ **Figure 9–4.** Supply of active registered nurses per 100,000 population in the United States. (Source: Auerbach DI, Buerhaus PI, Staiger DO. Will the RN workforce weather the retirement of the baby boomers? *Med Care.* 2015; 53:850−856.)

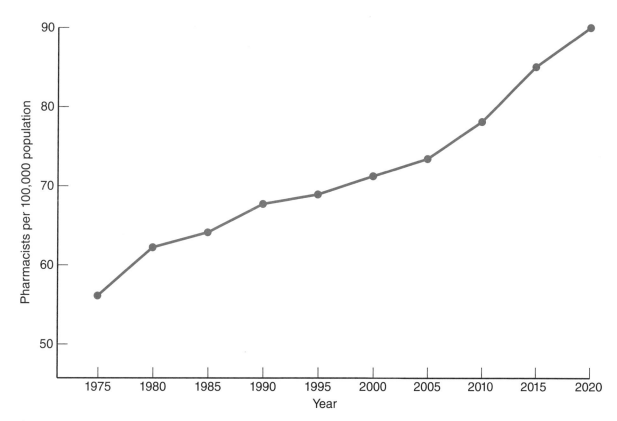

▲ **Figure 9–5.** Supply of active pharmacists per 100,000 population in the United States. (Source: Health Services and Resources Administration. The Adequacy of Pharmacist Supply: 2004 to 2030. December 2008.)

the adequacy of the workforce. The other part of the equation is a judgment about how many health workers are actually required. Even when the supply of health care professionals per capita is growing, there may be a workforce shortage if the requirements for these workers are judged to be increasing more rapidly than supply. For example, as people age they have more health care needs; a society like the United States with a growing proportion of older adults may require more health professionals per capita.

There are two general schools of thought about how to define health workforce requirements (Grumbach, 2002). One view considers market demand as the arbiter of workforce requirements. According to this view, if there is unmet market demand for, let us say, nurses, as indicated by many vacant nursing positions at hospitals, then a shortage exists. Or, to the contrary, if many nurses are unemployed or underemployed, a surplus exists. An alternative approach defines workforce requirements on the basis of population need rather than market demand. For example, a need-based approach for nursing would attempt to evaluate whether a certain level of nursing supply optimizes patient outcomes, such as by determining whether higher registered nurse staffing levels for a given volume and acuity of hospital inpatients result in fewer medication errors and hospital-acquired infections and better overall patient outcomes.

In the case of registered nursing, both demand and need perspectives converged to conclude that a shortage existed in the late 1990s (Bureau of Health Professions, 2002). As the intensity of hospital care increased and hospitals sought more highly trained registered nurses to staff their facilities, vacancy rates increased for hospital nurses. In response, hospitals began to increase wages to attract nurses into the workforce. Researchers around this time also began to produce evidence that lower levels of registered nurse staffing in hospitals were associated with worse clinical outcomes for hospitalized patients (Needleman et al., 2011), suggesting a true medical need for more registered nurses in hospitals. One state, California, proceeded to codify a need-based approach to nurse supply by enacting legislation requiring a minimum nurse staffing level per occupied hospital bed (Spetz, 2004).

The case of the physician workforce has been less straightforward. While most nurses work as employees

of hospitals or other employers, until recently most physicians were self-employed or part-owners of a medical group that acted as their employer, making vacancy rates or other typical labor market metrics less reliable indicators of the demand for physicians. Moreover, physicians' authority and influence over medical care give them considerable market power and create opportunities for supplier-induced demand (see Chapter 12), particularly when costs are covered by health insurance. In a health care environment like that in the United States, in which demand for physician labor may be almost limitless, physicians tend to keep busy even as supply continues to rise.

Although some groups have argued that the supply of physicians in the United States is not keeping up with rising demand driven by advances in medical care and an aging population (AAMC, 2019), research has raised questions about whether the health of the public benefits from more physicians. For example, mortality rates for high-risk newborns are worse in regions with a very low supply of neonatologists than in regions with a somewhat greater supply, but above that level, further increases in the supply of neonatologists are not associated with better clinical outcomes for newborns (Goodman et al., 2002). At the other age extreme, Medicare beneficiaries residing in areas with high physician supply do not report better access to physicians or higher satisfaction with care and do not receive better quality of care (Goodman & Grumbach, 2008). A recent study suggests that an increase in physician supply in a county may result in increased life expectancy for residents of the county, but that the effect is much greater from increasing primary care physician supply than from increasing the supply of specialists (Basu et al., 2019). The authors of this study expressed concern that the average supply of primary care physicians per capita in counties decreased during the decade studied, while the supply of specialists increased. In assessing the adequacy of health care professional supply, it is important not just to count the number of workers, but to examine how these workers are deployed.

The case of pharmacists provides a cautionary tale about boosting the number of graduates from a field without careful monitoring. In 2001, the Pharmacy Manpower Project predicted a shortfall of 157,000 pharmacists by 2020 (Covvey et al., 2015). In response, schools of pharmacy doubled the output of pharmacy students in a 20-year period. By 2020, the forecast had dramatically shifted, with an oversupply of 19,000 to 51,000 pharmacists predicted by 2030 (Brown, 2020). Why did the outlook change so drastically during this period? First, the rapid increase in supply of new pharmacists outpaced predictions. Moreover, although the original predictions were based on correct information about an aging population in need of greater pharmacy support, they failed to predict consolidation of community pharmacies by national retail drugstores and the dramatic reductions in pharmacists employed by those chains. In addition, training programs may be more forward-thinking than the current market. Schools of pharmacy are preparing graduates to work as experts in medication therapy and part of an interprofessional team, while many existing jobs still reflect an older model of "providing a commodity (medications) in reaction to the order of a prescriber" (Johnson, 2008).

Geographic Maldistribution of the Health Workforce

In addition to overall supply, it is important to consider whether there is misalignment of where health care personnel are located and where they are most needed. The Federal Government designates Healthcare Professional Shortage Areas (HPSAs) with a shortage of primary care, dental, or mental health care providers and services. In 2022, 97 million people in the United States were located in a primary care HPSA, 69 million in a dental HPSA, and 156 million in a mental health HPSA (Bureau of Health Workforce, 2022); rural communities are disproportionately represented among HPSAs.

As noted above, educational debt is a barrier to equitable distribution of health professionals. Physicians are more likely to practice in shortage areas if they have little or no debt than if they have significant debt (Goodfellow et al., 2016). Although government in the United States has done much less than governments in other high-income nations to lower educational costs for trainees, federal and state governments have attempted to mitigate the adverse impact of educational debt on public service by offering scholarship and loan repayment programs through the federal National Health Service Corps and similar state programs, tied to service in shortage areas after completing training. Most health professionals participating in these programs

continue to work in underserved communities after satisfying their service obligation (Negrusa et al., 2014). Training setting also impacts where health professionals ultimately practice. Graduates of medical and dental schools and residency programs with a rural focus, and family physicians trained in community health centers, are more likely to practice in HPSAs after their training (Goodfellow et al., 2016).

Reducing regulatory barriers to health personnel practicing across state lines may also alleviate geographic maldistribution. Traditionally, licensure of health care professionals has been the domain of states, and health professionals moving from one state to another faced significant time and expenses to apply for a license in a new state. The increasing amount of care provided through telehealth also argues for flexibility. During the COVID-19 pandemic, many states, needing assistance from medical personnel from other states, passed emergency licensing legislation allowing clinicians and nurses from other states to practice in their state. This natural experiment offered an opportunity to see the benefits of reducing barriers for interstate work, such as agreements across states to recognize licensing from another state (Frogner, 2022).

THE EPIDEMIC OF HEALTH WORKER BURNOUT

Levels of burnout among health professionals have long been much higher than those of workers in other occupations in the United States (Shanafelt et al., 2022). Driven by increasing expectations and decreasing control over work conditions, financial pressures, and escalating documentation requirements, burnout has been associated with both worker turnover (Hamidi et al., 2018) and reduction in work hours (Shanafelt et al., 2016).

The COVID-19 pandemic amplified these trends and brought new pressures to bear on the health workforce that may have long-term sequelae. Furloughs brought on by reductions in patient visits early in the pandemic, redeployment to different work and increased work hours, concerns for personal safety, exposure to death and grief, and mistreatment by people who objected to masking or vaccination were a few of the forces impacting health care workers (ASPH, 2022). The proportion of nurses reporting high emotional exhaustion increased from 41% in 2019 to 49%

in 2021. For physicians, the proportion reporting burnout increased from 32% in 2019 to 38% in 2021 (Sexton et al., 2022). Burnout and pandemic-related moral injury jeopardize the sustainability of the workforce. Almost a quarter of front-line nurses in 2021 reported plans to leave their position in the coming year, 60% of those because of the pandemic (US DHHS, 2022). In early 2022, one survey found that one-quarter of primary care physicians expected to leave primary care within the next 3 years (Larry Green Center, 2022).

Strategies to address burnout generally fall into two categories: those aimed at the individual and those seeking to change the organization. Strategies focused on the individual, such as classes to increase mindfulness or manage stress, have shown some benefit, but generally less than strategies aimed at changing organizational factors. Successful organizational strategies often include components such as reducing the documentation or messaging burden associated with electronic health records, reducing the number of patients that each clinician cares for, or providing additional team-based supports for patient care (Panagioti et al., 2017).

TEAMMATES OR COMPETITORS?

Health care is a team sport. A successful outcome for a patient undergoing a surgical operation requires team members with complementary skills—anesthesiologist or nurse anesthetist, surgeons, scrub nurses, surgical techs, and others—and teamwork among these personnel. The same is true in other settings, whether it be a small primary care office practice with a team of a physician, NP, medical assistants, and receptionist; a large behavioral health clinic with social workers, psychiatrists, substance use counselors, and community health workers; or a hospital medical ward with RNs, hospitalist and specialist physicians, clinical pharmacists, respiratory and physical therapists, and many other personnel. The growing complexity of health care requires that health professionals collaborate "in systems of inescapable interdependence" (Berwick & Finkelstein, 2010). Better teamwork, as measured by elements such as communication and cohesion, is associated with better quality of care (Rosen et al., 2018) and reduced health worker burnout (Willard-Grace et al., 2014).

Teams are also essential for enhancing access to care, particularly in settings with workforce shortages. New models of primary care recognize that many preventive and chronic care tasks traditionally performed by physicians may be delegated to medical assistants, nurses, and pharmacists, allowing more productive use of the work effort of the limited supply of primary care clinicians (Bodenheimer, 2022). Expanding the roles of staff may also provide a mechanism to enhance access to care and health equity. The Alaskan Dental Health Aide program engaged dentists to help train local Dental Assistants to progressively assume expanded care roles, beginning with applying fluoride varnish and sealants and progressing to performing cleaning and restorations. The program was motivated by a realization that traditional models of care delivery relying on dentists in very short supply were resulting in nearly 4 in 5 children having tooth decay in the Alaskan Native population. Early evaluation suggests that the model is effective at improving access to quality dental care and improving preventive services (Shoffstall-Cone & Williard, 2013).

The aspiration of collaborative teamwork confronts a lonstanding medical culture of rigid hierarchy that has positioned physicians as commanders issuing "orders" for nursing care, dispensing of medications, and related tasks to be completed by other personnel. And while health care is a team sport, it is also a business, with professional and labor associations often striving to protect their occupational "turf" against encroachment from competing occupations. Efforts by some professional groups to expand their licensed scope of practice are frequently met with resistance from groups that consider expansion a professional and economic threat. Ophthalmologist associations resist expanded scope of practice for optometrists, physician groups push back against increased scope for NPs and PAs, and RN organizations sometimes oppose medical assistants taking on duties viewed as belonging to the skill mix of nurses. The culture of hierarchy and guild protectionism is slowly changing as growing numbers of health workers recognize the imperative for teamwork and the need to value the contributions of all members of the health care team.

CONCLUSION

Health care in the United States relies on an array of health professionals skilled in different aspects of patient care. Although making definitive determinations about the "right" number of health care professionals often proves elusive, health systems should deploy their workers in a manner that makes the best use of their training and skills under regulatory rules and practice structures that allow health care professionals to operate at their fullest capability while ensuring high standards of quality and patient safety. The composition and deployment of the health workforce powerfully influences health care access, quality, costs, and equity. While many Americans benefit from timely access to superb teams of health workers, persistent geographic maldistribution results in workforce shortages in many rural and under-resourced urban communities, and the failure to achieve greater racial-ethnicity diversity among health professionals contributes to racial-ethnic health inequities. Health workers are a precious human resource. Growing burnout among health care workers is making it clear that the people who provide care also need to be cared for.

REFERENCES

American Association of Colleges of Nursing. 2020. Data tables. https://www.aacnnursing.org/Portals/42/News/Surveys-Data/EthnicityTbl.pdf.

American Association of Colleges of Pharmacy (AACP). Profile of pharmacy students. Fall 2017. https://www.aacp.org/node/1657.

American Association of Colleges of Pharmacy (AACP). National Pharmacist Workforce Study. 2019. https://www.aacp.org/article/national-pharmacist-workforce-studies.

American Association of Colleges of Pharmacy (AACP). Academic Pharmacy's Vital Statistics. 2023. https://www.aacp.org/article/academic-pharmacys-vital-statistics#.

American Association of Nurse Practitioners (AANP). State practice environment. 2018. https://www.aanp.org/advocacy/state. https://nursejournal.org/nurse-practitioner/np-practice-authority-by-state/.

American Association of Nurse Practitioners (AANP). NP Fact Sheet. 2022. https://www.aanp.org/about/all-about-nps/np-fact-sheet.

Association of American Medical Colleges (AAMC). Facts: applicants, matriculants, enrollment, graduates, MD-PhD, and residency applicants' data. Report. 2018. www.aamc.org/data/facts.

Association of American Medical Colleges (AAMC). The complexities of physician supply and demand: projections from 2017 to 2032. 2019. Association of American Medical Colleges › workforce-studies › reports.

Association of American Medical Colleges (AAMC). Physician specialty data report. 2020. https://www.aamc.org/about-us/mission-areas/health-care/workforce-studies/data/number-people-active-physician-specialty-2019.

Association of American Medical Colleges (AAMC). Facts: applicants, matriculants, enrollment, graduates, MD-PhD, and residency applicants data. Report. 2021. www.aamc.org/data/facts.

Auerbach DI, Staiger DO, Buerhaus PI. Growing ranks of advanced practice clinicians—implications for the physician workforce. *N Engl J Med*. 2018;378:2358–2360.

Basu S, Berkowitz SA, Phillips RL, Bitton A, Landon BE, Phillips RS. Association of primary care physician supply with population mortality in the United States, 2005–2015. *JAMA Intern Med*. 2019;179(4):506–514.

Bazemore A, Wilkinson E, Petterson S, Green LA. Proportional erosion of the primary care physician workforce has continued since 2010. *Am Fam Physician*. 2019;100(4):211–212.

Berwick DM, Finkelstein JA. Preparing medical students for the continual improvement of health and health care: Abraham Flexner and the new "public interest". *Acad Med*. 2010;85:S56–S65.

Block R. Behavioral health integration and workforce development. Milbank Memorial Fund issue brief. May 2018.

Bodenheimer T. Revitalizing primary care, Part 2: hopes for the future. *Ann Fam Med*. 2022;20:469–478.

Brown DL. Years of rampant expansion have imposed Darwinian survival-of-the-fittest conditions on US pharmacy schools. *Am J Pharm Educ*. 2020;84(10):ajpe8136.

Buerhaus PI, Staiger DO, Auerbach DI. Implications of an aging registered nurse workforce. *JAMA*. 2000;283:2948–2954.

Bureau of Health Professions. *Projected Supply, Demand, and Shortages of Registered Nurses, 2000–2020*. Rockville, MD: Health Resources and Services Administration; 2002.

Bureau of Health Workforce. US Department of Health and Human Services. Designated health professional shortage area statistics. Report. 30 September 2022.

Chapman S, Marks A, Chan M. The increasing role of medical assistants in small primary care physician practice: issues and policy implications. Center for the Health Professions Research Brief. February 2010.

Chen C. The redistribution of Graduate Medical Education positions in 2005 failed to boost primary care or rural training. *Health Aff (Millwood)*. 2013;32:102–110.

Chisholm-Burns MA, Kim Lee J, Spivey CA, et al. US pharmacists' effect as team members on patient care: systematic review and meta-analyses. *Med Care*. 2010;48:923–933.

Chisholm-Burns MA, Spivey CA, Stallworth S, Zivin JG. Analysis of educational debt and income among pharmacists and other health professionals. *Am J Pharm Educ*. 2019;83(9):7460.

Council on Graduate Medical Education (COGME). *Eighth Report: Patient Care Physician Supply and Requirements: Testing COGME Recommendations*. Rockville, MD: Council on Graduate Medical Education; 1996.

Council on Graduate Medical Education (COGME). *Sixteenth Report: Physician Workforce Policy Guidelines for the United States, 2000–2020*. Rockville, MD: Council on Graduate Medical Education; 2005.

Covvey JR, Cohron PP, Mullen AB. Examining pharmacy workforce issues in the United States and the United Kingdom. Statement. *Am J Pharm Educ*. 2015;79:17.

Dahrouge S, Seale E, Hogg W, et al. A comprehensive assessment of family physician gender and quality of care. *Med Care*. 2016;54:277–286.

Egenes KJ. History of nursing. Chapter in: Issues and trends in nursing: essential knowledge for today and tomorrow. 2017 January 10:1–26. United States: Jones & Bartlett Learning. E-book.

Frogner BK. Patients receive flexible and accessible care when state workforce barriers are removed. *Health Aff (Milwood)*. 2022.41:1139–1141.

Ganguli I, Sheridan B, Gray J, Chernew M, Rosenthal MB, Neprash H. Physician work hours and the gender pay gap—evidence from primary care. *N Engl J Med*. 2020;383:1349–1357.

Goodfellow A, Ulloa JG, Dowling PT, et al. Predictors of primary care physician practice location in underserved urban and rural areas in the United States. *Acad Med*. 2016;91:1313–1321.

Goodman D, Fisher ES, Little GA, Stukel TA, Chang CH, Schoendorf KS. The relation between the availability of neonatal intensive care and neonatal mortality. *N Engl J Med*. 2002;346:1538–1544.

Goodman D, Grumbach K. Does having more physicians lead to better health system performance? *JAMA*. 2008;299:335–337.

Grumbach K, Mendoza R. Disparities in human resources: addressing the lack of diversity in the health professions. *Health Aff (Millwood)*. 2008;27(2):413–422.

Grumbach K. Fighting hand to hand over physician workforce policy. *Health Aff (Millwood)*. 2002;21:13–17.

Hamidi MS, Bohman B, Sandborg C, et al. Estimating institutional physician turnover attributable to self-reported burnout and associated financial burden: a case study. *BMC Health Serv Res*. 2018;18(1):851.

Hooker RS, Cawley JF. Physician assistants/associates at 6 decades. *Am J Manag Care*. 2021;27:498–504.

Iglehart JK. Institute of Medicine report on GME—a call for reform. *N Eng J Med*. 2015;372:376–381.

Johnson TJ. Pharmacist workforce in 2020: implications of requiring residency training for practice. *Am J Health Sys Pharm*. 2008;65:166–170.

Kaiser Family Foundation (KFF). Total number of medical school graduates. Data table. 2021.

Karan A, DeUgarte D, Barry M. Medical "brain drain" and health care worker shortages. *AMA J Ethics*. 2016;18: 665–675.

Katakam SK, Frintner MP, Pelaez-Velez C, Chakraborty R. Work experiences and satisfaction of international medical school graduates. *Pediatrics*. 2019;143(1):e20181953.

King KM, Scott GA. Graduate medical education: trends in training and student debt. GAO-09-438R. 2009.

Larry A. Green Center. Quick COVID-19 primary care survey: Series 35 fielded February 25–March 1, 2022. https://www.green-center.org/covid-survey.

Lo Sasso AT, Armstrong D, Forte G, Gerber SE. Differences in starting pay for male and female physicians persist. *Health Affairs*. 2020;39:256–263.

Muench U, Sindelar J, Busch SH, Buerhaus PI. Salary differences between male and female registered nurses in the United States. *JAMA*. 2015;313:1265–1267.

National Commission on Certification of Physician Assistants. 2019 Statistical Profile of Recently Certified Physician Assistants. Annual Report. 2020.

National Council of State Boards of Nursing. National Nursing Workforce Study, 2017. https://www.ncsbn.org/workforce.htm.

Needleman J, Buerhaus P, Pankratz VS, Leibson CL, Stevens SR, Harris M. Nurse-staffing levels and inpatient hospital mortality. *N Engl J Med*. 2011;364:1037–1045.

Negrusa S, Ghosh P, Warner JT. Provider retention in high need areas. Final Report. 2014. https://aspe.hhs.gov/reports/provider-retention-high-need-areas-0.

Panagioti M, Panagopoulou E, Bower P, et al. Controlled interventions to reduce burnout in physicians. *JAMA Intern Med*. 2017;177:195–205.

Pew Health Professions Commission. *Critical Challenges. Revitalizing the Health Professions for the Twenty-First Century*. San Francisco, CA: UCSF Center for the Health Professions; 1995.

Pollack SW, Skillman SM, Frogner BK. Assessing the size and scope of the pharmacist workforce in the U.S. Report. Center for Health Workforce Studies. September 2020.

Pulcini J, Wagner M. Nurse practitioner education in the United States. *Clin Excel Nurse Pract*. 2002;6:1-8.

Rosen MA, DiazGranados D, Dietz AS, et al. Teamwork in healthcare: key discoveries enabling safer, high-quality care. *Am Psychol*. 2018;73:433–450.

Roter D, Hall JA, Aoki Y. Physician gender effects in medical communication: a meta-analytic review. *JAMA*. 2002;288:756–764.

Salsberg E, Richwine C, Westergaard S, et al. Estimation and comparison of current and future racial/ethnic representation in the US health care workforce. *JAMA Netw Open*. 2021;4(3):e213789.

Sexton JB, Adair KC, Proulx J, et al. Emotional exhaustion among US health care workers before and during the COVID-19 pandemic, 2019–2021. *JAMA Netw Open*. 2022;5(9):e2232748.

Shanafelt TD, Mungo M, Schmitgen J, et al. Longitudinal study evaluating the association between physician burnout and changes in professional work effort. *Mayo Clin Proc*. 2016; 91:422–431.

Shanafelt TD, West CP, Sinsky C, et al. Changes in burnout and satisfaction with work-life integration in physicians and the general US working population between 2011 and 2020. *Mayo Clin Proc*. 2022;97:491–506.

Shoffstall-Cone S, Williard M. Alaska dental health aide program. *Int J Circumpolar Health*. 2013;72(1):21198.

Simmons University. Evolution of Social Work: Historical Milestones. Updated 2023. https://online.simmons.edu/blog/evolution-social-work-historical-milestones/.

Spetz J. California's minimum nurse-to-patient ratios: the first few months. *J Nurs Adm*. 2004;34:571–578.

Staiger DO, Auerbach DI, Buerhaus PI. Registered nurse labor supply and the recession—are we in a bubble? *N Engl J Med*. 2012;366:1463–1465.

Stanik-Hutt J, Newhouse RP, White KM, et al. The quality and effectiveness of care provided by nurse practitioners. *J Nurse Pract*. 2013;9:492–500.

Starr P. *The Social Transformation of American Medicine*. New York, NY: Basic Books; 1982.

Taché S, Hill-Sakurai L. Medical assistants: the invisible "glue" of primary health care practices in the United States? *J Health Organ Manag*. 2010;24:288–305.

Thom DH, Hessler D, Willard-Grace R, et al. Health coaching by medical assistants improves patients' chronic care experience. *Am J Manag Care*. 2015a;21:685–691.

Thom DH, Willard-Grace R, Hessler D, et al. The impact of health coaching on medication adherence in patients with poorly controlled diabetes, hypertension, and/or hyperlipidemia. *J Am Board Fam Med*. 2015b;28:38–45.

US Bureau of Labor Statistics (BLS). Occupational outlook handbook. 2021. https://www.bls.gov/ooh/.

US Bureau of Labor Statistics (BLS). Labor force statistics from the current population survey. Data table. 2022. https://www.bls.gov/cps/cpsaat11.htm.

US Department of Health and Human Services. The rationale for diversity in the health professions: a review of the evidence. Health resources and services administration; 2006. http://bhpr.hrsa.gov/healthworkforce/reports/diversityreviewevidence.pdf.

US Department of Health and Human Services. Impact of the COVID-19 Pandemic on the Hospital and Outpatient Clinician Workforce. Issue Brief HP-2022-13. 3 May 2022. https://aspe.hhs.gov/reports/covid-19-health-care-workforce.

Valentin VL, Najmabadi S, Everett C. Cross-sectional analysis of US scope of practice laws and employed physician assistants. *BMJ Open*. 2021;11(5):e043972.

Walker KO, Moreno G, Grumbach K. The association among specialty, race, ethnicity, and practice location among California physicians in diverse specialties. *J Natl Med Assoc*. 2012;104(1–2):46–52.

Wheeler JS, Gray JA, Gentry CK, Farr GE. Advancing pharmacy technician training and practice models in the United States: historical perspectives, workforce development needs, and future opportunities. *Res Soc Admin Pharm*. 2020;16:587–590.

Willard-Grace R, Chen EH, Hessler D, et al. Health coaching by medical assistants to improve control of diabetes, hypertension, and hyperlipidemia in low-income patients: a randomized controlled trial. *Ann Fam Med*. 2015;13:130–138.

Willard-Grace R, Hessler D, Rogers E, Dubé K, Bodenheimer T, Grumbach K. Team structure and culture are associated with lower burnout in primary care. *J Am Board Fam Med*. 2014;27:229–238.

Yakusheva OR. Nurse value-added and patient outcomes in acute care. *Health Serv Res*. 2014;49:1767–1786.

Long-Term Care

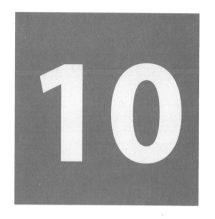

Eddie Taylor awoke one morning at his home in California unable to speak or to move the right side of his body, but able to understand other people around him. After 3 terrifying days in a hospital and 3 frustrating weeks in a stroke rehabilitation center, Eddie failed to improve. Because he no longer required hospital-level care, he became ineligible for Medicare hospital coverage. Since his spouse, James, was wheelchair-bound with crippling rheumatoid arthritis and unable to care for him, Eddie was transferred to a nursing home. Medicare did not cover the $297 per day cost. After 2 years, Medicaid began to pick up the nursing home bills. Much of the couple's life savings—earned during the 50 years Eddie worked in a men's clothing store—had been spent down to allow Medicaid eligibility. Because Medicaid paid only $182 per day, few recreational activities were offered, and Eddie spent each day lying in bed next to a demented patient, who screamed for hours at a time. Unable to voice his complaints at the inhuman conditions of his life, he became severely depressed, stopped eating, and within 3 months was dead.

On high school graduation night, Lyle celebrated with a few drinks, lost control of the car, hit a tree, and suffered a fractured cervical spine, unable to move his arms or legs. After 9 months in a rehabilitation unit, Lyle remained quadriplegic. He returned home, with a home care agency providing 24-hour-a-day care at $300 per day, not covered by insurance. Lyle's father became increasingly angry

at his wife, the principal flutist in the city's professional orchestra, because she refused to leave the orchestra to care for Lyle. One night Lyle's father awoke in a cold sweat; in his dream, he had placed a plastic bag over Lyle's head and suffocated him.

Time and again the tragedy of debilitating illness is compounded by the failure of the nation's health care system to meet the social needs created by the illness. The crisis of long-term care is twofold: Thousands of families each year lose their savings to pay for the illness of a family member, and long-term care often takes place in dehumanizing institutions that rob their occupants of their last remaining vestiges of independence.

Long-term care (also called long-term services and supports) includes those health, social, housing, transportation, and other supportive services needed by persons with physical, mental, or cognitive limitations sufficient to compromise independent living. The need for long-term care services is usually determined by evaluating a person's impairment of activities of daily living (ADLs; e.g., eating, dressing, bathing, toileting, and getting in or out of bed or a chair) and instrumental activities of daily living (IADLs; e.g., housework, meal preparation, grocery shopping, transportation, financial management, taking medications, and telephoning) (Table 10–1). Fourteen million people in the United States require assistance with one or more ADLs or IADLs, and can therefore be considered as needing long-term care services (Hado & Komisar, 2019).

Projections of growth for the older population in the United States are startling. In 2020, the population

Table 10–1. Activities requiring assistance in long-term care

Activities of daily living (ADLs) (basic human functions)
Feeding
Dressing
Bathing or showering
Getting to and from the toilet and caring for incontinence
Getting in and out of a bed or chair

Instrumental activities of daily living (IADLs) (activities necessary to remain independent)
Doing housework and laundry
Preparing meals
Shopping for groceries
Using transportation
Managing finances
Making and keeping appointments
Taking medications
Telephoning

65 years of age and older numbered 56 million; this figure is expected to reach 73 million by the year 2030. The number of people 85 years and older will grow from 6.5 million in 2020 to 11.8 million in 2035 (U.S. Census Bureau, 2020). Those 75 years and older are most likely to need long-term care because over 50% have disabilities (ADA National Network, 2018). As more and more people need long-term care, the answers to two questions become increasingly urgent: How shall the nation finance long-term care? Should most long-term care be delivered through institutions or in people's homes and communities?

WHO PAYS FOR LONG-TERM CARE?

The United States spent over $400 billion on long-term care in 2020, including $157 billion on nursing home care. In 2021, the median annual cost of a private room in a nursing home was $108,000 (Kaiser Family Foundation, 2022a).

In 2020, direct out-of-pocket payments by patients and their families financed 13% of long-term care services in the United States. A common scenario is that of Eddie Taylor: After a portion of their life savings are spent for long-term care, families finally become eligible for Medicaid long-term care coverage. In 2020, Medicaid paid for 54% of US long-term care expenditures and private insurance paid for 8% (Kaiser Family Foundation, 2022a). Many people expect the Medicare program to pay for nursing home stays, but are surprised and shocked when they find that Medicare will barely assist them. Only 18% of long-term care costs are financed by Medicare (Congressional Research Service, 2022).

What are the precise roles of Medicare, Medicaid, and private insurance in the financing of long-term care services?

▶ Medicare Long-Term Coverage

Glenn Whitehorse developed diabetes-related gangrene of his right leg requiring above-the-knee amputation. He was transferred to the hospital's skilled nursing facility, where he received physical therapy services. Because he was generally frail, he was unable to move from bed to chair without assistance. Mr. Whitehorse's physical and occupational therapists felt he might do better at home, where he could receive home physical therapy and nursing care. All these services were covered by Medicare.

Ms. Whitehorse had Parkinson's disease and was unable to assist her husband in bathing, getting out of bed, and going to the bathroom; she was forced to hire an aide for these custodial functions, not covered by Medicare. When Mr. Whitehorse no longer showed any potential for improvement, Medicare discontinued coverage of his home health services. Moreover, the aide developed COVID and no one was available to replace her. Mr. Whitehorse was placed in a nursing home for custodial care. Medicare did not cover the nursing home costs.

Which services provided in a nursing facility or at home are covered by Medicare? The key distinction is between "skilled care," for which Medicare pays, and "custodial care," usually not covered. A related issue is that of post-acute versus chronic care. Medicare usually covers services needed for a few weeks or months after an acute hospitalization but often does not pay for care required by a stable chronic condition.

Nurses in a nursing home or home care agency provide a wide variety of services, such as changing the dressing on a wound, taking blood pressures, and listening to the heart and lungs to detect heart failure or pneumonia. Physical and occupational therapists work with stroke, hip fracture, and other patients to help them reach their maximum potential level of functioning. Speech therapists teach stroke patients with speech deficits how to communicate. These are all skilled services, usually covered by Medicare.

Custodial services involve assistance with ADLs and IADLs, tasks such as cooking, cleaning house, shopping, or helping a patient to the toilet. These services, sometimes provided by home health aides but more commonly by unpaid family members, are considered unskilled and often not covered by Medicare.

Medicaid Long-Term Coverage

Juan Robles, who lived alone, had deforming degenerative arthritis and was unable to do anything more active than sitting in a chair. Because Mr. Robles had no skilled care medical needs, Medicare would not provide any assistance. Mr. Robles lived in a state that supported Medicaid home and community-based services, enabling Mr. Robles to remain at home. His cousin, in a different state, was forced to enter a nursing home when her condition became disabling; within 2 weeks she died of COVID, which had infected half the nursing home residents.

Medicaid differs from Medicare in paying the costs of nursing home care. To qualify for Medicaid nursing home coverage, families may be forced to spend their savings down to low levels. When a person with disabilities spends down to become Medicaid eligible, their spouses are allowed to retain some of their assets.

Medicaid's coverage of home health services has increased as a result of home- and community-based care 1915(c) waivers, initially authorized in 1981. This program, which attempts to prevent nursing home admissions, varies widely from state to state. In 2020, about 5 million Medicaid recipients benefited from the program (Kaiser Family Foundation, 2022a). However, caregiver shortages, worsened by the COVID pandemic, have limited the program's reach.

Private Long-Term Care Insurance

Sue and Lew MacPherson, both aged 72, were worried about their future. They remembered their cousin, who was turned down for private long-term care insurance because of his high blood pressure and later spent his entire savings on nursing home bills. Hoping to protect their $32,000 in savings, they decided to apply for long-term care insurance before an illness would make them uninsurable. Their insurance agent calculated the cost of two policies at $15,000 per year, or 50% of their $30,000 per year income. At that price, Sue and Lew would spend most of their savings on insurance premiums within a few years. They declined the insurance.

Private insurance plays a minor role in long-term care financing; only 7.5 million people have private long-term care insurance. Experience rating (see Chapter 2), with premiums increasing with age, has had a profound effect on the dynamics of private long-term care insurance. Under experience-rated insurance, older adults are charged high premiums because they are at considerable risk of requiring long-term care services. Purchasing long-term care insurance at age 40 is far less expensive, but only a tiny fraction of younger people are interested because the prospects of needing such care are so remote. From 2015 to 2020, premiums rose about 40%. In 2020, the annual premium for a policy purchased at age 65 was between $1,500 and $3,000, depending on the health of the insured person and the benefit package (American Association for Long-Term Care Insurance, 2020).

People purchasing long-term care insurance may find it to be a poor investment. Private policies may specify that a policyholder must be dependent in two or three ADLs before receiving benefits. Long-term care policies usually have a deductible (measured in days), and most policies pay a fixed daily fee rather than reimbursing actual charges. A typical policy might provide $150 per day after a 60-day deductible (no benefits for the first 60 days). The 2020 average daily nursing home charge was about $300, meaning that $150 per day would be the patient's responsibility. Thus, a year's stay would require out-of-pocket expenditures totaling $63,750 (60 days × $300 = $18,000 plus 305 days × $150 = 45,750) over and above the insurance premium. Policies may limit their coverage to a few years, which places a cap on how much the insurance will pay.

WHO PROVIDES LONG-TERM CARE?

▶ Informal Caregivers

Since her husband died, Mrs. Dora Whitney has lived alone. At age 71, she became forgetful and one day left the gas stove on, causing a fire in the kitchen. Two months later, she was unable to find her way home after going to the store and was found by the police wandering in the streets. Her daughter, Kimberly, took her to the community health center where she was diagnosed with Alzheimer's dementia. After a team conference with her mother's physician, occupational therapist, and social worker, Kimberly reluctantly abandoned her career as a teacher to care for her mother. Kimberly refused to place her mother in a nursing home, and funds were not available to hire 24-hour-a-day home help.

Most people needing long-term care services receive them from their family and friends. In 2019, about 53 million people served as unpaid family caregivers, 61% of whom are women. For men, their wives often provide long-term care, and for women, their daughters are frequently caregivers. A growing number of older adults do not have family living near enough to provide informal care; the absence of an informal caregiver is a common reason for nursing home placement. Informal caregivers of adults provide an average of 24 hours of care per week. In 2019, 26% of family caregivers quit their job or reduced their work hours. Twenty-one percent report fair or poor health and health often declines during the caregiving years; 36% consider their caregiving situation to be highly stressful (AARP and National Alliance for Caregiving, 2020). The estimated economic value of caregivers' unpaid work was approximately $470 billion in 2013 (Reinhard et al., 2019).

▶ Home and Community-Based Services

Ana Dominguez insisted that her daughter Juana accept the Yale scholarship. Though at age 49 Ms. Dominguez was bed and wheelchair bound with multiple sclerosis, she would feel too guilty if Juana remained in San Antonio, TX, just to care for her. But Ms. Dominguez needed someone at home 24 hours a day, a service not covered by Medicare. For $15 a day, Juana was able to hire Vilma, an undocumented teenager from El Salvador, to live at home. Adding Vilma's pay and the cost of her food, Juana figured they would spend $35,000 of their $42,000 in savings by the time she graduated from Yale.

Community-based long-term care is delivered through a variety of programs, such as home care, adult day care, assisted living settings, home-delivered meals, board and care homes, hospice care for the terminally ill, mental health programs, and others. During the 1970s, the independent living movement among people with disabilities created a strong push away from institutional (hospital and nursing home) care toward community-based and home care that fostered the greatest possible independence. During the 1980s, AIDS activists furthered the development of hospice programs that provide intensive home care services for people with terminal cancer and AIDS. The home is a more therapeutic, comforting environment than the hospital or nursing home.

As a product of the intersection of the popular movement toward home care and the DRG-created incentive to reduce Medicare hospital stays, home health services expanded rapidly after 1980. In 2000, Medicare instituted a prospective payment system for home care based on the episode-of-illness model (see Chapter 4) in an effort to contain home care costs. Home care agencies are paid a lump sum (which, like DRG hospital payments, varies with the severity of the illness) for each 30 days of care.

Health caregivers function in teams to perform home care, including nurses, physical, occupational, speech, and respiratory therapists, social workers, home health aides, case managers, and drivers delivering meals-on-wheels. Yet home care, designed to help fill the once low-tech niche in the health care system that assists people who have disabilities with ADLs and IADLs, has become increasingly specialized. Home care agencies now offer intravenous antibiotic infusions, morphine pumps, indwelling central venous lines, and home kidney dialysis, administered by skilled intravenous and wound care nurses, respiratory therapists, and other health care professionals. These developments are a major advance in shifting medical care from hospital to home, but they have not been matched by growth in paid custodial care needed to allow people with disabilities to remain safely in their homes. Similarly, home hospice care, while providing excellent nursing services for patients with terminal illnesses, does not provide 24-hour coverage for ADL support.

Assisted living, which provides housing with a graded intensity of services depending on the functional capabilities of its residents, has been growing rapidly. However, the average annual cost in 2020 was $54,000, most of which comes from out-of-pocket payments, thereby pricing assisted living out of the reach of low- and moderate-income families.

Nursing Homes

In 1980, health policy expert Bruce Vladeck wrote:

Each morning, more than one and a quarter million Americans awaken in nursing homes. Most of them are very old and very feeble. Most will stay in the nursing home for a long time. For most, it will be the last place they ever live. . . . [Nursing home] residents live out the last of their days in an enclosed society without privacy, dignity, or pleasure, subsisting on minimally palatable diets, multiple sedatives, and large doses of television— eventually dying, one suspects at least partially of boredom.

Vladek's observation unfortunately remains apt 40 years later. In 2020, 1.3 million people resided in US nursing homes. Sixty-six percent of nursing home residents are women, who more often outlive their spouses. Frequently, after caring for a sick husband at home, women will themselves fall ill and be placed in a nursing home because no one is left to care for them at home. Sixty-one percent of nursing home residents have moderate or severe cognitive impairment, and 65% are incontinent; 92% have difficulty walking and 87% need assistance transferring in and out of bed (National Academies of Sciences, Engineering, and Medicine, 2022).

The Omnibus Budget Reconciliation Act of 1987 set standards for nursing home quality and mandated surveys to enforce these standards. Yet, nursing homes often fail to provide high-quality care and underappreciate and underprepare nursing home staff for their critical responsibilities. From 2011 to 2018, the number of resident and family complaints per 1,000 nursing home residents increased by 60%. Low staff salaries and benefits combined with inadequate training has made the nursing home an undesirable place of employment. Research reveals inequities in care, such as lower flu vaccination rates, higher hospital readmission rates, and greater feelings of social isolation among people of color than White residents in the same facility (National Academies of Sciences, Engineering, and Medicine, 2022). Commonly cited deficiencies are failure to prevent falls, failure to prevent or treat pressure ulcers, and inadequate infection control (U.S. Department of Health and Human Services, 2019).

Residents are housed in close quarters with other patients and become dependent on an underpaid, inadequately trained staff. Hour after hour may be spent lying in bed or sitting in a chair in front of a TV. While quality of life varies between one nursing home and another, placement in a nursing home almost always thwarts the human yearning for some degree of independence of action and for companionship. A sense of futility overwhelms many nursing home residents, and the desire to live often wanes (Vladeck, 1980).

To keep down costs, most care in nursing homes is provided by nurse's aides, who are paid little, receive minimal training, are inadequately supervised, and are required to care for more residents than they can properly serve. The job of the nursing home aide is difficult, involving bathing, feeding, walking residents, cleaning them when they are incontinent, lifting them, and hearing their complaints. In 2022, 71% of all nursing homes were under for-profit ownership, many operated by large corporate chains (Kaiser Family Foundation, 2022b). For-profit ownership has been associated with lower staffing levels and poorer quality of care compared with nonprofit ownership (Boccuti et al., 2015).

February 28, 2020 was a day of reckoning for the nation's nursing homes. In the ensuing days, 81 residents, 34 staff members, and 14 visitors were diagnosed with coronavirus disease (COVID-19) at a Washington State nursing home; 23 persons died. As of October 2021, despite nursing home residents making up less than one-half of 1 percent of the population, they accounted for approximately 19% of COVID-19 deaths. As of February 2022, more than

149,000 nursing home residents and more than 2,200 staff members had died of COVID-19. During the midst of the pandemic, nursing home work was one of the most dangerous jobs in the country. Burnout and turnover among the nursing home workforce (prevalent even before the pandemic) exacerbated preexisting staff shortages across the country (National Academies of Sciences, Engineering, and Medicine, 2022).

Offering a humane existence to people with severe disabilities who are housed together in close quarters is a nearly impossible task. One view of nursing home reform holds that only the abolition of most nursing homes and the development of adequately financed home and community-based care can solve the nursing home problem.

IMPROVING LONG-TERM CARE

Financing Long-Term Care

Boomer was mad. As a self-employed person, his family's health insurance coverage was costing $1,600 each month, in addition to his out-of-pocket dental bills. To make matters worse, a big chunk of his social security payments went to Medicare each year, not to mention federal and state taxes going to finance Medicare and Medicaid, so that other people could get health care. While spending all this money, Boomer was healthy and had not seen a physician for 6 years.

One day Boomer's father, Abraham, suffered a devastating stroke. After weeks in the hospital, largely paid by Medicare, Abraham was transferred to a nursing home. Because Medicare does not cover most long-term care, Boomer's mother paid the bills out of her savings until most of the money ran out. Abraham then became eligible for Medicaid, which took care of the nursing home bills. After Abraham's illness, Boomer stopped complaining about his social security and tax payments going to medical care. Even though Boomer was paying more than he was receiving, Abraham was receiving far more than he was paying. Boomer was grateful for the care his father received and figured that he might be in Abraham's shoes someday.

In the early 1960s, it was recognized that private insurance was unable to solve the problem of health care financing for people older than 65. The costs of health care for older adults were too great, making experience-rated health insurance premiums unaffordable for most of them. Accordingly, Medicare, a social insurance program, was passed (see Chapter 2). An identical problem confronts long-term care financing: As shown earlier in this chapter, Medicare covers few long-term care costs and most people who might wish to purchase long-term care insurance are unable to afford an adequate policy. Table 10–2 lists some proposals for improving long-term care.

The Pepper Commission (1990) recommended that the nation institute a social insurance program to finance long-term care. This program, like Medicare Part A, could be financed by an increase in the rate of social security contributions by employers and employees. It would pay for caregivers to provide those services not currently covered by Medicare, especially in-home help in feeding, dressing, bathing, toileting, housework, grocery shopping, transportation, and other assistance with ADLs and IADLs. A similar proposal was offered by Physicians for a National Health Program (Harrington et al., 1991). Neither came into being.

Providing Long-Term Care

Mei Soon Wang was desperate to go home. Since a brain tumor had paralyzed her left side, she had been confined to a nursing home because she had no family in San Francisco to care for her. Her daughter, visiting from Portland, heard of On Lok Senior Health Services, which cared for the frail older adults in their homes. On Lok accepted Ms. Wang, placed her in adult day care, arranged for meals to be delivered to her home, and paid for part-time help on evenings and weekends.

Table 10–2. Proposals for improving long-term care

Developing social insurance to finance long-term care
Shifting from nursing home care to home and community-based care
Training and paying for family members as caregivers
Expanding the number of comprehensive long-term care organizations modeled on On Lok Senior Health Services

Long-term care reformers advocate that most long-term care be provided at home. The first step toward deinstitutionalizing long-term care is a financing mechanism that pays for more home and community-based services.

The ideal long-term caregivers are the patient's family and friends; thus, it can be argued that long-term care reform should support, assist, and pay informal caregivers, not replace them. Teams of nurses, physical and occupational therapists, physicians, social workers, and attendants can train and work with informal caregivers, and personnel can be available to provide respite care so informal caregivers can have some relief from the 24-hours-a-day, 7-days-a-week burden.

An innovative long-term care program in the United States that has achieved great success has been the On Lok program. Translated from Chinese, On Lok means peaceful, happy abode. Begun in 1971 in San Francisco's Chinatown, On Lok merges adult day services, in-home care, home-delivered meals, housing and transportation assistance, comprehensive medical care, respite care for caregivers, hospital care, and skilled nursing care into one program. Persons eligible for On Lok have chronic illness sufficiently severe to qualify them for nursing home placement, but few spend time in a nursing home. Services for each participant are organized by a multidisciplinary team, including physicians, nurses, social workers, rehabilitation and recreation therapists, and nutritionists.

In 1983, On Lok became the first organization in the United States to assume full financial risk for the care of a frail older population, receiving monthly capitation payments from Medicare and Medicaid to cover all services. Whereas 47% of US personal health care expenditures go to hospital and nursing home services, On Lok spent a mere 17% on these items, making 83% of the health care dollar available for ambulatory home- and community-based services (Bodenheimer, 1999). In 2022, 149 On Lok "look alikes" existed in 32 states under the Program of All-Inclusive Care for the Elderly (PACE). However, PACE sites care for only 64,000 of the 8 million frail older and disabled people in the United States. Overall, PACE programs have reduced nursing home use compared to a similar non-PACE population, but Medicare and Medicaid costs appear to be somewhat higher for PACE participants (Ghosh et al., 2015).

The United States has not implemented a social insurance program for long-term care. In contrast, most industrialized nations have adopted long-term care social insurance programs (OECD, 2020). A major expansion of the PACE concept combined with comprehensive social insurance for long-term care could provide a badly needed solution to the problems of long-term care in the United States.

REFERENCES

AARP and National Alliance for Caregiving. Caregiving in the U.S. May 2020.

ADA National Network. Aging and the ADA. 2018.

American Association for Long-Term Care Insurance. Long-Term Care Insurance Facts. 2020. https://www.aaltci.org/long-term-care-insurance/learning-center/ltcfacts-2020.php#2020costs.

Boccuti C, Casillas G, Neuman T. Reading the stars: nursing home quality star ratings, nationally and by state. Kaiser Family Foundation Issue Brief, May 14, 2015.

Bodenheimer T. Long-term care for frail elderly people—the On Lok model. *N Engl J Med.* 1999;341:1324–1328.

Congressional Research Service. Who pays for long-term services and supports? June 15, 2022. https://crsreports.congress.gov/product/pdf/IF/IF10343.

Ghosh A, Schmitz R, Brown R. Effect of PACE on costs, nursing home admissions, and mortality 2006–2011. U.S. Department of Health and Human Services, March 2015. https://aspe.hhs.gov/report/effect-pace-costs-nursing-home-admissions-and-mortality-2006-2011.

Hado E, Komisar H. Long-Term Services and Supports. AARP Public Policy Institute, August 26, 2019.

Harrington C, Cassel C, Estes CL, Woolhandler S, Himmelstein DU. A national long-term care program for the United States: a caring vision. *JAMA.* 1991;266: 3023–3029.

Kaiser Family Foundation. 10 Things about Long-Term Services and Supports. September 12, 2022a.

Kaiser Family Foundation. A Look at Nursing Facility Characteristics Through July 2022. August 24, 2022b.

National Academies of Sciences, Engineering, and Medicine. *The National Imperative to Improve Nursing Home Quality.* The National Academies Press; 2022. https://doi.org/10.17226/26526.

OECD. Long-term Care and Health Care Insurance in OECD and Other Countries, 2020. https://www.oecd.org/daf/fin/insurance/Long-Term-Care-Health-Care-Insurance-in-OECD-and-Other-Countries.pdf.

Pepper Commission. *A Call for Action*. Washington, DC: US Government Printing Office; 1990.

Reinhard SC, Feinberg LF, Houser A, Choula R, Evans M. Valuing the Invaluable: 2019 Update. AARP Public Policy Institute, November 2019.

U.S. Census Bureau. Demographic Turning Points for the United States: Population Projections for 2020 to 2060. February 2020.

U.S. Department of Health and Human Services. Office of Inspector General. Trends in Deficiencies at Nursing Homes Show That Improvements Are Needed to Ensure the Health and Safety of Residents. April 2019. https://oig.hhs.gov/oas/reports/region9/91802010.pdf.

Vladeck BC. *Unloving Care: The Nursing Home Tragedy*. New York, NY: Basic Books; 1980.

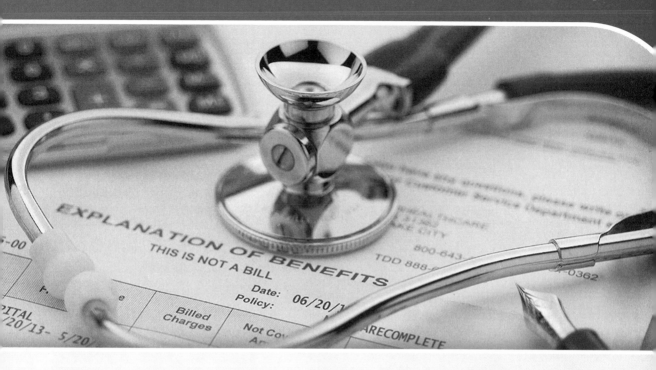

COST, QUALITY, AND VALUE

Painful Versus Painless Cost Control

Dr. Joshua Worthy is chief of neurology at Dollars'n'Sense Health System and serves as the physician representative to the health system's executive committee. The federal government has just taken the unprecedented step of imposing mandatory cost controls. The health system's budget for the coming year will be frozen at the current year's level. In past years, the annual growth in the budget has averaged 8%.

The health system's CEO begins the committee meeting by groaning, "These cuts are draconian! To meet these new budget limits we'll have to cut staff and ration life-saving technologies. Patients will suffer." A consumer member responds, "We all know there's fat in the system. Why, in the newspaper just the other day there was an article about how rates of back surgery in our city are twice the national average. And if we're going to talk about cuts, maybe we should start by looking at your salary and the number of administrators working here. I'm not so sure patients have to suffer just because we're adopting the kind of reasonable spending limits that they have in most countries."

Dr. Worthy remains silent for much of the meeting. He wonders to himself, "Is the CEO right? Is cost containment inevitably a painful process that will deprive our patients of valuable health services? Or, could we be doing a better job with the resources we're already spending? Is there a way that our health system could implement these cost controls in a relatively painless fashion as far as

our patients' health is concerned?" Interpreting Dr. Worthy's silence as an indication of great wisdom and judgment, the committee assigns him to chair a task force charged with developing a cost-control strategy to meet the new budgetary realities.

With the United States spending $4.1 trillion on health care in 2020, concerns over health care costs feature prominently in the nation's health policy agenda. The lack of adequate insurance and access to care for millions of people—which spawned the Affordable Care Act—is in part attributable to the problem of rising costs. Health care inflation has made health insurance and health services unaffordable to many families and employers.

Private and public payers in the United States have taken aim at health care cost increases and discharged volleys of innovative strategies attempting to curb expenditure growth, such as creating new approaches to utilization review, encouraging Accountable Care Organization (ACO) enrollment, making patients pay more out-of-pocket for care, and a multitude of other measures. Yet national health expenditures per capita increased more than tenfold between 1980 and 2020, rising from $1,110 to $12,530 (Fig. 11–1). Viewed as a percentage of gross domestic product (GDP), US health expenditures increased from 9.2% in 1980 to 19.7% in 2020 (Fig. 11–2). By 2030, national health expenditures per capita are projected to increase from $12,530 to $19,294 (Hartman et al., 2022; Poisal et al., 2022).

Health care providers must consider the prospect of practicing in an era of finite resources. Like Dr. Worthy, physicians and other health caregivers

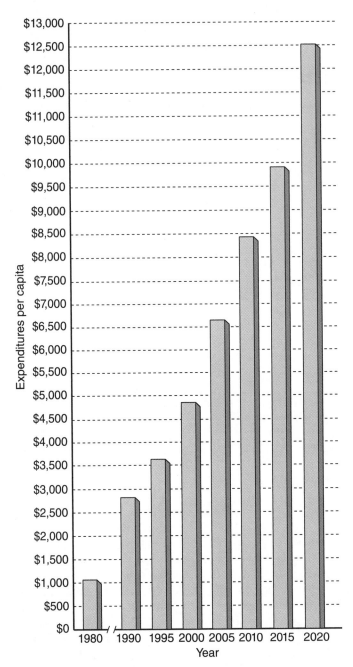

▲ **Figure 11–1.** US per capita health care expenditures. (Source: Hartman M, Martin AB, Washington B, Catlin A, The National Health Expenditure Accounts Team. National health care spending in 2020. *Health Aff (Millwood)*. 2022;41:13–25.)

need to deliberate about how constraints on expenditure growth may affect patients' health. Must cost control necessarily be painful, leading to rationing of beneficial services? Or, is there a painless route to containing costs, reached by eliminating unnecessary medical treatments and administrative expenses?

This chapter explores the painful–painless cost-control debate. First, a model will be constructed

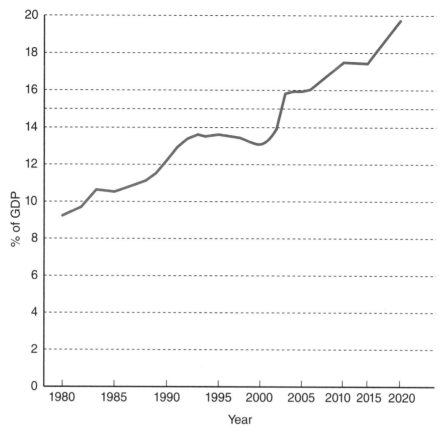

▲ **Figure 11–2.** US health care expenditures as a percentage of the gross domestic product.

describing the relationship between health care costs and benefits in terms of improved health care outcomes. Then different approaches to cost containment and their potential for achieving painless cost control will be discussed. Chapter 12 will describe specific cost-control measures in more detail.

HEALTH CARE COSTS AND HEALTH CARE OUTCOMES

Before entering medical school, Dr. Worthy worked in the Peace Corps in a remote area in Central America. At the time he first arrived in the region, the infant mortality rate was quite high, with many deaths due to infectious gastroenteritis. Dr. Worthy participated in the creation of a sewage treatment system and clean well-water sources for the region, as well as a program for implementing oral rehydration techniques for infants. By the end of Dr. Worthy's 2-year stay, the infant mortality

rate had dropped by nearly 25%. The cost for the entire program amounted to 15 cents per capita, paid for by the World Health Organization.

Conditions have been very different for Dr. Worthy as a practicing neurologist in the United States. Over 30 new magnetic resonance imaging (MRI) scanners have been installed in the city where Dollars'n'Sense Health System is located, an urban area with a population of 800,000. Dr. Worthy has found that MRI scans allow him to more accurately diagnose conditions such as multiple sclerosis in earlier stages. But many MRI scans in the city are underutilized, and Dr. Worthy wonders if half as many scanners in the city would suffice.

From society's point of view, the value of health care expenditures lies in purchasing better health for the population. The concept of "better health" is a broad one, encompassing improved longevity and quality of life, reduced mortality and morbidity rates from specific diseases, relief of pain and suffering, enhanced ability to function independently for those with chronic illnesses, and reduction in fear of illness and death. It is important to know whether investing more resources in health care buys improved health care outcomes for society, and if so, the magnitude of the improvement in outcomes relative to the amount of resources invested.

Figure 11–3, drawn from the work of the health economist Robert Evans (1984), illustrates a theoretic relationship between health care resource input and health care outcomes. Initially, as health care resources increase, these outcomes improve, but above a certain level, the slope of the curve diminishes, signifying that increasing investments in health care yield more marginal benefits. In terms of Dr. Worthy's experiences, the Central American region in which he worked lay on the steep slope of this cost–benefit curve: A small investment of resources to create more sanitary water supplies and to administer inexpensive rehydration therapy yielded dramatic improvements in health. On the other hand, purchasing more MRI scanners represents a health care system operating on the flatter portion of the curve: Large investments of resources in new technologies may produce few or no improvements in the overall health of a population.

Different medical interventions lie on steeper (e.g., childhood immunizations) or on flatter (e.g., the costly prolongation of life for an anencephalic infant) portions of the curve. The curve in Fig. 11–3 may be viewed as an aggregate cost–benefit curve for the functioning of a health care system as a whole. The system may be an entire nation or a smaller entity such as a multispecialty medical group with its defined patient population.

Overall, the US health care system currently operates along the flatter portion of the curve. Let us assume that Dr. Worthy's organization lies at point A on the curve in Fig. 11–3, with average total health care expenditures per patient being the same as the average overall per capita health care cost in the United States ($12,530 in 2020). If stringent new cost containment policies forced the health system to virtually freeze spending at point A rather than increasing annual expenditures at their usual clip to move to point B, then Fig. 11–3 implies that it would sacrifice improving the health of its enrollees by an amount equal to the distance between points A and B on the vertical axis.

Such an analysis would confirm the opinion of those who argue that cost containment requires painful choices that affect the health of the population. Proponents of this view are Aaron and Schwartz (1984

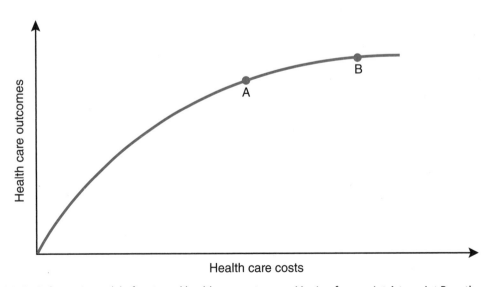

▲ **Figure 11–3.** A theoretic model of costs and health care outcomes. Moving from point A to point B on the curve is associated with both higher costs and better health outcomes.

and 1990), who described cost containment as a "painful prescription" requiring rationing of beneficial care. In Fig. 11–3, the distance between points A and B on the y-axis measures how much health "pain" accompanies the decision to limit spending at point A instead of advancing to point B. Some degree of pain is inherent in the curve. As Evans (1984) observes, "if its slope is everywhere positive, then in a world of finite resources, unmet needs are inevitable." No matter where we sit on the curve, it will always be true that if we spent more we could do a little better.

In Fig. 11–3, the distance between points A and B on the y-axis is small, given the relatively flat slope of the curve at these points. But reassurances about relatively mild cost containment pain bring to mind the physician, scalpel in hand, hovering over a patient and declaring that "it will only hurt a little bit." A little pain, necessary as it may be, is not the same as no pain; or as Fuchs (1993) puts it, "'low yield' medicine is not 'no yield' medicine."

Before allowing ourselves (and Dr. Worthy) to become overly chagrined at the inevitable painfulness of cost containment, let us add the new dimension of efficiency. We can picture a point C (Fig. 11–4) at which spending is the same as that at point A, but outcomes are better. How does the model account for point C, a point off the curve?

The move to point C requires a shifting of the curve (Fig. 11–5), signifying a new, more efficient (or productive) relationship between costs and health care outcomes (Donabedian, 1988). Another way of stating this is that point C represents higher value care. There are numerous possible routes to greater efficiency. For example, diagnostic radiographic imaging services are a rapidly inflating expenditure in the United States. An estimated 30% to 50% of CT scans may be unnecessary and CT radiation exposure is responsible for causing 2% to 5% of all cancers in the United States (Smith-Bindman, 2018). Eliminating unnecessary diagnostic radiographic procedures, such as CT scans for patients with low-risk abdominal pain, could simultaneously decrease health care costs and improve health. In the remainder of this chapter, we will examine in greater detail the various possible methods that Dr. Worthy's cost-control task force could consider to achieve more health "bang" for the health care "buck." Before turning to this discussion, however, it is necessary to make explicit three assumptions about this model of costs and outcomes.

1. Implicit in the model is the notion that the relevant outcome of interest is the overall health of a population rather than of any one individual patient. A number of authors have emphasized the need for

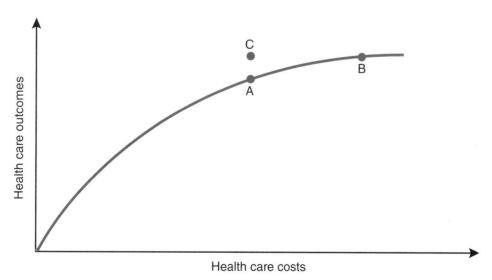

▲ **Figure 11–4.** Moving off the curve. Point C represents achievement of better health care outcomes without increased costs.

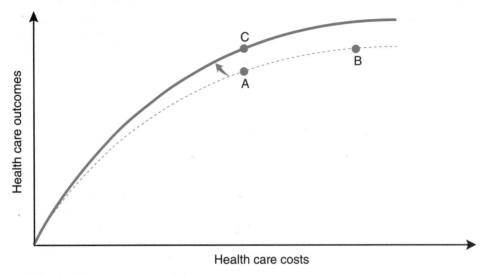

▲ **Figure 11–5.** Shifting the curve. The shift of the curve represents moving to a more efficient relationship between costs and health care outcomes.

health professionals to broaden their perspective to encompass the health of a general population, as well as their narrower traditional focus on providing the best possible care for each patient (Eddy, 1991; Krieger, 2012). The population-oriented model of costs and outcomes depicted in Figs. 11–3 to 11–5 may not fit easily with many health professionals' experiences of caring for a particular patient. At the level of the individual patient, the outcome may be all or nothing (e.g., the patient will almost certainly live if he or she receives an operation and die without it) and not easily thought about in terms of curves and slopes. Rather than focusing on any one particular intervention or patient, the curve attempts to represent the overall functioning of a health care system in the aggregate for the population under its care. (The ethical issues of the population health perspective were discussed in Chapter 6.)

2. The model assumes that it is possible to quantify health at a population level. Traditionally, health status at this level has been measured relatively crudely, using vital statistics such as life expectancy and infant mortality rates. While an index such as infant mortality rates may be a sensitive, meaningful way of evaluating the impact of health care and

public health programs in rural Central America, many analysts have questioned whether such crude indicators accurately gauge the impact of health care services in wealthier industrialized nations. In these latter nations, much of health care focuses on "softer" health care outcomes such as enhancement of functional status and quality of life in individuals with chronic diseases—aspects more difficult to monitor at the population level than death rates and related vital statistics. In other words, it may be difficult to conceptualize a scale on the y-axis of Figs. 11–3 to 11–5 that can register both the effects of managing gastroenteritis in a low-income nation and the addition of MRI scanners in a US city.

3. When evaluating population health, it is difficult to disentangle the effects of health care on health from the effects of such basic social factors as poverty, education, lifestyle, and social cohesiveness (see Chapters 5 and 14). For the purpose of our discussion of cost control, we view the curves depicted in Figs. 11–3 to 11–5 as representing the workings of the health care system (including public health) per se rather than of the broader economic and social milieu. We therefore use the term *health care outcomes* to describe the y-axis, a term intended

to suggest that we are evaluating those aspects of health status directly under the influence of health care. The *x*-axis correspondingly represents expenditures for formal health care services.

Prices and Quantities

We have shown that painless cost control is theoretically possible. But can efficiency be improved in the real world? What strategies could Dr. Worthy's task force propose to move Dollars'n'Sense Health System from point A to point C on the curve? An answer to these questions requires further scrutiny of resource costs in the health care sector.

Costs may be described by the equation

$$Cost = Price \times Quantity$$

Price refers to such items as the hospital daily room charge or the physician fee for a routine office visit. *Quantity* represents the volume and intensity of health service use (e.g., the length of stay in an intensive care unit, or the number of visits to an orthopedic surgeon). Lomas and colleagues (1989), noting this distinction between prices (Ps) and quantities (Qs), refer to cost containment as "minding the Ps and Qs" of health care costs.

Let us look at an example of the $C = P \times Q$ equation:

Blue Shield pays Dr. Morton $1,000 for 10 office visits at a fee of $100 per visit. The next year, the insurer pays Dr. Morton $1,200 for 10 visits at $120 per visit.

United Healthcare pays Dr. Norton $1,000 for 10 office visits, and the next year pays $1,200 for 12 visits at the same $100 fee. An identical cost increase is a price rise for Dr. Morton but an increase in quantity of care for Dr. Norton.

Changes in prices and quantities have different implications for patients and providers (Reinhardt, 1987). In the preceding example, both physicians increase their income (and both insurance plans increase their expenditures) by $200, though in the case of the price increase, the additional income does not require a higher volume of work. To the patient, however, only the additional $200 spent on a greater number of visits purchases more health care services. (For simplicity's sake, we assume that all visits are identical and that the price rise does not reflect increased quality of service, but simply a higher price for the same product.) A cost increase that merely represents higher prices without additional quantities of health care is an inefficient use of resources from the patient's point of view. Returning to the diagrams in Figs. 11–3 and 11–4, if real costs in a health care system were rising only because medical price inflation was exceeding general price inflation while the quantity of care per capita remained static, then increased health costs would not bring about improved health care outcomes, and the overall curve would become absolutely flat.

COST-CONTROL STRATEGIES

Controlling Price Inflation

After intense deliberation, Dr. Worthy's task force submits a plan for "painless cost containment" to the executive committee. The first proposal calls for aggressive discounts on the prices paid for supplies, equipment, and pharmaceuticals by selectively contracting with suppliers for bulk purchases and stocking a more limited variety of product lines and drugs within the same therapeutic class. The proposal also calls for a 10% reduction in salaries for all employees earning over $275,000 per year, as well as a 10% reduction in the capitation fee paid to the health system's physician group. The executive committee never gets beyond this part of the plan, as furious argument erupts over the proposed income cuts.

Price inflation has been a major contributor to the rise of health care costs in recent decades. The rapid rise of health care prices manifests itself in such ways as prices for prescription drugs in the United States often being more than 50% higher than prices for the same products sold in other nations. Specialist physician incomes are high and continue to rise. Higher prices explain much of the higher costs of health care in the United States compared with the costs in other industrialized nations (Anderson et al., 2019). Limiting price inflation is one way to restrain expenditures without inflicting "pain" on the public's health (Table 11–1).

Table 11–1. Examples of painless cost control

Controlling fees and provider incomes
Cutting the price of pharmaceuticals and other supplies
Reducing administrative waste
Eliminating medical interventions of no benefit
Substituting less costly technologies that are equally effective
Increasing the provision of those preventive services that cost less than the illnesses they prevent

Eliminating Ineffective and Inappropriate Care

After a brief hiatus to let the furor subside, the executive committee reconvenes. Dr. Worthy introduces his task force's second recommendation—developing appropriateness of care guidelines—by recounting one of his own clinical experiences. When Dr. Worthy first arrived, the neurologists were keeping their stroke patients at bed rest for 1 week before initiating physical therapy. Dr. Worthy, in contrast, began physical therapy and discharge planning for stroke patients the moment their neurologic status was stable. The average length of stay in the acute hospital for his stroke patients was 3 days, compared with 9 days for other neurologists. Dr. Worthy gave a grand rounds presentation demonstrating that 4 days of exercise are required to regain the strength lost from each day of bed rest, meaning that stroke patients would have better outcomes and use fewer resources—shorter acute hospital stays and less rehabilitation—under his care than under the care of his colleagues. Dr. Worthy cites this as just one example of how resources are being diverted to ineffective, or even harmful, care.

If controlling prices is one approach to painless cost control, are there also ways to contain the "Q" (quantity) factor in a manner that does not sacrifice beneficial care? Earlier, we cited unnecessary diagnostic imaging studies as an example of inefficient resource use in terms of quantities of services that add to costs and may cause harm. A number of researchers have found convincing evidence of substantial amounts of unnecessary care in the United States (Brownlee, 2007; Kilo & Larsen, 2009; Berwick & Hackbarth, 2012; Lyu et al., 2017). Physicians in the United States perform large numbers of inappropriate procedures (Deyo et al., 2009), and physicians may inappropriately and harmfully accept new technologies as a result of industry influence rather than proven efficacy (Avorn, 2007; Moynihan & Bero, 2017).

Persuasive evidence comes from the work of Fisher, Wennberg, and colleagues, who found that per capita Medicare costs were three times as high in some cities (e.g., Miami) than in others (e.g., Salem OR and Honolulu HI) (Gottlieb et al., 2010). This difference was explained not by prices or degree of illness but was related to the quantity of services provided, which in turn is associated with the predominance of specialists in the higher-cost areas (Fisher et al., 2003). Moreover, residents of areas with a greater per capita supply of hospital beds were up to 30% more likely to be hospitalized than those in areas with fewer beds, after controlling for socioeconomic characteristics and disease burden (Fisher et al., 2000). As for the value of this spending, quality of care and health care outcomes were, if anything, worse in the highest spending regions than in areas with less intensive use of services. These findings suggest that a great deal of unnecessary care is taking place in the high-cost areas.

The slope of the cost–benefit curve would become more favorable if a system could eliminate those wasteful components of rising expenditures that have flat slopes (no medical benefit) or negative slopes (harm exceeding benefit, as in the case of inappropriate surgical procedures or prolonged bed rest after strokes). However, inducing physicians and patients to selectively eliminate unnecessary care is no easy matter.

Administrative Waste

The third item on Dr. Worthy's painless cost containment plan targets the health system's administrative costs. The task force proposes eliminating the TV and radio advertising budget, laying off 25% of all administrative personnel, and reassigning 25 of the 50 staff members in the department that handles contracts with employers to a new department designed to develop a program to ensure that the system provides up-to-date child immunizations and adult preventive care services for 100% of patients. The marketing director patiently explains to Dr. Worthy that although he, in principle, agrees with these recommendations, he does not consider it wise to cut costs in a way that jeopardizes the health system's ability to attract more patients.

Not all quantities in the health care cost equation are clinical in nature. The tremendous administrative overhead of the US health care system has come under increasing scrutiny in recent years as a source of inefficiency in health care expenditures. Administrative expenses account for between 15% and 25% of total US health expenditures—an estimated $600 billion to $1 trillion in 2019 (Chernew & Mintz, 2021)—far higher than other nations such as Canada (Woolhandler et al., 2003; Himmelstein et al., 2014). While some level of administrative service is necessary for health care finance management and related activities such as quality assurance, few argue that the burgeoning administrative and marketing activities translate into meaningful improvement in patient health. Reducing administrative services is another route to painless cost containment.

Eliminating purely wasteful quantities of health care services, be they ineffective clinical services or unnecessary administrative activities, is a relatively straightforward approach to painless cost control. The motto of this approach is: Stop doing things of no clinical benefit. More complicated are approaches to efficiency that involve not simply ceasing completely unproductive activities, but doing things differently. Examples of this latter approach include innovations that substitute less costly care of equal benefit, preventive care, and redistribution of resources from services with some benefit to services with greater benefit relative to cost. Let us examine each of these examples in turn.

Innovation and Cost Savings

Innovation in health care includes the search for less costly ways of producing the same or better health care outcomes. A new drug is developed that is less expensive but is equally efficacious and well tolerated as a conventional medication. Services provided by highly paid physicians can often be delivered with the same quality by nurses, nurse practitioners, or physician assistants.

Infusion of chemotherapy for many cancer treatments may be done safely on an outpatient basis, averting the expense of hospitalization. Often new technologies are introduced in hopes that they will ultimately prove to be less costly than existing treatment methods.

However, new technologies often fail to live up to cost-saving expectations (Bodenheimer, 2005). A case in point is that of laparoscopic cholecystectomy. Through the use of fiberoptic technology, the gallbladder may be surgically removed using a much smaller abdominal incision than that required for traditional open cholecystectomy, lowering days in the hospital, reducing the cost of each operation, and improving outcomes due to less postoperative pain and disability—seemingly a classic case of "efficient substitution" that lowers costs and improves health outcomes. There's a catch, however. The necessity of gallbladder surgery is not always clear-cut for patients with gallstones. Many patients have only occasional, mild symptoms, and prefer to tolerate these symptoms rather than undergo an operation. Rates of cholecystectomy increased dramatically following the advent of the laparoscopic technique, apparently because more patients with milder symptoms were undergoing gallbladder surgery. In one study, 21% of the surgeries were unnecessary (Pulvirenti et al., 2013). In one HMO, the cholecystectomy rate increased by 59% between 1988 and 1992 after the introduction of the laparoscopic technique. Even though the average cost per cholecystectomy declined by 25%, the total cost for all cholecystectomies in the HMO rose by 11% because of the increased number of procedures done (Legorreta et al., 1993).

Ounces of Prevention

If an ounce of prevention is worth a pound of cure, then replacement of expensive end-stage treatment with low-cost prevention would appear to be an ideal candidate for the "painless cost controller award." Investing in prevention sometimes generates this type of efficiency in health care spending (e.g., many childhood vaccinations cost less than caring for children who experience severe and disabling infections) (Zhou et al., 2014).

However, the prevention story is not always so simple. In many cases, the cost of implementing a widespread prevention program may exceed the cost of caring for the illness it aims to prevent (Cohen et al., 2008). For example, screening the general population for elevated blood pressure and providing long-term treatment for those with mild-to-moderate hypertension to prevent strokes and other cardiovascular complications has been found to cost more than the expense of treating the eventual complications themselves (Russell, 2009). For some diseases, this is the case because the complications are rapidly and inexpensively fatal, while successful prevention leads to a long life with high medical costs, perhaps for a different illness, required at some point. Blood pressure screening programs result in the improved health of the population but require a net investment in additional resources.

▶ Prioritization and Analysis of Cost-Effectiveness

A fourth recommendation of Dr. Worthy's task force involves the diagnosis and treatment of colon cancer. Screening colonoscopy is associated with a 68% reduction in colon cancer mortality (Ladabaum et al., 2020). All the health system's oncologists strongly recommend chemotherapy for patients who develop widespread metastatic colon cancer.

Analysis of cost-effectiveness has demonstrated that screening colonoscopy saves many more years of life per dollar spent than chemotherapy for metastatic colon cancer. Yet chemotherapy allows patients with widespread metastatic disease to enjoy some extra months of life. The task force takes the position that the health system's physicians should do screening colonoscopies, but that the system's insurance plan should not cover chemotherapy for widespread metastatic colon cancer.

The most controversial strategy for making health care more efficient is the redistribution of resources from services with some benefit to services with greater benefit relative to cost. This approach is commonly guided by cost-effectiveness analysis, which calculates the net cost of the health care service divided by a defined outcome such as years of life saved (Eisenberg, 1989). For example, a study comparing a comprehensive smoking cessation program with standard tobacco use counseling found that the new program cost $4,137 per

additional patient who quit smoking and $7,301 per additional life saved (Levy et al., 2017). Another study of patients with stable coronary artery disease comparing treatment with medication alone versus medication plus coronary artery angioplasty or stenting (procedures to mechanically open the arteries) found that medication plus procedure cost about $150,000 per additional patient relieved of symptoms and more than $200,000 per additional year of life saved (Weintraub et al., 2008). To get the most "bang" for the health care "buck," these studies suggest that a system operating under limited resources would do better by maximizing resources for smoking cessation than by performing invasive procedures on patients with stable coronary artery disease.

Cost-effectiveness analysis must be used with caution. If the data used are inaccurate, the conclusions may be incorrect. Moreover, cost-effectiveness analysis may discriminate against people with disabilities. Researchers are likely to assign less worth to a year of life of a person with disabilities than does the person himself or herself; thus, analyses using "quality-adjusted life years (QALYs)" may have a built-in bias against persons with less capacity to function independently (Sinclair, 2012). The disability-adjusted life year concept has been proposed to address this bias (Neumann et al., 2018), but QALYs are likely to remain an important metric for cost-effectiveness analysis (Neumann & Cohen, 2018).

Dr. David Eddy (1991, 1992, 1993), in a series of provocative articles in the *Journal of the American Medical Association,* has discussed the practical and ethical challenges of applying cost-effectiveness analysis to medical practice. Two of the essays involve the case of an HMO trying to decide whether to adopt routine use of low-osmolar contrast agents, a type of dye for special x-ray studies that carries a lower risk of provoking allergic reactions than the cheaper conventional dye. With the use of this agent for all x-ray dye studies, 40 nonfatal allergic reactions would be avoided annually and the cost to the HMO would be $3.5 million more per year, compared with costs for use of the older agent in routine cases and use of the low-osmolar dye only for patients at high risk of allergy. The same $3.5 million dollars invested in an expanded cervical cancer screening program in the HMO would prevent approximately 100 deaths from cervical cancer per year.

In discussing how best to deploy these resources, Eddy highlights several points of particular relevance to clinicians:

1. It must be agreed upon that resources are truly limited. Although the cost-effectiveness of low-osmolar contrast dye and cervical cancer screening is quite different, both programs offer some benefit (i.e., they are not flat-of-the-curve medicine). If no constraints on resources existed, the best policy would be to invest in both services.

2. If resources are limited and trade-offs based on cost-effectiveness considerations are to be made, these trade-offs will have professional legitimacy only if it is clear that resources saved from denying services of low cost-effectiveness will be reinvested in services with greater cost-effectiveness, rather than siphoned off for ineffective care or higher profits.

3. Ethical tensions exist between maximizing health outcomes for a group or population as opposed to the individual patient. The radiologist experiences the trauma of patients having severe allergic reactions to the injection of contrast dye. Preventing future deaths from cervical cancer in an unspecified group of patients not directly under the radiologist's care seems an abstract and remote benefit from his or her perspective—one that may be perceived as conflicting with the radiologist's obligation to provide the best care possible to his or her patients.

Many analysts, including those who question the methods of cost-effectiveness analysis, share Eddy's conclusion: health professionals must broaden their perspective to balance the needs of individual patients directly under their care with the overall needs of the population served by the health care system, whether the system is a local health care institution or the nation's health care system as a whole (see Chapter 6). Professional ethics will have to incorporate social accountability for resource use and population health, as well as clinical responsibility for the care of individual patients (Hiatt, 1975; Greenlick, 1992).

The final recommendation of Dr. Worthy's task force is to hire a consultant to advise on the relative cost-effectiveness of different services in order to prioritize the most cost-effective activities. While waiting for the consultant's report, the task force suggests that the health system begin implementing this strategy by allocating an extra 5 minutes to every routine medical appointment for patients who smoke, so that a member of the practice team has time to counsel patients on smoking cessation, as well as by setting up two dozen new community-based group classes in smoking cessation. Since many invasive coronary artery procedures are inappropriate (Chan et al., 2011; Maron et al., 2020), the smoking cessation costs are to be funded from the existing budget for invasive coronary artery procedures, and the number of these procedures is to be restricted to 30 fewer than the number performed during the current year. The day following the executive committee meeting, the health system's health education director buys Dr. Worthy lunch and compliments him on his "enlightened" views. On the way back from lunch, the chief of cardiology accosts Dr. Worthy in the corridor and says, "Why don't you just take a few dozen of my patients with severe coronary artery disease out and shoot them? Get it over with quickly, instead of denying them the life-saving stents they need."

CONCLUSION

The relationship between health care outcomes and health care costs is not a simple one. The cost–benefit curve has a diminishing slope as increasing investment of resources yields more marginal improvements in the health of the population. The curve itself may shift up or down, depending on the efficiency with which a given level of resources is deployed.

The ideal cost containment method is one that achieves progress in overall health care outcomes through the "painless" route of making more efficient use of an existing level of resources. Examples of this approach include restricting price increases, reducing administrative waste, and eliminating inappropriate and ineffective services. "Painful" cost containment represents the other extreme—sacrificing quantities of medically beneficial services. Making trade-offs in services based on relative cost-effectiveness may be felt as painless or painful, depending on one's point of view; some individuals may experience the pain of being denied potentially beneficial services, but at a net gain in health for the overall population through more efficient use of the resources at hand.

Cost containment in the real world tends to fall somewhere between the entirely painless paragon and the completely painful pariah. As the experiences of Dr. Worthy reveal, putting painless cost control into practice may be impeded by political, organizational, and technical obstacles. Price controls may make economic sense but risk intense opposition from providers. Administrative savings may be largely beyond the control of any single health institution or group of providers and require an overhaul of the entire health care system. Identifying and modifying inappropriate clinical practices is a daunting task, as is prioritizing services on the basis of cost effectiveness. But while painless cost control may be difficult to achieve, few would argue that the US health care system currently operates anywhere near a maximum level of efficiency. Regions in the nation with higher health care spending do not have better health care outcomes (Fisher et al., 2003). The nation's lackluster performance on indices such as infant mortality and life expectancy rates suggests that the prolific degree of spending on health care in the United States has not been matched by a commensurate level of excellence in the health of the population (Schneider et al., 2017). Making better use of existing resources must be the priority of cost-control strategies in the United States.

REFERENCES

Aaron H, Schwartz WB. Rationing health care: the choice before us. *Science.* 1990;247:418–422.

Aaron H, Schwartz WB. *The Painful Prescription: Rationing Hospital Care.* Washington, DC: Brookings Institution; 1984.

Anderson GF, Hussey P, Petrosyan V. It's still the prices, stupid: why the US spends so much on health care and a tribute to Uwe Reinhardt. *Health Aff (Millwood).* 2019;38:87–95.

Avorn J. Keeping science on top in drug evaluation. *N Engl J Med.* 2007;357:633–635.

Berwick DM, Hackbarth AD. Eliminating waste in US health care. *JAMA.* 2012;307:1513–1516.

Bodenheimer T. High and rising health care costs. Part 2: Technologic innovation. *Ann Intern Med.* 2005;142:932–937.

Brownlee S. *Overtreated.* New York, NY: Bloomsbury; 2007.

Chan PS, Patel MR, Klein LW, et al. Appropriateness of percutaneous coronary intervention. *JAMA.* 2011;306:53–61.

Chernew M, Mintz H. Administrative costs in the US health care system. Why so high? *JAMA.* 2021;326:1679–1680.

Cohen JT, Neumann PJ, Weinstein MC. Does preventive care save money? *N Engl J Med.* 2008;358:661–663.

Deyo RA, Mirza SK, Turner JA, Martin BI. Overtreating chronic back pain: time to back off. *J Am Board Fam Med.* 2009;22:62–68.

Donabedian A. Quality and cost: choices and responsibilities. *Inquiry.* 1988;25:90–99.

Eddy DM. The individual vs. society: is there a conflict? *JAMA.* 1991;265:1446–1450.

Eddy DM. Applying cost-effectiveness analysis. *JAMA.* 1992;268:2575–2582.

Eddy DM. Broadening the responsibilities of practitioners. *JAMA.* 1993;269:1849–1855.

Eisenberg JM. Clinical economics. *JAMA.* 1989;262:2879–2886.

Evans RG. *Strained Mercy: The Economics of Canadian Health Care.* Toronto, Ontario, Canada: Butterworths; 1984.

Fisher ES, Wennberg DE, Stukel TA, Gottlieb DJ, Lucas FL, Pinder EL. The implications of regional variation in Medicare spending. *Ann Intern Med.* 2003;138:273–287.

Fisher ES, Wennberg JE, Stukel TA, et al. Associations among hospital capacity, utilization, and mortality of US Medicare beneficiaries, controlling for sociodemographic factors. *Health Serv Res.* 2000;34:1351–1362.

Fuchs VR. No pain, no gain: perspectives on cost containment. *JAMA.* 1993;269:631–633.

Gottlieb DJ, Zhou W, Song Y, Andrews KG, Skinner JS, Sutherland JM. Prices don't drive regional Medicare spending variations. *Health Aff (Millwood).* 2010;29:537–543.

Greenlick MR. Educating physicians for population-based clinical practice. *JAMA.* 1992;267:1645–1648.

Hartman M, Martin AB, Washington B, Catlin A, The National Health Expenditure Accounts Team. National health care spending in 2020. *Health Aff (Millwood).* 2022;41:13–25.

Hiatt HH. Protecting the medical commons: who is responsible? *N Engl J Med.* 1975;293:235–241.

Himmelstein DU, Jun M, Busse R, et al. A comparison of hospital administrative costs in Eight Nations: US costs exceed all others by far. *Health Aff (Millwood).* 2014;33:1586–1594.

Kilo CM, Larsen EB. Exploring the harmful effects of health care. *JAMA.* 2009;302:89–91.

Krieger N. Who and what is a "population"? *Milbank Q.* 2012;90:634–681.

Ladabaum U, Dominitz JA, Kahi C, Schoen RE. Strategies for colorectal cancer screening. *Gastroenterology.* 2020;158:418–432.

Legorreta AP, Silber JH, Costantino GN, Kobylinski RW, Zatz SL. Increased cholecystectomy rate after the introduction of laparoscopic cholecystectomy. *JAMA.* 1993;270:1429–1432.

Levy DE, Klinger EV, Linder JA, et al. Cost-effectiveness of a health system-based smoking cessation program. *Nicotine Tob Res.* 2017;19:1508–1515.

Lomas J, Fooks C, Rice T, Labelle RJ. Paying physicians in Canada: minding our Ps and Qs. *Health Aff (Millwood).* 1989;8(1):80–102.

Lyu H, Xu T, Brotman D, et al. Overtreatment in the United States. *PLoS One.* 2017;12(9):e0181970.

Maron DJ, Hochman JS, Reynolds HR, et al. Initial invasive or conservative strategy for stable coronary disease. *NEJM.* 2020;382:1395–1407.

Moynihan R, Bero L. Toward a healthier patient voice: more independence, less industry funding. *JAMA Internal Med.* 2017;177:350–351.

Neumann PJ, Anderson JE, Panzer AD, et al. Comparing cost-per QALYs gained and cost per DALYs averted analysis. *Value in Health.* 2018;21(suppl 1):S118.

Neumann PJ, Cohen JT. QALYs in 2018—advantages and concerns. *JAMA.* 2018;319:2473–2474.

Poisal JA, Sisko AM, Cuckler GA, et al. National health expenditure projections, 2021–30. *Health Aff (Millwood).* 2022;41:474–486.

Pulvirenti E, Toro A, Gagner M, Mannino M, Di Carlo I. Increased rate of cholecystectomies performed with doubtful or no indications after laparoscopy introduction. *BMC Surgery.* 2013;13:17.

Reinhardt UE. Resource allocation in health care: the allocation of lifestyles to providers. *Milbank Mem Fund Q.* 1987;65:153–176.

Russell LB. Preventing chronic disease: an important investment, but don't count on cost savings. *Health Aff (Millwood).* 2009;28:42–45.

Schneider EC, Sarnak DO, Squires D, Shah A, Doty MM. Mirror, mirror 2017: international comparison reflects flaws and opportunities for better U.S. health care. The Commonwealth Fund, July 14, 2017. https://www.commonwealthfund.org/publications/fund-reports/2017/jul/mirror-mirror-2017-international-comparison-reflects-flaws-and.

Sinclair S. How to avoid unfair discrimination against disabled patients in healthcare resource allocation. *J Med Ethics.* 2012;38:158–162.

Smith-Bindman R. Use of advanced imaging tests and the not-so-incidental harms of incidental findings. *JAMA Internal Med.* 2018;178:227–228.

Weintraub WS, Boden WE, Zhang Z, et al. Cost-effectiveness of percutaneous coronary intervention in optimally treated stable coronary patients. *Circ Cardiovasc Qual Outcomes.* 2008;1:12–20.

Woolhandler S, Campbell T, Himmelstein DU. Costs of health care administration in the United States and Canada. *N Engl J Med.* 2003;349:768–775.

Zhou F, Shefer A, Wenger J, et al. Economic evaluation of the routine childhood immunization program in the United States, 2009. *Pediatrics.* 2014;133:577–585.

Mechanisms for Controlling Costs

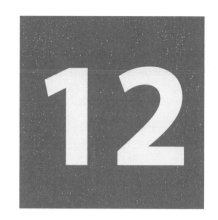

In Chapter 11, we discussed the general relationship between costs and health outcomes and explored the tension between painful and painless approaches to cost containment. In this chapter, we examine specific methods for controlling costs. We briefly cite evidence about how these mechanisms may affect cost and health outcomes.

Financial transactions under private or public health insurance (see Chapter 2, Figs. 2–2, 2–3, and 2–4) may be divided into two components:

1. *Financing*, the flow of dollars (premiums from individuals and employers or taxes) to the health insurance plan (private health insurance or government programs), and
2. *Payment*, the flow of dollars from insurance plans (private or public) to physicians, hospitals, and other providers.

Cost-control strategies can be divided into those that target the financing side versus those that impact the payment side of the funding stream (Fig. 12–1 and Table 12–1).

FINANCING CONTROLS

Cost controls aimed at the financing of health insurance attempt to limit the flow of funds into health insurance plans, with the expectation that the plans will then be forced to limit the outflow of payment to providers. Financing controls come in two basic flavors—regulatory and competitive.

▶ Regulatory Strategies

Dieter Arbeiter, a carpenter in Berlin, Germany, is enrolled in one of his nation's health insurance plans, the "sick fund" operated by the Carpenter's Guild. Each month, Dieter pays 7.3% of his wages to the sick fund and his employer contributes another 7.3%. The German federal government regulates these payroll tax rates. When the government proposes raising the employee rate to 8.3%, Dieter and his coworkers march to the parliament building to protest the increase. The government backs down and as a result, physician fees do not increase that year.

In nations with tax-financed health insurance, government regulation of taxes serves as a control over public expenditures for health care. This regulatory control is most evident when certain tax funds are earmarked for health insurance, as in the case of the German health insurance plans (see Chapter 15) or Medicare Part A in the United States. Under these types of social insurance systems, an increase in expenditures for health care requires explicit legislation to raise the rate of earmarked health insurance taxes. Public antipathy to tax hikes may serve as a political anchor against health care inflation.

A somewhat different model of financing regulation was offered by President Clinton's 1994 health care proposal (which never passed). That proposal called for government regulation of premiums paid to private health insurance plans.

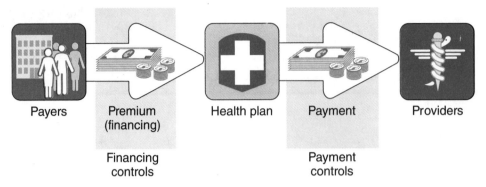

▲ Figure 12–1. Cost-control mechanisms may be applied to both the financing and payment components of health care spending.

▶ Competitive Strategies

An alternative strategy for containing costs would control the financing flow through competition rather than regulation. The basic premise of competitive financing is to make employers, employees, and individuals more cost-conscious in their health insurance purchasing decisions. Health insurance plans would be encouraged to compete on the basis of price, with lower-cost plans being rewarded with a greater number of enrollees. Instead of having a government agency regulate financing, the competitive market would pressure plans to restrain their premium prices and overall costs.

Giovanni Costa works for General Auto (GA). It is 1995, and he and his family have Blue Cross health insurance that covers most services provided by the health care provider of his choice, with no deductible. Giovanni does not know how much his health plan costs, because GA pays the total premium. Once Giovanni asked his friend in the employee benefits department whether the company was worried about the costs of health insurance. "It's a problem," Giovanni was told, "but it's not too bad because our health insurance premiums are tax deductible for the company. When it comes right down to it, the government's paying a portion of those premiums."

This vignette suggests that in 1995, no cost-restraining financing strategy existed for employer-based insurance. When considering competitive strategies to make purchasers more price sensitive, it is important to consider who the purchaser of health insurance really is. For employment-based health insurance, is the purchaser the employer selecting which health plans to offer employees, or is it the individual employee deciding to enroll in a specific plan? As in the case of Giovanni Costa and GA, the answer is often both: GA selects which plans to offer employees and what

Table 12–1. Categories of cost controls

Financing controls
Regulatory: limits on taxes or premiums
Competitive
Payment controls
Price controls
Regulatory
Competitive
Utilization (quantity) controls
Aggregate units of payment: capitation, diagnosis-related groups (DRGs), global budgets
Patient cost-sharing
Utilization management
Supply limits
Mixed controls

portion of the premium to subsidize, and Giovanni chooses a particular plan from those offered by GA.

For employers, inflation of health insurance premiums in the 1950s and 1960s was an acceptable part of doing business when the economy was booming and health insurance costs consumed only a small portion of overall business expenses. However, as health insurance costs continued to spiral upward and economic growth slowed, employers became more active in limiting their health insurance costs.

It is 2018, and GA now offers Giovanni Costa three choices of health insurance plans: The health maintenance organization (HMO) plan costs $1,600 per month for family coverage, the preferred provider organization (PPO) plan is worth $1,800 per month, and the fee-for-service plan runs $2,000 a month. In all three choices, GA pays 70% of the lowest cost plan, and Giovanni pays the rest. If Giovanni chooses the HMO plan, GA pays $1,120 (70%) and Giovanni pays $480 (30%). If Giovanni signs up for the $1,800 PPO plan, GA still pays $1,120 (70% of the lowest-cost plan) and Giovanni must pay the rest—$680. If Giovanni wants to choose the fee-for-service plan, GA pays $1,120 and Giovanni pays $880. GA negotiated with all three of its health plans that premium levels would be frozen at their 2018 rates for the next 3 years. A fourth plan previously offered by GA refused to agree to this stipulation, and GA dropped this plan from its portfolio of employee benefits. After 2021, however, the three health plans can demand yearly premium increases, increasing health insurance costs for both GA and Giovanni.

The competitive approach to health insurance financing is intended to encourage price-sensitive purchasing by both employer and employee. For employers, the competitive strategy calls for businesses to be more aggressive in their negotiations with health plans over premium rates. Employers bargain actively with health plans and offer employees only plans that keep their rates below a certain level. Moreover, employers make employees more cost aware when selecting a health plan by limiting the amount of the insurance premium that the employer will pay. Rather than paying all or most of the premium, many employers offer a fixed amount of insurance subsidy—often indexed to the cost of the cheapest health plan—and compel employees selecting more costly plans to pay the extra amount. Economist Alain Enthoven, one of the chief proponents of the competitive approach, has called this strategy "managed competition" (Enthoven, 2003). The strategy is also known as the "defined contribution" approach.

Is the evolving competitive approach succeeding at controlling costs? From 2000 to 2010, employer—sponsored health insurance premiums rose by over 10% per year, a major cost-control failure (Claxton et al., 2010). From 2010 to 2022, these premiums grew more slowly, about 5% per year, in part due to the economic recession and the COVID-19 pandemic (Claxton et al., 2018; Claxton et al., 2022). However, competition has never been truly instituted in the United States; 94% of metropolitan markets are controlled by one or two large commercial insurance companies, and this level of consolidation is increasing, allowing insurers to extract increasing premiums from employers (American Medical Association, 2020). Moreover, insurance plans find it easier to compete by "gaming" the market through selection of low-cost enrollees rather than by disciplining providers to deliver a lower-cost, higher-quality product. Studies have shown that competing Medicare HMOs have utilized precisely that strategy (Mehrotra et al., 2006).

If competition could succeed at containing costs, would the outcome be painful or painless cost control? Whatever pain may be produced would be experienced most acutely by individuals with lower incomes. Under competition, individuals with higher incomes would be the ones most likely to pay the extra premium costs to enroll in more expensive health plans, while individuals of lesser means could not afford the extra premiums and would be relegated to the lower-cost plans. Enrollees in low-cost plans might experience inferior quality of care and health outcomes.

The Weaknesses of Financing Controls

For cost controls—whether regulatory or competitive—on the financing side of the health care equation to be successful, these strategies ultimately must produce reductions in the flow of funds on the payment side. A government may try to limit the level of taxes earmarked for health care. However, if payments to physicians, hospitals, and other providers continue to grow at a rapid clip, the imbalance between the level of financing and level of payment will ultimately force the government to raise taxes. Similarly, under competition, health insurers will attempt to hold down premium increases in order to gain more customers, but if these health plans cannot successfully control what they pay to hospitals, physicians, pharmacies, and other providers, then insurers will be forced to raise their premiums, and competitive relief from health care inflation will prove elusive. It is on the payment side that the rubber meets the road in health care cost containment. Governments in nations with publicly financed insurance programs do not simply regulate health care financing, but are actively involved in controlling provider payment. We now turn to an examination of the options available to private insurers or government for controlling the flow of funds in the payment transaction.

PAYMENT CONTROLS

In Chapter 11, we distinguished between the "Ps" and "Qs" of health care costs: prices and quantities. Cost equals price multiplied by quantity

$$C = P \times Q$$

Strategies to control costs on the payment side can primarily target either prices or quantities (see Table 12–1).

▶ Price Controls

Under California's fee-for-service Medicaid program, Dr. Vincent Lo's reimbursement for a routine office visit is set by California's government.

The Medicare program reduced Dr. Ernesto Ojo's fee for cataract surgery from $900 to $780.

Instead of paying all hospitals in the area the going rate for magnetic resonance imaging (MRI) brain scans ($1,400), Apple a Day HMO contracts only with those hospitals that agree to perform scans for $1,000, and will not allow its patients to receive MRIs at any other hospital.

Metropolitan Hospital wants a contract with Apple a Day HMO at a per diem rate of $2,000.

Because Apple a Day can hospitalize its patients at Crosstown Hospital for $1,700 a day, Metropolitan has no choice but to reduce its per diem rate to Apple a Day to $1,700 in order to get the contract. In turn, to make up the $300 per day shortfall, Metropolitan increases its charges to several other private insurers.

Reference PPO asks each hospital in its market region to submit a bid for the total charge for a knee replacement. Most bids are at least $40,000, but High Value Hospital, which has a reputation for good quality care, submits a bid of $33,000. Reference PPO informs the patients enrolled in the plan that they can choose any hospital for a knee replacement, but that the PPO will only pay the hospital $33,000 and the patient will be responsible for paying any charges above that amount. After this policy is put into effect, most Reference PPO patients needing knee replacement get their operations at High Value Hospital.

In Canada and most European nations, a public or quasipublic agency regulates a uniform fee schedule for physician and hospital payments. Often, negotiations occur between the payers and professional organizations in establishing these fee schedules. In the United States, as discussed in Chapter 4, Medicare, Medicaid, and many private insurance plans have replaced "usual, customary, and reasonable" physician payment with predetermined prices for particular services. Competitive approaches to controlling prices have also been attempted in the United States. In the 1980s, California initiated competitive bidding among hospitals for Medicaid contracts, with contracts awarded to hospitals offering lower per diem charges. Private insurance plans have also used competitive bidding to bargain for reductions in physician and hospital fees. A recent variation on competitive payment strategies is "reference pricing," such as the approach used by Reference PPO. In theory, public disclosure of prices—price transparency—might deter hospitals and physicians from setting excessively high prices, but such transparency is rarely found in the United States (Mehrotra et al., 2018).

Prices explain much of the difference in health expenditures between the United States and other nations (Anderson et al., 2019). For example, in 2012, the regulated fee for coronary artery bypass surgery in European nations ranged from $14,000 to $23,000; the average fee paid by private insurance plans in the United States was $73,420 (Klein, 2013). A study of reference pricing implemented by one large purchaser in California for joint replacements found that it reduced payments by about 30%, although the purchaser saved only 0.26% in total costs because joint replacements are a relatively small contributor to total costs (Lechner et al., 2013). Two major problems limit the potency of price controls for containing overall costs, particularly when prices are regulated at the fee-for-service level.

1. The first problem occurs when price controls are implemented in a piecemeal fashion by different payers. Providers, like Metropolitan Hospital, often respond to price controls imposed by one payer by increasing charges to other payers with less restrictive policies on fees—a phenomenon known as cost shifting. The cost-shifting problem may be avoided when a uniform fee schedule is used by all payers (as in Germany) or by a single payer (as in Canada).
2. The quantity of services provided often surges when prices are strictly controlled, leading analysts to conclude that providers respond to fee controls by inducing higher use of services in order to maintain earnings (Bodenheimer, 2005).

Price controls have the appeal of being a relatively painless form of cost control insofar as they do not limit the quantity of services provided. However, variations in fee schedules may compromise access to care for certain populations; Medicaid fee-for-service rates to physicians are far below private insurance rates in most states, making it difficult for Medicaid patients to find private physicians who will accept Medicaid payment. In nations with uniform fee schedules, concerns have been voiced that ratcheting down of fees may result in "patient churning" (high volumes of brief visits), with a deterioration in quality of care and patient satisfaction.

Utilization (Quantity) Controls

Because the effectiveness of price controls may be limited by increases in quantity, payers need to consider methods for containing the actual use of services. As indicated in Table 12–1, there are a variety of methods for attempting to control use. We begin by examining

one strategy, changing the unit of payment, that we introduced in Chapter 4. We then describe additional mechanisms that attempt to restrain the quantity of services.

Changing the Unit of Payment

Dr. John Wiley is upset when the PPO reduces his fee from $125 to $110 per visit. In order to maintain his income, Dr. Wiley lengthens his day by half an hour so he can schedule more patient visits.

Dr. Jane Stuckey is angry when the HMO reduces her capitation payment from $35 to $30 per patient per month. She is unable to maintain her income by providing more visits because more patient visits do not bring her more money. She hopes that more HMO patients will enroll in her practice so that she can receive more capitation payments.

One simple way to get a handle on the quantity factor is by redefining the unit of payment. In Chapter 4, we discussed how services may be bundled into more aggregate units of payment, such as capitated physician payment, diagnosis-related group (DRG) episode-of-care hospital payment, and bundled payments that combine both physician and hospital payment for an episode of care.

The more aggregated the unit of payment, the more predictable the quantity tends to be. For example, in the case of Dr. Wiley receiving fee-for-service payment, there is a great potential for costs to rise due to increases in the number of physician visits, surgical procedures, and diagnostic tests. When the unit of payment is capitation, as in the case of Dr. Stuckey, the quantity factor is not the number of visits but rather the number of individuals enrolled in a practice or plan. From a health plan's perspective, the $C = P \times Q$ formula still applies when paying physicians by capitation, but now the P is the capitation fee and the Q is the number of individuals covered. Other than by raising birth rates, physicians have little discretion in inducing a higher volume of "quantities" at the capitation level for the health care system as a whole. Similarly, under global budgeting of hospitals, P represents the average global budget per hospital and Q is the number of hospitals.

Shifting payment to a more aggregated unit has obvious appeal as a way for payers to counter cost inflation due to the quantity factor. Life is never so simple, however. In Chapter 4, we discussed how more aggregate units of payment shift financial risk to providers of care. Another way of describing this shifting of risk is that one person's solution to the quantity problem becomes another person's new quantity problem. A hospital paid by global budget instead of by fee-for-service now must monitor its own internal quantities of service lest these quantities drive hospital operating costs over budget. To the extent that providers are unsuccessful in managing resources under more aggregated forms of payment, pressures mount to raise the prices paid at these more aggregated payment units.

Changes in policies for units of payment rarely occur independent of other reforms in cost-control strategies, making it difficult to isolate the specific effects of changing the unit of payment. For example, physician capitation usually occurs in the context of other organizational and cost-control features within a managed care plan. Group practice HMOs receiving capitation payments from employers and paying physicians by salary have been shown to reduce costs by reducing the quantity of services provided, in particular by reducing rates of hospitalization (Hellinger, 1996; Bodenheimer, 2005). Compared with group practice HMOs, network model HMOs (see Chapter 8), which often pay physicians fee-for-service, do not significantly control health care costs (Draper et al., 2002).

For hospitals, changing Medicare payments from a fee-for-service to an episode-of-care unit under the DRG-based system in 1983 resulted in a modest slowing of the rate of increase in Medicare Part A expenditures. However, hospitals were able to shift costs to private payers to make up for lower DRG revenues, and national health expenditures as a whole were not affected by Medicare's new payment mechanism (Rice, 1996). Medicare's use of bundled episode-based payments for physicians and hospitals is a more recent development. Bundled Medicare payments for a mixture of cardiovascular and orthopedic inpatient services found no cost reduction (Chen et al., 2018), but payments for hip or knee replacement surgery found modest reductions in cost without an increase in complications (Barnett et al., 2019). Global hospital budgeting in Canada has been a key element of that nation's relative success at containing hospital costs (Commonwealth Fund, 2016).

The health care system in Germany and in some Canadian provinces has countered the open-ended dynamic of fee-for-service payment by introducing global budgeting, called expenditure caps, for physician payment (Bodenheimer, 2005). Under Canadian expenditure caps, a budget is established for all physician services in a province. Although individual physicians continue to bill the provincial health plan on a fee-for-service basis, if increases in the use of services cause overall physician costs to exceed the budget, fees are reduced (or fee increases for the following year are sacrificed) to stay within the expenditure cap. Evidence from Canada suggests that implementation of expenditure caps was associated with stabilization of physician costs in the mid-1990s (Barer et al., 1996). In the United States, Medicare adopted a less-stringent version of an expenditure cap for physician fees, known as the "sustainable growth rate," that was abandoned in 2015 (Aaron, 2015). Expenditure caps for physician payments allow the payer to focus on the aggregate C part of the equation—in this case, the total physician budget. ACO shared savings programs, discussed in Chapter 4, are a related strategy attempting to provide a global expenditure feedback loop to modulate fee-for-service payments. A 2019 evaluation of the Medicare Shared Savings Program found that through 2014, the ACO program had not reduced costs nor improved quality (Markovitz et al., 2019). A separate review of Medicare, Medicaid, and private insurance ACO contracts found that they were associated with some reduction in hospital and emergency department use (Kaufman et al., 2019).

Patient Cost-Sharing

Randy Payton has an insurance policy with a $2,000 deductible and 20% copayment for all services; if he incurs medical expenses of $6,000, he pays the first $2,000 plus 20% of $4,000, for a total of $2,800.

Joseph Mednick's health plan requires that he pay $20 each time he fills a prescription for a medication, with the health plan paying the cost above $20; because he suffers from diabetes, hypertension, and coronary artery disease, copayments for his multiple medications cost him $1,200 per year.

Cost-sharing makes patients pay directly out of pocket for some portion of their health care and is a major cause of underinsurance (Chapter 3). In managed competition, cost-sharing occurs as part of the financing transaction *at the point of purchasing a health insurance plan*. In this section, we discuss the more traditional notion of cost-sharing—using deductibles, copayments, and uncovered services as part of the payment transaction to make patients pay a share of costs *at the point of receiving health care services*.

The primary intent of cost-sharing at the point of service is to discourage patient demand for services. (Cost-sharing also shifts some of the overall bill for health care from third party payers to individuals in the form of greater out-of-pocket expenses.) Cost-sharing at the point of service has been one of the few cost-containment devices subjected to the rigorous evaluation of a randomized controlled experiment (Chapter 3). In the Rand Health Insurance Experiment conducted in the 1970s, individuals were randomly assigned to health insurance plans with varying degrees of cost-sharing. Individuals with cost-sharing plans made about one-third fewer visits and were hospitalized one-third less often than individuals randomized to the plan with no cost-sharing (Newhouse et al., 1981).

Although the randomized controlled trial provides an excellent laboratory for scrutinizing the effect of a single cost-containment mechanism, analyses based on controlled research designs cannot be generalized to the real world of health policy. For example, the United States has a greater level of cost-sharing than many industrialized nations, but also the highest overall costs. Seventy percent of health care expenditures are incurred by 10% of the population—people who are extremely ill and generate huge costs through lengthy ICU stays and other major expenses. Cost-sharing has little influence over this component of care. Compared to the microworld of one not-very-sick patient deciding whether to spend some money on a physician visit, patient cost-sharing in the macro-world may remove only a thin slice from a large, expanding pie (Bodenheimer, 2005).

Patients were less likely to purchase needed medications under cost-sharing policies, for example Medicare Part D (see Chapter 2), leading to worse control of chronic illnesses and more emergency hospitalizations (Hsu et al., 2006; Goldman et al., 2007; Schneeweiss et al., 2009). Even small copayments were associated with reduced medication adherence in lower income, but not in higher income, populations (Aznar-Lou et al., 2018). These studies suggest that cost-sharing is not painless cost control.

Cost-sharing for emergency department care may reduce inappropriate use of emergency services without adversely affecting appropriate use or patient health outcomes. Cost-sharing may be a painless form of cost control when used in modest amounts, not applied to low-income patients, and designed to encourage patients to use lower-cost alternative sources of care (e.g., clinics instead of emergency departments) rather than to discourage use of services altogether.

Utilization Management

Thelma Graves suffers from a severe hyperthyroid condition. Before scheduling thyroid surgery, the physician has to call Ms. Graves' insurance company to obtain preauthorization, without which the insurer will not pay for the surgery.

Fred Brady is hospitalized for an acute myocardial infarction. The hospital contacts the utilization management firm for Mr. Brady's insurer, which authorizes 5 hospital days. On the fourth day, Mr. Brady develops a heart rate of 36 beats/min, requiring the insertion of a temporary pacemaker and prolonging the hospital stay for 10 extra days. After the fifth hospital day, Mr. Brady's physician has to call the utilization management (UM) firm every 2 days to justify why the insurer should continue to pay for the hospitalization.

Derek Jordan has type 1 diabetes and at age 42 becomes eligible for Medicare due to his permanent disability from complications of his diabetes. He is admitted to the hospital for treatment of a gangrenous toe. Under Medicare's DRG method of payment, the hospital receives the same payment for Derek's hospitalization regardless of whether it lasts 2 days or 12 days. Therefore, the hospital wants Derek's physician to discharge Derek as soon as possible. Each day, a hospital nurse reviews Derek's chart and suggests to the physician that Derek no longer requires acute hospitalization.

Utilization management (UM) involves the surveillance of and intervention in the clinical activities of physicians for the purpose of controlling costs (Grumbach & Bodenheimer, 1990). In contrast to cost-sharing, which attempts to influence patient behavior, UM seeks to influence physician behavior. The mechanism of influencing physician decisions is simple and direct: denial of payment for services deemed unnecessary.

UM is related to the unit of payment in the following way: Whoever is at financial risk (see Chapter 4) performs UM. Under fee-for-service reimbursement, insurance companies perform UM to reduce their payments to hospitals and physicians. The DRG system induces hospitals, at risk for losing money if their patients stay too long, to perform UM. Under an HMO capitation contract with a primary physician group, the physician group conducts UM so that it does not pay more to physicians than it receives in capitation payments. If an insurance plan pays a hospital a per diem rate, the insurer may send a UM nurse to the hospital each day to review whether the patient is ready to go home.

Micromanage, Inc., performs UM for several insurance companies. Each day, Rebecca Hasselbach reviews the charts of each patient hospitalized by these insurers to determine whether the patients might be ready for discharge. By pushing for early discharges, Ms. Hasselbach and her Micromanage colleagues around the country save their insurers about $1,000,000 each year. The annual cost of administering UM is $900,000.

There is little evidence that UM yields substantial savings, particularly when the overhead of administering the UM program is taken into account (Wickizer, 1990). UM would appear to be a painless form of cost control because it intends to selectively reduce inappropriate or unnecessary care. However, reviewers often make decisions on a case-by-case basis without explicit guidelines or criteria, with the result that decisions may be inconsistent both between different reviewers for the same case and among the same reviewer for different cases (Light, 1994).

UM has come under fire as a process of micromanagement of clinical decisions that intrudes into the physician–patient relationship and places an unwelcome administrative burden on physicians and other caregivers. Physicians in the United States have been called the most "second-guessed and paperwork-laden physicians in western industrialized democracies" (Lee

& Etheredge, 1989). Substantial physician time goes into appealing denials and persuading insurers about the appropriateness of services delivered.

Several approaches to UM have been developed that attempt to avoid some of the onerous features of case-by-case utilization review. Practice profiling, rather than focusing on individual cases, uses summary data on practice patterns to identify physicians whose overall use of services significantly deviates from the standards set by other physicians in the community. These outlier physicians can be made subject to strict UM monitoring with denials.

The strategy of "narrow networks" takes UM to its logical conclusion: denying any payments to providers with high-cost profiles by eliminating them from the insurer's provider network. Narrow network plan premiums are 6.7% less than premiums for broad network plans (Polsky et al., 2016). While narrow networks may control costs, a concern has arisen that the networks may lower health care quality by excluding high-quality providers (Corlette et al., 2014).

Supply Limits

Bob is a patient in the Canadian province of Alberta. He develops back pain and his family physician requests an MRI of his spine to rule out disk disease. His physician, who does not suspect a disk herniation, agrees to place him on the waiting list for an MRI, which for nonurgent cases is 5 months long.

Rob lives in Alberta, and after lifting an 80-lb load at work, experiences severe lower back pain radiating down his right leg. His family physician calls the radiologist and obtains an emergency MRI scan within 3 days.

Supply limits are controls on the number of physicians and other caregivers and on material resources such as the number of hospital beds or MRI scanners. Supply limits can take place within an organized delivery system in the United States, or for an entire geographic region such as a Canadian province.

The number of elective operations and invasive procedures, such as cardiac catheterization, performed per-capita increases with the per-capita supply of surgeons and cardiologists, respectively (Bodenheimer, 2005).

This phenomenon is sometimes called "supplier-induced demand" (Evans, 1984; Rice & Labelle, 1989; Phelps, 2003). Controlling physician supply may reduce the use of physician services and thereby contribute to cost containment.

Supplier-induced demand pertains to material capacity as well as to physician supply. Per-capita spending for fee-for-service Medicare patients is over twice as high in some regions of the United States than in others (Gawande, 2009, www.dartmouthatlas.org). This remarkable cost variation is not explained by differences in demographic characteristics of the population, prices of services, or levels of illness, but is due to the quantity of services provided. Residents of areas with a greater per-capita supply of hospital beds are up to 30% more likely to be hospitalized than those in areas with fewer beds (Fisher et al., 2000). The maxim that "empty beds tend to become filled" has been known as Roemer's law (Roemer & Shain, 1959). Conversely, strictly regulating the number of centers allowed to perform heart surgery establishes a limit for the total number of cardiac operations that can be performed. In situations of limited supply, physicians must determine which patients are most in need of the limited supply of services. Ideally, those truly in need gain access to appropriate services, with physicians possessing the wisdom to distinguish those patients truly in need (Rob) from those not requiring the service (Bob).

There are clear instances in which limitations of capacity restrain use. For example, international comparisons in 2013 demonstrate large variations in use of coronary revascularization procedures (coronary artery bypass surgery and angioplasty), with the United Kingdom's rate of these procedures only 57%, and Canada's 78%, of the US rate (OECD, 2013). These rates correspond to the degree to which these nations regulate (minimally in the case of the United States) the number of centers performing cardiac surgery. In spite of doing more procedures, US coronary heart disease mortality is slightly higher than that of the UK and Canada (OECD, 2013).

A "natural experiment" provides an illustration of how restricting the supply of a high cost resource may be implemented in a relatively painless manner for patients' clinical outcomes. A US hospital experiencing a nursing shortage abruptly reduced the number of staffed intensive care unit beds from 18 to 8 (Singer et al.,

1983). For patients admitted to the hospital for chest pain, physicians became more selective in admitting to the intensive care unit only those patients who actually suffered heart attacks. Limiting the use of ICU beds did not result in any adverse health outcomes for patients admitted to nonintensive care unit beds, including those few nonintensive care unit patients who actually sustained heart attacks. This study suggests that when faced with supply limits, physicians may be able to prioritize patients on clinical grounds in a manner that selectively reduces unnecessary services. Establishing supply limits that require physicians to prioritize services represents a very different (and less intrusive) approach to containing costs than UM, which relies on external parties to authorize or deny individual services in a setting of unconstrained capacity.

Controlling the Type of Supply

A specific form of supply control is regulation of the *types* (rather than the total number) of providers. Chapter 7 explored the balance between the number of generalist and specialist physicians in a health care system. Increasing the proportion of generalists may yield savings for two reasons. First, generalists earn lower incomes than specialists. Second, generalists practice a less resource-intensive style of medicine and generate lower overall health care expenditures (Bodenheimer & Grumbach, 2007).

CONCLUSION

In the real world, cost-containment strategies are applied not as isolated phenomena in a static system, but as an array of policies concerned with modes of financing, organization of health care delivery, and cost control all mixed together. Managed care is a strategy that utilizes a mixture of cost-control mechanisms: changing the unit of payment, utilization management, price discounts, and in some cases supply controls. The Canadian health care system (see Chapter 15) also relies on regulation of prices, global budgets and supply controls.

There is no perfect mechanism for controlling health care costs. Strategies must be judged by their relative success at containing costs and doing so in as painless a manner as possible—without compromising health outcomes. In the view of Dr. John Wennberg, the key to cost control in the United States.

is not in the micromanagement of the doctor–patient relationship but the management of capacity and budgets. The American problem is to find the will to set the supply thermostat somewhere within reason (Wennberg, 1990).

Although US-managed care plans and Canadian provincial health plans are often viewed as diametrically opposed paradigms for health care reform, both the Canadian plans and US group practice HMOs base their cost-control approaches on what Wennberg terms "the management of capacity and budgets." In Canada, this management is under public control through regulation of physician supply, physician and hospital budgets, and technology. In the United States, private group practice HMOs adjust their own "thermostats" by setting their own budgets and numbers of physicians, hospital beds, and high-cost equipment.

If there is a lesson to be learned from attempts to control health care costs in the United States over the past decades, it is that cost-containment policies affecting provider payment need to focus more on macromanagement and less on micromanagement. Trying to manage costs at the level of individual patient encounters (i.e., regulating fees for each service, reviewing daily practice decisions, or imposing cost-sharing for every prescription and physician visit) is a cumbersome and largely ineffectual strategy for containing overall expenditures. Moreover, one payer lowering its costs by shifting expenses to another payer does not produce systemwide cost savings. Those systems that have been most successful in moderating the inexorable increase in health care costs have tended to emphasize global cost-containment tools, such as paying by capitation or other aggregate units, limiting the size and specialty mix of the physician workforce, and concentrating high-technology services in regional centers. The future debate over cost containment in the United States will center on whether these cost-containment tools are best wielded by private health care plans operating in the health care market or by public regulation of health care providers and suppliers.

REFERENCES

Aaron HJ. Three cheers for logrolling–the demise of the SGR. *N Engl J Med.* 2015;372(21):1977–1979.

American Medical Association. Competition in Health Insurance. 2020. https://www.ama-assn.org/system/files/2020-10/competition-health-insurance-us-markets.pdf.

Anderson GF, Hussey P, Petrosyan V. It's still the prices, stupid: why the US spends so much on health care and a tribute to Uwe Reinhardt. *Health Aff (Millwood).* 2019;38:87–95.

Aznar-Lou I, Pottegård A, Fernández A, et al. Effect of copayment policies on initial medication non-adherence according to income: a population-based study. *BMJ Qual Saf.* 2018;27:878–891.

Barer ML, Lomas J, Sanmartin C. Re-minding our Ps and Qs: cost controls in Canada. *Health Aff (Millwood).* 1996;15(2):216–234.

Barnett ML, Wilcock A, McWilliams JM, et al. Two-year evaluation of mandatory bundled payments for joint replacement. *N Engl J Med.* 2019;380:252–262.

Bodenheimer T. High and rising health care costs. *Ann Intern Med.* 2005;142:847–854, 932, 996.

Bodenheimer T, Grumbach K. Improving primary care. *Strategies and Tools for a Better Practice.* New York, NY: McGraw-Hill; 2007.

Chen LM, Ryan AM, Shih T, Thumma JR, Dimick JB. Medicare's acute care episode demonstration: effects of bundled payments on costs and quality of surgical care. *Health Serv Res.* 2018;53:632–648.

Claxton G, DiJulio B, Whitmore H, et al. Health benefits in 2010. *Health Aff (Millwood).* 2010;29:1942–1950.

Claxton G, Rae M, Long M, Damico A, Whitmore H. Health benefits in 2018: modest growth in premiums, higher worker contributions at firms with more low-wage workers. *Health Aff (Millwood).* 2018;37:1892–1900.

Claxton G, Rae M, Damico A, Wager E, Young G, Whitmore H. Health benefits in 2022: premiums remain steady. *Health Aff (Millwood).* 2022;41:1670–1680.

Commonwealth Fund. International Profiles of Health Care Systems 2015, January 2016. https://www.commonwealthfund.org/publications/fund-reports/2016/jan/international-profiles-health-care-systems-2015.

Corlette S, Volk JA, Berenson R, Feder J. Narrow provider networks in new health plans: balancing affordability with access to quality care. Georgetown University Health Policy Institute, 2014. https://www.urban.org/sites/default/files/publication/22601/413135-Narrow-Provider-Networks-in-New-Health-Plans.PDF.

Draper DA, Hurley RE, Lesser CS, Strunk BC. The changing face of managed care. *Health Aff (Millwood).* 2002;21:11–23.

Enthoven AC. Employment-based health insurance is failing: now what? *Health Aff (Millwood).* 2003;(suppl web exclusives):W3–W237.

Evans RG. *Strained Mercy: The Economics of Canadian Health Care.* Toronto, Ontario, Canada: Butterworths; 1984.

Fisher ES, Wennberg JE, Stukel TA, et al. Associations among hospital capacity, utilization, and mortality of U.S. Medicare beneficiaries, controlling for sociodemographic factors. *Health Serv Res.* 2000;34:1351–1362.

Gawande A. The cost conundrum. *The New Yorker*. June 1, 2009.

Goldman DP, Joyce GF, Zheng Y. Prescription drug cost sharing: associations with medication and medical utilization and spending and health. *JAMA*. 2007;298:61–69.

Grumbach K, Bodenheimer T. Reins or fences: a physician's view of cost containment. *Health Aff (Millwood)*. 1990;9(3):120–126.

Hellinger FJ. The impact of financial incentives on physician behavior in managed care plans: a review of the evidence. *Med Care Res Rev*. 1996;53:294.

Hsu J, Price M, Huang J, et al. Unintended consequences of caps on Medicare drug benefits. *N Engl J Med*. 2006;354:2349.

Kaufman BG, Spivack BS, Stearns SC, Song PH, O'Brien EC. Impact of Accountable Care Organizations on utilization, care and outcomes: a systematic review. *Med Care Res Rev*. 2019;76:255–290.

Klein E. 21 graphs that show America's health-care prices are ludicrous. *Washington Post Blog*. March 26, 2013. http://www.washingtonpost.com/blogs/wonkblog/wp/2013/03/26/21-graphs-that-show-americas-health-care-prices-are-ludicrous/.

Lechner AE, Gourevitch R, Ginsburg PB. The potential of reference pricing to generate health care savings: lessons from a California pioneer. Research Brief No. 30, 2013. Center for Studying Health System Change. http://www.hschange.org/CONTENT/1397/1397.pdf.

Lee PR, Etheredge L. Clinical freedom: two lessons for the UK from US experience with privatisation of health care. *Lancet*. 1989;1:263–265.

Light DW. Life, death, and the insurance companies. *N Engl J Med*. 1994;330:498–500.

Markovitz AA, Hollingsworth JM, Ayanian JZ, Norton EC, Yan PL, Ryan AM. Performance in the Medicare Shared Savings Program after accounting for nonrandom exit. *Ann Intern Med*. 2019;171(1):27–36.

Mehrotra A, Grier S, Dudley RA. The relationship between health plan advertising and market incentives: evidence of risk-selective behavior. *Health Aff (Millwood)*. 2006;25:759–765.

Mehrotra A, Schleifer D, Shefrin A, Ducas AM. Defining the goals of health care price transparency. *NEJM Catalyst*, June 26, 2018.

Newhouse JP, Manning WG, Morris CN, et al. Some interim results from a controlled trial of cost sharing in health insurance. *N Engl J Med*. 1981;305:1501–1507.

OECD. Health at a glance 2013. Organization for Economic Cooperation and Development, 2013. www.oecd.org/els/health-systems/Health-at-a-Glance-2013.pdf.

Phelps CE. *Health Economics*. Boston, MA: Addison Wesley; 2003.

Polsky D, Cidav Z, Swanson A. Marketplace plans with narrow physician networks feature lower monthly premiums than plans with larger networks. *Health Aff (Millwood)*. 2016;35:1842–1848.

Rice TH. Containing health care costs. In: Andersen RM, Rice TH, Kominski GF, eds. *Changing the U.S. Health Care System*. San Francisco, CA: Jossey-Bass; 1996.

Rice TH, Labelle RJ. Do physicians induce demand for medical services? *J Health Polit Policy Law*. 1989;14:587–600.

Roemer MI, Shain M. *Hospital Utilization Under Insurance*. Chicago, IL: American Hospital Association; 1959.

Schneeweiss S, Patrick AR, Pedan A, et al. The effect of Medicare Part D coverage on drug use and cost sharing among seniors without prior drug benefits. *Health Aff (Millwood)*. 2009;28:w305–w316.

Singer DE, Carr PL, Mulley AG, Thibault GE. Rationing intensive care: physician responses to a resource shortage. *N Engl J Med*. 1983;309:1155–1160.

Wennberg JE. Outcomes research, cost containment, and the fear of health care rationing. *N Engl J Med*. 1990;323:1202–1204.

Wickizer TM. The effect of utilization review on hospital use and expenditures: a review of the literature and an update on recent findings. *Med Care Rev*. 1990;47:327–363.

Quality of Health Care

Each year in the United States, millions of people visit hospitals, physicians, and other caregivers and receive medical care of superb quality. But that's not the whole story. Many patients' interactions with the health care system fall short (Institute of Medicine, 2001). A prominent Institute of Medicine report (2001) concluded that between what we *know* and what we *do* lies not just a gap, but a chasm. A 2016 study estimated that over 250,000 people each year die as a result of preventable medical errors in hospitals, meaning that medical errors are the third leading cause of death in the United States (Makary & Daniel, 2016). A Medicare patient has a 1 in 4 chance of experiencing injury, harm, or death when admitted to a hospital (The Leapfrog Group, 2018).

As of 2020, concerted efforts had reduced medication errors, falls, and infections in hospital settings, and new requirements were holding health care organizations accountable for quality. Yet serious inequities exist, affecting minority and low-income populations (Dzau & Shine, 2020).

Hospitals vary greatly in their risk-adjusted mortality rates for Medicare patients; during 2009 to 2012, risk-adjusted deaths from heart failure and pneumonia were three times higher for lower-quality compared with higher-quality hospitals (Medicare Hospital Quality Chartbook, 2013). A previous study showed that if low-quality hospitals reduced mortality rates to the level of high-quality hospitals, 17,000 to 21,000 fewer deaths per year would have occurred (Schoen et al., 2006).

Outpatient care also has quality problems. A 2003 study found that adults in the United States received just over half of recommended health services (McGlynn et al., 2003). A 2016 follow-up concluded, "Despite more than a decade of efforts, the clinical quality of outpatient care delivered to American adults has not consistently improved" (Levine et al., 2016). Medication errors are the third leading cause of death in the United States and cause injury to an estimated 1.3 million people annually (Hodkinson et al., 2020). In some primary care practices, patients are not informed about abnormal laboratory results more than 20% of the time (Casalino et al., 2009).

Two million lives would have been saved in 2006 if preventive services had been regularly delivered to the entire population (Maciosek et al., 2010). Only 53% of people with hypertension are adequately treated (Yoon et al., 2015) and only 14% of people with diabetes meet their targets for glycemic, blood pressure, and cholesterol control (American Diabetes Association, 2019). Racial and ethnic minority patients experience an inferior quality of care compared with White patients (US Department of Health and Human Services, 2018).

Chassin and Loeb (2011) summarized, "Health care quality and safety today are best characterized as showing pockets of excellence on specific measures or in particular services .... The pockets of excellence ... coexist with enormously variable performance across the delivery system."

The quality chasm described in the 2001 Institute of Medicine report remains a fundamental concern. In this chapter we will examine the factors affecting quality and then explore what can be done to elevate all health care to the highest possible level.

THE COMPONENTS OF HIGH-QUALITY CARE

High-quality health care assists healthy people to stay healthy, cures acute illnesses, and allows chronically ill people to live as long and fulfilling a life as possible. What are the components of high-quality health care (Table 13–1)?

▶ Adequate Access to Care

Lydia and Laura were friends at a rural high school; both became pregnant. Lydia's middle-class parents took her to a nearby obstetrician, while Laura, from a lower income family, could not find a physician who would take Medicaid. Lydia became the mother of a healthy infant, but Laura, going without prenatal care, delivered a low–birth-weight baby with severe lung problems.

People with reduced access to care suffer worse health outcomes in comparison to those enjoying full access—the quality problem of underuse (see Chapter 3). Quality requires equality of access (Schiff et al., 1994). Access is impacted by insurance, having a sufficient number of health care providers, cultural and linguistic concordance, and distance. For some health needs, the challenge of distance may be overcome by telehealth, which may alleviate the need to find transportation or take time off work or school (Meyer et al., 2020). However, access to stable internet and experience using digital platforms are not universal, and data from the COVID-19 pandemic has shown that increased use of telehealth can increase inequities for non-English speakers, rural populations, people of color, older people, and people with limited resources. Digital navigators to help people overcome the digital divide could help enable access to care (Rodriguez et al., 2023).

▶ Adequate Scientific Knowledge

Brigitte Levy, a professor of family law, was started on estrogen replacement in 1960 when she reached menopause. Her physician prescribed the hormone pills for 10 years. In 1979, she was diagnosed with invasive cancer of the uterus, which spread to her entire abdominal cavity in spite of surgical treatment and radiation. She died in 1980 at age 68, at the height of her career.

A body of knowledge must exist that informs physicians what to do for the patient's problem. If clear scientific knowledge fails to distinguish between effective and ineffective or harmful care, quality may be compromised. During the 1960s, medical science taught that estrogen replacement, without the administration of progestins, was safe. Sadly, cases of uterine cancer caused by estrogen replacement did not show up until many years later. Brigitte Levy's physician was relying on inadequate scientific knowledge.

▶ Competent Health Care Providers

Ceci Yu, age 77, was waking up at night with shortness of breath and wheezing. Her physician told her she had asthma and prescribed albuterol, a bronchodilator. Two days later, Ms. Yu was admitted to the coronary care unit with a heart attack. Her physician had misdiagnosed the wheezing of congestive heart failure and had treated Ms. Yu incorrectly for asthma. The bronchodilator treatment may have precipitated the heart attack.

Where an adequate body of knowledge exists, the clinician must have the skills to diagnose problems and choose appropriate treatments. An inadequate level of competence resulted in poor quality care for Ms. Yu. Medical injuries can be classified as negligent or not negligent.

Jack was given a prescription for a sulfa drug. When he took the first pill, he turned beet red, began to wheeze, and fell to the floor. Jack was

Table 13–1. Components of high-quality health care

Access to care
Adequate scientific knowledge
Competent health care providers
Separation of financial and clinical decisions
Organization of health care institutions to maximize quality

*treated in the emergency department for anaphy-
lactic shock, a potentially fatal allergic reaction.
The emergency medicine physician learned that
Jack had developed a rash the last time he took
sulfa. Jack's physician had never asked him if he
was allergic to sulfa, and Jack did not realize that
the prescription contained sulfa.*

*Mack was prescribed a sulfa drug, following which
he developed anaphylactic shock. Before writing
the prescription, Mack's physician asked whether
he had a sulfa allergy. Mack had said "No."*

Medical negligence is defined as failure to meet the
standard of practice of an average qualified physician
practicing in the same specialty. Jack's drug reaction
would be considered negligence, while Mack's was not.
Of the medical injuries discovered in the 1984 Harvard
Malpractice Study, 28% resulted from negligence. In
those injuries that led to death, 51% involved negligence. The most common injuries were drug reactions
(19%) and wound infections (14%). Eight percent of
injuries involved failure to diagnose a condition, of
which 75% were negligent. Seventy percent of patients
suffering all forms of medical injury recovered completely in 6 months or less, but 47% of patients in
whom a diagnosis was missed suffered serious disabilities (Brennan et al., 1991; Leape et al., 1991).

Negligence cannot be equated with incompetence.
Any good health care professional may have a mental
lapse, may be overtired after a long night in the intensive care unit, or may have failed to learn an important
new research finding.

Money and Quality of Care

*Nina Brown, a 56-year-old woman with diabe-
tes, arrived at her primary care physician's office
complaining of chest pain over the past month.
Her physician examined Ms. Brown, performed
an electrocardiogram (ECG), which showed no
abnormalities, diagnosed musculoskeletal pain,
and recommended ibuprofen. Five minutes later
in the parking lot, Ms. Brown collapsed of a heart
attack.*

*Completely healthy at age 45, Henry Fung reluc-
tantly submitted to a treadmill exercise test at
the local YMCA. The study was inconclusive and*

*Mr. Fung, who had fee-for-service insurance,
sought the advice of a cardiologist. The cardiologist
knew that treadmill tests are sometimes positive in
healthy people. Yet he ordered a coronary angiogram, which was perfectly normal. Three hours
after the study, a clot formed in the femoral artery
at the site of the catheter insertion, and emergency
surgery was required to save Mr. Fung's leg.*

The quantity and quality of medical care are inextricably interrelated. Too much or too little can be injurious.
No one can know for certain what motivated the physician to send Ms. Brown home when unstable coronary
heart disease was one possible diagnosis (underuse);
nor can one be sure what led the fee-for-service cardiologist to perform an invasive coronary angiogram of
questionable appropriateness on Mr. Fung (overuse).
One factor that bears close attention is the impact of
financial considerations on the quantity (and thus the
quality) of medical care (Relman, 2007). As noted in
Chapter 4, fee-for-service payment encourages physicians to perform more services, whereas capitation
payments are sometimes structured to reward those
who perform fewer services.

More than 50 years ago, Bunker (1970) found that
the United States performed twice the number of surgical procedures per capita than Great Britain. He postu-
lated that this difference could be accounted for by the
greater number of surgeons per capita in the United
States and concluded that "the method of payment
appears to play an important, if unmeasured, part."
Most surgeons in the United States are compensated by
fee-for-service, whereas most in Great Britain are paid
a salary. An analysis of the National Practitioner Data
Base suggests that 10% to 20% of all surgeries in several
specialties are unnecessary (Eisler & Hansen, 2013).

Back surgery provides one case study. Even though
surgery for lumbar spine disc disease often has poorer
outcomes than medications and physical therapy, such
surgeries more than doubled from 2000 to 2009 in
the United States (Yoshihara & Yoneoka, 2015). From
2002 to 2007, Medicare patients undergoing surgery
for lumbar spinal stenosis experienced a doubling of
complex rather than simple operations resulting in a
major increase in surgical complications, rehospital-
izations, and costs. Rates of reoperation (because of
worsening pain) are high. Payment for this procedure

is greater than that provided for most other procedures performed by orthopedists and neurosurgeons (Deyo et al., 2004, 2010), which may be a driver of this excess.

Moving to the other side of the overuse–underuse spectrum, payment by capitation, or salaried employment by a for-profit business, may create a climate hostile to the provision of adequate services. In the 1970s, a series of HMOs called prepaid health plans (PHPs) sprang up to provide care to California Medicaid patients. The PHPs received a lump sum for each patient enrolled, meaning that the lower the cost of the services actually provided, the greater the PHP's profits (US Senate, 1975). The quality of care in several PHPs became a major scandal in California. At one PHP, administrators wrote a message to health care providers: "Do as little as you possibly can for the PHP patient," and charts audited by the California Health Department revealed many instances of undertreatment. More recent approaches to capitation payment have attempted to mitigate incentives for undertreatment by requiring providers to achieve quality of care targets and risk-adjusting capitation payments, with payments for patients at greater risk for needing medical services higher than payments for low-risk patients.

It was a nice dinner, hosted by the hospital radiologist and paid for by the company manufacturing magnetic resonance imaging (MRI) scanners. After the meal came the pitch: "If you physicians invest money, we can get an MRI scanner near our hospital; if the MRI makes money, you all share in the profits." One internist explained later, "After I put in my $10,000, it was hard to resist ordering MRI scans. With headaches, back pain, and knee problems, the indications for MRIs are kind of fuzzy. You might order one or you might not. Now, I do."

Another threat to quality of care arises from conflicts of interest. Relman (2007) writes about the commercialization of medicine: "The introduction of new technology in the hands of specialists, expanded insurance coverage, and unregulated fee-for-service payments all combined to rapidly increase the flow of money into the health care system, and thus sowed the seeds of a new, profit-driven industry."

During the 1980s, many physicians formed partnerships and joint ventures, giving them part ownership in laboratories, MRI scanners, and outpatient surgicenters. By 1990, 93% of diagnostic imaging facilities, 76% of ambulatory surgery centers, and 60% of clinical laboratories in Florida were owned wholly or in part by physicians. In a national study, physicians who received payment for performing x-rays and sonograms within their own offices obtained these examinations four times as often as physicians who referred the examinations to radiologists and received no payment for the studies (Hillman et al., 1990). Physicians who acquire MRI equipment order substantially more scans once they are able to bill for the imaging procedure (Baker, 2010). Surgeons who own and profit from ambulatory surgical centers operate more frequently than those who do not (Morgan et al., 2015).

Profitable diagnostic, imaging, and surgical procedures have rapidly migrated from the hospital to free-standing physician-owned ambulatory surgery centers, endoscopy centers, and imaging centers, with rapid increases in the number of tests and procedures performed (Berenson et al., 2006). The number of CT scans performed for Medicare patients increased by 300% from 1997 to 2017; 30% to 50% may be unnecessary, increasing patients' risk of radiation-induced cancer (Smith-Bindman, 2018).

▶ Health Care Systems and Quality of Care

The personnel cutbacks were terrible; staffing had diminished from four RNs per shift to two, with only two aides to provide assistance. Shelley Rush, RN, was barely able to administer the medications, including five insulin injections, with complicated dosing schedules. A family member rushed to the nursing station saying, "The lady in my mother's room looks bad." Shelley ran in and found the patient unconscious. She quickly checked the blood sugar, which was disastrously low at 20 mg/dL. Shelley gave 50% glucose, and the patient woke up. Then it hit her—she had injected the insulin into the wrong patient.

Health care institutions must be well organized, with an adequate number of competent staff. Shelley Rush was a superb nurse, but understaffing caused her to make a serious error. Nurse understaffing is associated with higher hospital mortality rates (McHugh et al., 2021).

The book *Curing Health Care* by Berwick et al. (1990) opens with a heartbreaking case:

She died, but she didn't have to. The senior resident was sitting, near tears, in the drab office behind the nurses' station in the intensive care unit. It was 2:00 AM, and he had been battling for 32 hours to save the life of the 23-year-old graduate student who had just suffered her final cardiac arrest.

*"Routine screening chest x-ray, taken 10 months ago. The tumor is right there, and it was curable—then. By the time the second film was taken 8 months later, because she was complaining of pain, it was too late. The tumor had spread everywhere, and the odds were hopelessly against her. We missed our chance. She missed her chance."
Exhausted, the resident put his head in his hands and cried.*

Two months later, the Quality Assurance Committee completed its investigation.... "We find the inpatient care commendable in this tragic case," concluded the brief report, "although the failure to recognize the tumor in a potentially curable stage 10 months earlier was unfortunate. . . . " Nowhere in this report was it written explicitly why the results of the first chest x-ray had not been translated into action. No one knew.

One year later . . . it was 2:00 AM, and the night custodian was cleaning the radiologist's office. As he moved a filing cabinet aside to sweep behind it, he glimpsed a dusty tan envelope that had been stuck between the cabinet and the wall. The envelope contained a yellow radiology report slip, and the date on the report—nearly 2 years earlier—convinced the custodian that this was, indeed, garbage.... He tossed it in with the other trash, and 4 hours later it was incinerated along with other useless things.

This patient may have had perfect access to care for an illness whose treatment is scientifically proved; she saw a physician who knew how to make the diagnosis and deliver the appropriate treatment; and yet the quality of her care was disastrously deficient. Dozens of people and hundreds of processes influence the care of one person with one illness. In her case, one person—perhaps a file clerk with a near-perfect record in handling thousands of radiology reports—lost track of one report, and the physician's office had no system to monitor whether or not x-ray reports had been received. The result was the most tragic of quality failures—the unnecessary death of a young person.

Oliver Hart lived in a city with a population of 80,000. He was admitted to Neighborhood Hospital with congestive heart failure caused by a defective mitral valve. He was told he needed semiurgent heart surgery to replace the valve. The cardiologist said "You can go to University Hospital 30 miles away or have the surgery done here." The cardiologist did not say that Neighborhood Hospital performed only seven cardiac surgeries last year. Mr. Hart elected to remain for the procedure. During the surgery, a key piece of equipment failed, and he died on the operating table.

Quality of care must be viewed in the context of regional systems of care (see Chapter 8), not simply within each health care institution. Hospitals performing more surgical procedures have lower mortality rates for that surgical procedure (Gonzalez et al., 2014). In addition, surgeons performing more procedures have better outcomes (Morche et al., 2016). Had Mr. Hart been told the relative surgical mortality rates at University Hospital, which performed 500 cardiac surgeries each year, and at Neighborhood Hospital, he would have chosen to be transferred 30 miles down the road.

The Components of Quality: Summary

Good-quality care can be compromised at a number of steps along the way.

Angie Roth has coronary heart disease and may need CABG surgery. (1) If she is uninsured or cannot get to a physician, high-quality care is impossible to obtain. (2) If clear evidence-based guidelines do not exist regarding who benefits from CABG and who does not, Ms. Roth's physician may make the wrong choice. (3) Even if clear guidelines exist, if Angie Roth's physician fails to evaluate her illness correctly or sends her to a surgeon with poor operative skills, quality may suffer. (4) If indications for surgery are not clear in Ms. Roth's case but the surgeon will benefit economically from the procedure, the surgery may be inappropriately performed. (5) Even if the surgery is appropriate and performed by an excellent surgeon, faulty equipment in the operating room or poor teamwork among the operating room surgeons, anesthesiologists, and nurses may lead to a poor outcome.

The 2001 Quality Chasm report conceptualized six core dimensions of quality: safe, effective, patient-centered, timely, efficient, and equitable. These dimensions, defined in greater detail in Table 13–2, are consistent with the components of quality discussed earlier.

PROPOSALS FOR IMPROVING QUALITY

▷ Traditional Quality Assurance: Licensure, Accreditation, and Peer Review

Traditionally, the health care system has placed great reliance on educational institutions and licensing and accrediting agencies to ensure the competence of individuals and institutions in health care. Health care professionals undergo rigorous training and pass special licensing examinations intended to ensure that caregivers have at least a basic level of knowledge and competence. However, clinicians may have been competent practitioners at the time they took their examinations, but their skills lapsed or they developed impairment

Table 13–2. Quality aims as defined by the Institute of Medicine

- *Safe*—avoiding injuries to patients from the care that is intended to help them
- *Effective*—providing services based on scientific knowledge to all who could benefit and refraining from providing services not likely to benefit (avoiding underuse and overuse, respectively)
- *Patient-centered*—providing care that is respectful of and responsive to individual patient preferences, needs, and values and ensuring that patient values guide all clinical decisions
- *Timely*—reducing waits and harmful delays
- *Efficient*—avoiding waste, including waste of equipment, supplies, ideas, and energy
- *Equitable*—providing care that does not vary in quality because of personal characteristics such as gender, ethnicity, geographic location, and socioeconomic status

Source: Institute of Medicine. *Crossing the Quality Chasm: A New Health System for the 21st Century.* Washington, DC: National Academies Press; 2001.

from alcohol or drug use, depression, or other conditions (Leape & Fromson, 2006). Many organizations that confer specialty board certification require physicians to pass examinations on a periodic basis.

The traditional approach to quality assurance has also relied heavily on physician self-regulation. Peer review is the evaluation by health care practitioners of the appropriateness and quality of services performed by other practitioners, usually in the same specialty (Edwards, 2018). Medicare anointed the Joint Commission on Accreditation of Hospitals (now named the Joint Commission) with the authority to terminate hospitals from the Medicare program if quality of care was found to be deficient. The traditional quality assurance strategies of licensing and peer review have not been effective tools (Chassin & Baker, 2015). Peer review often adheres to the theory of bad apples, attempting to discipline physicians (to remove them from the apple barrel) for mistakes rather than to improve their practice through education. With the hundreds of decisions physicians make each day, often in time-constrained situations, serious errors are relatively common in medical practice. One-third of physicians surveyed in 2009 did not agree with disclosing serious errors to patients and 20% had not disclosed errors to their patients (Iezzoni et al., 2012).

Even if sanctions against the truly bad apples had more teeth, these measures would not solve the quality problem. Removing the incontrovertibly bad apples from the barrel does not address all the quality problems that emanate from competent caregivers who are not performing optimally. Health care systems do need to forcefully sanction caregivers who, despite efforts at remediation, cannot operate at a basic standard of acceptable practice. But measures are also needed to "shift the curve" of overall clinical practice to a higher level of quality, not just to trim off the poor-quality outliers. Efforts are underway to formalize standards of care using clinical practice guidelines and to move from individual case review to more systematic monitoring of overall practice patterns (Table 13–3).

▷ Clinical Practice Guidelines

Dr. Denise Drier learned about urinary incontinence in family medicine residency but did not feel secure about caring for the problem. On the

Table 13–3. Proposals for improving quality

Licensure, accreditation, peer review
Clinical practice guidelines
Measuring practice patterns
Continuous quality improvement
Electronic Health Records
Artificial intelligence
Interdisciplinary teams
Public reporting of quality
Pay for performance
Balancing payment incentives

web, she found "Urinary Incontinence in Adults: Clinical Practice Guideline Update." She studied the material and applied it to her incontinence patients. After a few successes, she and the patients were feeling better about themselves.

Clinical practice guidelines make specific recommendations to physicians on how to treat clinical conditions such as diabetes, osteoporosis, or urinary incontinence. However, many guidelines are unreliable and tainted by monetary interests (Graham et al., 2011). Moreover, guidelines developed based on research on a narrowly defined population, such as adult patients with a single chronic condition, may not be applicable to different patient populations, such as older patients with multiple diseases (Boyd et al., 2005). The US Preventive Services Task Force and other respected professional organizations seek to improve the quality of clinical guidelines by applying rigorous and objective review of scientific evidence.

In 2012, the American Board of Internal Medicine Foundation and Consumer Reports launched the Choosing Wisely campaign, which called on professional societies and health care providers to reduce the unnecessary and potentially harmful health services that cost about $200 billion in wasteful spending in the United States in 2011 (www.choosingwisely.org). Choosing Wisely can be effective in reducing low-value care (Cliff et al., 2021).

Practice guidelines are not appropriate for many clinical situations. Uncertainty pervades clinical medicine, and practice guidelines are applicable only for those cases in which we enjoy "islands of knowledge in our seas of ignorance." Practice guidelines can assist but not replace clinical judgment in the quest for high-quality care.

Pedro Urrutia, age 59, was waking up frequently to urinate. His friend had prostate cancer, and he became concerned. The urologist said that his prostate was only slightly enlarged, and surgery was not needed. Mr. Urrutia wanted surgery and found another urologist to do it.

At age 82, James Chin was waking up at night and having difficulty urinating. He had two glasses of wine on his wife's birthday and later that night was unable to urinate. He went to the emergency department, was found to have a large prostate without nodules, and was catheterized. The urologist strongly recommended a transurethral resection of the prostate. Mr. Chin refused, thinking that the urinary retention was caused by the alcohol. Five years later, he was in good health with his prostate intact.

Some, like Mr. Urrutia, want prostate surgery, even though it is not needed; others, like Mr. Chin, have strong indications for surgery but do not want it. Practice guidelines must take into account not only scientific data, but also patient preferences (Montori et al., 2013).

Measuring Practice Patterns

Quality improvement requires systematic monitoring of how well individual caregivers, institutions, and organizations are performing. Two types of indicators used to evaluate clinical performance are process measures and outcome measures. *Process* of care refers to the types of services delivered by caregivers. Examples are prescribing aspirin to patients with coronary heart disease or turning immobile patients in hospital beds on a regular schedule to prevent bed sores. *Outcomes*—e.g., death, symptoms, physical functioning, laboratory studies, and health status—are the gold standard for measuring quality. However, outcomes (particularly those dealing with quality of life) may be difficult to measure. More easily counted outcomes such as mortality may be rare events, and therefore uninformative for evaluating quality of care for many conditions that are not immediately life-threatening. Also, outcomes may be heavily influenced by the underlying severity of illness and related patient characteristics, and not just by the quality of health care that patients received (King, 2016). When measuring patient outcomes, it is necessary to "risk adjust" these outcome measurements for differences in the underlying characteristics of different groups of patients. Because of these challenges in using outcomes as measures to monitor quality of care, process measures are commonly used. For process measures to be valid indicators of quality, there must be solid research demonstrating that the processes do in fact influence patient outcomes.

Dr. Susan Cutter felt horrible. It was supposed to have been a routine hysterectomy. Somehow she had inadvertently lacerated the large intestine of the patient, a 45-year-old woman with symptomatic fibroids of the uterus but otherwise in good health prior to surgery. After a protracted battle in the ICU the patient died of septic shock.

Dr. Cutter met with the Chief of Surgery at her hospital. The Chief reviewed the case with Dr. Cutter, but also pulled out a report showing the statistics on all of Dr. Cutter's surgical cases over the previous 5 years. The report showed that Dr. Cutter's mortality and complication rates were among the lowest of surgeons on the hospital's staff. However, the Chief did note that another surgeon, Dr. Dehisce, had a complication rate that was much higher than that of all the other staff surgeons. The Chief of Surgery asked Dr. Cutter to serve on a departmental committee to review Dr. Dehisce's cases and to meet with Dr. Dehisce to consider ways to address his poor performance.

The contemporary approach to quality monitoring moves beyond examining a few isolated cases toward measuring processes or outcomes for a large population of patients. Reviewing an individual case may help a surgeon and the operating team understand where errors may have occurred—a process known as "root cause" analysis. However, it does not indicate whether the case represented an aberrant bad outcome for a surgeon or team that usually has good surgical outcomes, or whether the case is indicative of more widespread

problems. To answer these questions requires examining data on all the patients operated on by the surgeon and the operating team to measure the overall rate of surgical complications, and having benchmark data that indicate whether this rate is higher than expected for similar types of patients.

▶ Continuous Quality Improvement (CQI)

In LDS Hospital in Salt Lake City, variation in wound infection rates by different surgeons was related to the timing of the administration of prophylactic antibiotics. Patients who received antibiotics 2 hours before surgery had the lowest infection rates. The surgery department adopted a policy that all patients receive antibiotics precisely 2 hours before surgery; the rate of postoperative wound infections dropped from 1.8% to 0.9%. (Burke, 2001)

Maximizing excellence for individual health care professionals is only one ingredient in the recipe for high-quality health care. Improving institutions is the other, through CQI—the identification of concrete problems and the formation of interdisciplinary teams to gather data and implement solutions to the problems. Successes such as that described at LDS dot, but do not dominate, the health care quality landscape (Solberg, 2007). The Institute for Healthcare Improvement (IHI) has led efforts to spread CQI by sponsoring "collaboratives" to assist institutions and groups of institutions to improve health care outcomes. Hundreds of health care organizations have participated in collaboratives concerned with such topics as improving the care of chronic illness, reducing waiting times, improving care at the end of life, and reducing adverse drug events. Collaboratives have shown modest improvement in patient outcomes (Burton et al., 2018).

▶ Electronic Health Records (EHRs)

The HITECH Act of 2009 resulted in nearly 90% adoption of EHRs by hospitals and physicians. Evidence supports their impact on medication safety by alerting clinicians about inappropriate medication doses or medications to which the patient is known to be allergic. EHRs have improved preventive care by alerting clinicians to overdue care, such as cervical screening, influenza vaccines, or cardiovascular risk assessment. Protocols for sharing electronic medical record data across practices and health systems allow key clinical information to flow with patients across the care continuum. While EHRs hold promise for improving care quality, large studies of their impact have been mixed (McCullough et al., 2013; Atasoy et al., 2019). Moreover, widespread implementation has had unintended consequences, such as the disruption of workflows, increasing documentation burden, and negative impacts on communication with patients (Atasoy et al., 2019; Forde-Johnston et al., 2023). Electronic health records are a tool that can improve care, but transformation of practice organization is required to take full advantage of this tool (Wachter, 2015).

Artificial Intelligence (AI)

The digital revolution in health care is opening up vistas for the application of artificial intelligence to mine the massive amounts of data in electronic medical records, digital radiographic images, genomic assays, and other health data repositories (Rajkomar et al., 2019). AI can assist interpretation of diagnostic imaging, improve the ability to detect pathologies, and alert health care personnel to emergency situations (such as bleeding in the brain). In some studies, AIs matched or outperformed human pathologists in the detection of certain early cancers. AI systems in EHRs have been successful at identifying a number of underdiagnosed conditions, such as hyperparathyroidism, based on information in the medical record (Mintz & Brodie, 2019) or to predict the risk of acute coronary disease or heart failure. Many concerns remain about the broader application of artificial intelligence to the very human work of care and healing.

Interdisciplinary Teams

Interprofessional team-based care has become integral to ensuring quality and access. Team-based care is associated with higher quality of care for patients with chronic conditions (Reiss-Brennan et al., 2016; Pany et al., 2021) and reduced use of high-cost care such as emergency departments (Kiran et al., 2022). Behavioral health clinicians, nurses, pharmacists, navigators, and health coaches can expand capacity, enabling clinicians to attend to the needs of additional patients or to

focus on complex medical decision making. Registered nurses or pharmacists managing chronic conditions have achieved as good or better clinical outcomes compared to physicians (Denver et al., 2003; Fazel et al., 2017). Medical assistants trained in population health have improved provision of preventive care and patient self-management of chronic conditions (Willard-Grace et al., 2015). Community health workers have bridged the gap between clinics and underserved communities, helping to address barriers to care such as transportation or food insecurity (O'Brien et al., 2010).

A number of prominent team-based models of care have achieved extraordinary outcomes. Southcentral Foundation in Alaska redesigned care teams and was able to achieve a 36% reduction in hospital days, 42% reduction in emergency department usage, and quality metrics in the top quartile of performers (Gottlieb, 2013). Homeless Patient Aligned Care Teams at the Veteran's Administration showed a 19% reduction in emergency department use and a 35% reduction in hospitalizations six months after enrollment (O'Toole et al., 2016).

Public Reporting of Quality

Public reporting directs quality data to the public through "report cards" that could empower health care consumers to select higher-quality caregivers and institutions. In 2003, Medicare initiated public reporting for hospitals, called Hospital Compare, focusing on risk-adjusted quality of care for heart attacks, heart failure, and pneumonia. In 2010, Medicare added a Physician Compare website. It is uncertain whether these public reports have significantly improved quality (Ryan et al., 2012; Findlay, 2015).

In 1990, the New York State Department of Health released data on risk-adjusted mortality rates for coronary bypass surgery performed at each hospital in the state, and in 1992, mortality rates were also published for each cardiac surgeon. Each year's list was big news and highly controversial. Difficulties in measurement were highlighted by the fact that within 1 year, 46% of the surgeons had moved from one-half of the ranked list to the other half.

Several fascinating results came of this project: (1) Patients did not switch from hospitals with high mortality rates to those with lower mortality rates.

(2) With the release of each report, one in five bottom quartile surgeons relocated or ceased practicing. (3) In 4 years, overall risk-adjusted coronary artery bypass mortality dropped by 41% in New York State. Mortality for this operation also dropped in states without report cards, but not as much. In summary, the New York State experiment had less effect on changing the market decisions of patients and purchasers than on motivating quality improvements in hospitals (Marshall et al., 2000; Jha & Epstein, 2006).

Report cards are based on a philosophy that says "if you can't count it, you can't improve it." Albert Einstein expressed an alternative philosophy that might illuminate the report card enterprise: "Not everything that can be counted counts, and not everything that counts can be counted." In recent years, there have been concerns about the proliferation of questionable quality metrics. Increasingly, the focus on quality is switching to a focus on value, with value referring to quality divided by cost. Thus, an increase in a quality measure associated with a growth in cost may not improve value, where improved quality with a stable or reduced cost increases value (Owens et al., 2011).

▶ Pay for Performance

Pay-for-performance (P4P) programs provide financial rewards or penalties to health care providers, groups of providers, or institutions according to their performance on measures of quality (Mendelson et al., 2017). One of the oldest P4P programs is the Integrated Healthcare Association (IHA) program in California with performance measures including clinical care, patient satisfaction, use of information technology, and health care costs. In 2017, 9 health plans and 200 physician organizations—impacting 9.6 million patients—participated in the IHA program. From 2001 to 2015, physician organizations received over $500 million in performance-based payments (Integrated Healthcare Association, 2016). Overall performance improved an average of 3% annually but varied substantially among physician organizations (Chee et al., 2016).

The IHA program is unique in that all major health plans collaborate in choosing the measures upon which performance bonuses are based. If only one health plan sets up a P4P program with physicians, there may not be enough patients from that health plan to accurately measure the physician's quality; with all health plans participating, a substantial portion of a physician's patient panel is included in the measures. The ability of the California experience to aggregate a large number of patients allows for more accurate performance evaluation.

Medicare has initiated three hospital P4P programs, reducing payments to low-quality hospitals and rewarding those with high quality (NEJM Catalyst, 2018). These programs have not achieved significant quality improvement or readmission reduction (Joshi et al., 2019). A P4P program described as "the world's largest pay-for-performance healthcare scheme" was launched in the United Kingdom in 2004 (Chapter 15).

P4P programs could encourage physicians and hospitals to avoid high-risk patients in order to keep their performance scores up (McMahon et al., 2007). Many patients see a large number of physicians in a given year, making it impossible to determine which physician should receive a performance bonus (Pham et al., 2007). Moreover, P4P programs could increase disparities in quality by preferentially rewarding physicians and hospitals caring for higher-income patients and having greater resources available to invest in quality improvement, and penalizing those institutions and physicians attending to more vulnerable populations in resource-poor environments (Casalino et al., 2007).

▶ Balancing Payment Incentives

The quest for quality care encompasses a search for a financial structure that does not reward over- or undertreatment and that separates physicians' personal incomes from their clinical decisions. Balanced incentives (see Chapter 4), combining elements of capitation or salary and fee-for-service, may have the best chance of minimizing the payment–treatment nexus, encouraging physicians to do more of what is truly beneficial for patients while not inducing inappropriate and harmful services.

WHERE DOES MALPRACTICE REFORM FIT IN?

A set of institutions called the malpractice liability system forms an important part of US health care

(Mello et al., 2014). The goals of the malpractice system are twofold: To financially compensate people who in the course of seeking medical care have suffered medical injuries and to deter physicians and other health care personnel from negligently causing harm to their patients. The malpractice system has scored miserably on both counts. According to the Harvard Medical Practice Study, only 2% of patients who suffer from medical negligence file malpractice claims that would allow them to receive compensation, meaning that the malpractice system fails in its first goal. And the system does not address 98% of negligent acts performed by physicians, making it difficult to attain its second goal. More recent research has confirmed the findings of the Harvard study (Localio et al., 1991; Sage & Kersh, 2006).

The malpractice system has serious negative side effects on medical practice (Localio et al., 1991).

1. The system assumes that punishment—which usually involves physicians paying large amounts of money to a malpractice insurer plus enduring the stress of a malpractice jury trial—is a reasonable method for improving the quality of medical care. In fact, fear of a lawsuit closes physicians' minds to improvement and leads to unnecessary and costly diagnostic testing (Carrier et al., 2013).
2. The system is wasteful. For every dollar in compensation received by patients, legal costs and fees consume 40 to 60 cents (Mello et al., 2010; Shepherd, 2013).
3. The system is based on the belief that trial by jury is the best method of determining whether there has been negligence, a questionable assumption.
4. People with lower incomes generally receive smaller awards (because wages lost from a medical injury are lower) and are therefore less attractive to lawyers. Accordingly, low-income patients, who suffer more medical injury, are less likely than wealthier people to receive compensation (McClellan et al., 2012).

In summary, the malpractice system is burdened with expensive, unfounded litigation that harasses physicians who have done nothing wrong, fails to discipline or educate most physicians committing actual medical negligence and does not compensate most true victims of negligence.

CONCLUSION

Each year people in the United States make 1.5 billion ambulatory care visits and have more than 33 million hospital admissions. While quality of care provided during most of these encounters is excellent, the goal of the health care system should be to deliver high-quality care every day to every patient. This goal presents an unending challenge to each health caregiver and health care institution. Health professionals make hundreds of decisions each day, including which questions to ask in the patient history, which parts of the body to examine in the physical examination, which laboratory tests and x-rays to order and how urgently, which diagnoses to entertain, which treatments to offer, and whether other clinicians need to be consulted. It is humanly impossible to make all of these decisions correctly every day. For health care to be of high quality, mistakes should be minimized, mistakes with serious consequences should be avoided, and systems should be in place that reduce, detect, and correct errors to the greatest extent possible. Even when all decisions are technically accurate, if caregivers are insensitive or fail to provide the patient with a full range of informed choices, quality is impaired.

To safeguard and improve quality of care, a culture must pervade health systems that strives to identify, understand, and change structures and processes that lead to poor quality care. The culture can be supported through laws and regulations; licensure, and measurement to inform institutions, practitioners, and patients about the quality of their care. Improvement of health care quality cannot solely rely on regulators in Washington, DC, in state capitals, or across town; it must come from within each institution, whether a huge academic center, a community hospital, or a small medical office.

REFERENCES

American Diabetes Association. Standards of medical care in diabetes—2019 abridged for primary care providers. *Clin Diabetes*. 2019;37:11–34.

Atasoy H, Piri Cinar B, Aciman Demirel E, et al. The digitization of patient care: a review of the effects of electronic health records on health care quality and utilization. *Ann Review Public Health*. 2019;40:487–500.

Baker LC. Acquisition of MRI equipment by doctors drives up imaging use and spending. *Health Aff (Millwood)*. 2010;29:2252–2259.

Berenson RA, Ginsburg PB, May JH. Hospital–physician relations: cooperation, competition, or separation? *Health Aff (Millwood)*. 2006;26:w31–W43.

Berwick DM, Godfrey AB, Roessner J. *Curing Health Care*. San Francisco, CA: Jossey-Bass; 1990.

Boyd CM, Darer J, Boult C, Fried LP, Boult L, Wu AW. Clinical practice guidelines and quality of care for older patients with multiple comorbid diseases. *JAMA*. 2005;294:716–724.

Brennan TA, Leape LL, Laird NM, et al. Incidence of adverse events and negligence in hospitalized patients. *N Engl J Med*. 1991;324:370–376.

Bunker J. Surgical manpower. *N Engl J Med*. 1970;282:135–144.

Burke JP. Maximizing appropriate antibiotic prophylaxis for surgical patients. *Clin Infect Dis*. 2001;33(suppl 2):S78–S83.

Burton RA, Peters RA, Devers KJ. Perspectives on implementing quality improvement collaboratives effectively. *Joint Commission J Qual Safety*. 2018;44:12–22.

Carrier ER, Reschovsky JD, Katz DA, Mello MM. High physician concern about malpractice risk predicts more aggressive diagnostic testing in office-based practice. *Health Aff (Millwood)*. 2013;32:1383–1391.

Casalino LP, Dunham D, Chin MH, et al. Frequency of failure to inform patients of clinically significant outpatient test results. *Arch Intern Med*. 2009;169:1123–1129.

Casalino LP, Elster A, Eisenberg A, Lewis E, Montgomery J, Ramos D. Will pay-for-performance and quality reporting affect health care disparities? *Health Aff (Millwood)*. 2007;26:w405–w414.

Chassin MR, Baker DW. Aiming higher to enhance professionalism. *JAMA*. 2015;313:1795–1796.

Chassin MR, Loeb J. The ongoing quality improvement journey: next stop, high reliability. *Health Aff (Millwood)*. 2011;30:559–568..

Chee TT, Ryan AM, Wasfy JH, Borden WB. Current state of value-based purchasing programs. *Circulation*. 2016;133:2197–2205.

Cliff BQ, Avanceña ALV, Hirth RA, Lee SD. The impact of Choosing Wisely interventions on low-value medical services. *Milbank Q*. 2021;99:1024–1058.

Denver EA, Barnard M, Woolfson RG, Earle KA. Management of uncontrolled hypertension in a nurse-led clinic compared with conventional care for patients with type 2 diabetes. *Diabetes Care*. 2003;26:2256–2260.

Deyo RA, Mirza SK, Martin BI, Kreuter W, Goodman DC, Jarvik JG. Trends, major medical complications, and charges associated with surgery for lumbar spinal stenosis in older adults. *JAMA*. 2010;303:1259–1265.

Deyo RA, Nachemson A, Mirza SK. Spinal fusion surgery—the case for restraint. *N Engl J Med*. 2004;350:722–726.

Dzau VJ, Shine KI. Two decades since To Err is Human: progress, but still a "chasm." *JAMA*. 2020;324:2489–2490.

Edwards MT. In pursuit of quality and safety: an 8-year study of clinical peer review best practices in US hospitals. *Intern J Qual in Health Care*. 2018;30:602–607.

Eisler P, Hansen B. Doctors perform thousands of unnecessary surgeries. *USA Today*, June 20, 2013.

Fazel MT, Bagalagel A, Lee JK, Martin JR, Slack MK. Impact of diabetes care by pharmacists as part of health care team in ambulatory settings. *Ann Pharmacother*. 2017;51:890–907.

Findlay S. Physician compare. *Health Affairs Health Policy Brief*. October 29, 2015.

Forde-Johnston C, Butcher D, Aveyard H. An integrative review exploring the impact of electronic health records on the quality of nurse–patient interactions and communication. *J Adv Nurs*. 2023;79:48–67.

Gonzalez AA, Dimick JB, Birkmeyer JD, Ghaferi AA. Understanding the volume-outcome effect in cardiovascular surgery: the role of failure to rescue. *JAMA Surg*. 2014;149:119–123.

Gottlieb K. The Nuka System of Care: improving health through ownership and relationships. *Int J Circumpolar Health*. 2013;31;72:21118.

Graham R, Mancher M, Wolman DM, Greenfield S, Steinberg E. *Clinical Practice Guidelines We Can Trust*. Washington, DC: National Academies Press; 2011. https://www.ncbi.nlm.nih.gov/books/NBK209539/.

Hillman BJ, Joseph CA, Mabry MR, Sunshine JH, Kennedy SD, Noether M. Frequency and costs of diagnostic imaging in office patients: a comparison of self-referring and radiologist-referring physicians. *N Engl J Med*. 1990;323:1604–1608.

Hodkinson A, et al. Preventable medication harm across health care settings: a systematic review and meta-analysis. *BMC Med*. 2020;18(1):313.

Iezzoni LI, Rao SR, DesRoches CM, Vogeli C, Campbell EG. Survey shows that at least some physicians are not always open or honest with patients. *Health Aff (Millwood)*. 2012;31:383–391.

Institute of Medicine. *Crossing the Quality Chasm: A New Health System for the 21st Century*. Washington, DC: National Academies Press; 2001. http://www.nationalacademies.org/hmd/~/media/Files/Report%20Files/2001/Crossing-the-Quality-Chasm/Quality%20Chasm%202001%20%20report%20brief.pdf.

Integrated Healthcare Organization. Value Based Pay for Performance in California. September 2016. Integrated Healthcare Association › files › vbp4p-fact-sheet-final-2016.

Jha AK, Epstein AM. The predictive accuracy of the New York State coronary artery bypass surgery report-card system. *Health Aff (Millwood)*. 2006;25:844–855.

Joshi S, Nuckols T, Escarce J, Huckfeldt P, Popescu I, Sood N. Regression to the mean in the Medicare Hospital Readmissions Reduction Program. *JAMA Intern Med.* 2019;179:1167–1173.

King T. *The Medical Management of the Vulnerable and Underserved Patient.* New York, NY: McGraw-Hill; 2016.

Kiran T, Moineddin R, Kopp A, Glazier RH. Impact of team-based care on emergency department use. *Ann Fam Med.* 2022;20:24–31.

Leape LL, Brennan TA, Laird N, et al. The nature of adverse events in hospitalized patients. *N Engl J Med.* 1991;324:377–384.

Leape LL, Fromson JA. Problem doctors: is there a system-level solution? *Ann Intern Med.* 2006;144:107–115.

Levine DM, Linder JA, Landon BE. The quality of outpatient care delivered to adults in the United States, 2002–2013. *JAMA Intern Med.* 2016;176:1778–1790.

Localio AR, Lawthers AG, Brennan TA, et al. Relation between malpractice claims and adverse events due to negligence. *N Engl J Med.* 1991;325:245–251.

Maciosek MV, Coffield AB, Flottemesch TJ, Edwards NM, Solberg LI. Greater use of preventive services in U.S. health care could save lives at little or no cost. *Health Aff (Millwood).* 2010;29:1656–1660.

Makary M, Daniel M. Medical error—the third leading cause of death in the US. *BMJ.* 2016;353:i2139.

Marshall MN, Shekelle PG, Leatherman S, Brook RH. The public release of performance data. *JAMA.* 2000;283:1866–1874.

McClellan FM, White AA 3rd, Jimenez RL, Fahmy S. Do poor people sue doctors more frequently? *Clin Orthop Relat Res.* 2012;470:1393–1397.

McCullough JS, Christianson J, Leerapan B. Do electronic medical records improve diabetes quality in physician practices? *Am J Manag Care.* 2013;19:144–149.

McGlynn EA, Asch SM, Adams J, et al. The quality of health care delivered to adults in the United States. *N Engl J Med.* 2003;348:2635–2645.

McHugh MD, Aiken LH, Sloane DM, Windsor C, Douglas C, Yates P. Effects of nurse-to-patient ratio legislation on nurse staffing and patient mortality, readmissions, and length of stay. *Lancet.* 2021;397:1905–1913.

McMahon LF Jr, Rize K, Irby-Johnson N, Chopra V. Physician-level P4P—DOA? *Am J Manag Care.* 2007;13:233–236.

Medicare Hospital Quality Chartbook. Center for Medicare and Medicaid Services. September, 2013. https://www.cms.gov/Medicare/Quality-Initiatives-Patient-Assessment-Instruments/HospitalQualityInits/Downloads/-Medicare-Hospital-Quality-Chartbook-2013.pdf.

Mello MM, Chandra A, Gawande AA, Studdert DM. National costs of the medical liability system. *Health Aff (Millwood).* 2010;29:1569–1577.

Mello MM, Studdert DM, Kachalia A. The medical liability climate and prospects for reform. *JAMA.* 2014;312:2146–2155.

Mendelson A, Kondo K, Damberg C, et al. The effects of pay-for-performance programs on health, health care use, and processes of care: a systematic review. *Ann Intern Med.* 2017;166:341–353.

Meyer C, Becot F, Burke R, Weichelt B. Rural telehealth use during the COVID-19 pandemic: how long-term infrastructure commitment may support rural health care systems resilience. *J Agromedicine.* 2020;25:362–366.

Mintz Y, Brodie R. Introduction to artificial intelligence in medicine. *Minim Invasive Ther Allied Technol.* 2019;28:2, 73–81.

Montori VM, Brito JP, Murad MH. The optimal practice of evidence-based medicine. *JAMA.* 2013;310:2503–2504.

Morche J, Mathes T, Pieper D. Relationship between surgeon volume and outcomes. *Syst Rev.* 2016;5:204.

Morgan DJ, Wright SM, Dhruva S. Update on medical overuse. *JAMA Intern Med.* 2015;175:120–124.

NEJM Catalyst. What is pay for performance in healthcare? March 1, 2018.

O'Brien MJ, Halbert CH, Bixby R, Pimentel S, Shea JA. Community health worker intervention to decrease cervical cancer disparities in Hispanic women. *J Gen Intern Med.* 2010;25:1186–1192.

O'Toole TP, Johnson EE, Aiello R, Kane V, Pape L. Tailoring care to vulnerable populations by incorporating social determinants of health: the Veterans Health Administration's "Homeless Patient Aligned Care Team" Program. *Prev Chronic Dis.* 2016;31;13:E44.

Owens DK, Qaseem A, Chou R, Shekelle P; Clinical Guidelines Committee of the American College of Physicians. High-value, cost-conscious health care. *Ann Intern Med.* 2011;154:174–180.

Pany MJ, Chen L, Sheridan B, Huckman RS. Provider teams outperform solo providers in managing chronic diseases and could improve the value of care. *Health Aff (Millwood).* 2021;40:435–444.

Pham HH, Schrag D, O'Malley AS, Wu B, Bach PB. Care patterns in Medicare and their implications for pay for performance. *N Engl J Med.* 2007;356:1130–1139.

Rajkomar A, Dean J, Kohane I. Machine learning in medicine. *N Engl J Med.* 2019;380:1347–1358.

Reiss-Brennan B, Brunisholz KD, Dredge C, et al. Association of integrated team-based care with health care quality, utilization, and cost. *JAMA.* 2016;316:826–834.

Relman AS. *A Second Opinion: Rescuing America's Health Care*. New York, NY: Public Affairs; 2007.

Rodriguez JA, Charles JP, Bates DW, Lyles C, Southworth B, Samal L. Digital healthcare equity in primary care: implementing an integrated digital health navigator. *J Am Med Inform Assoc*. 2023;30(5):965–970.

Ryan AM, Nallamothu BK, Dimick JB. Medicare's public reporting initiative on hospital quality had modest or no impact on mortality from three key conditions. *Health Aff (Millwood)*. 2012;31:585–592.

Sage WM, Kersh R. *Medical Malpractice and the US Health Care System*. New York, NY: Cambridge University Press; 2006.

Schiff GD, Bindman AB, Brennan TA. A better-quality alternative. Single-payer national health system reform. *JAMA*. 1994;272:803–808.

Schoen C, Davis K, How SK, Schoenbaum SC. US health system performance: a national scorecard. *Health Aff Web Exclusive*. 2006;25(6):w457.

Shepherd J. Uncovering the silent victims of the American medical liability system. *Vanderbilt Law Review*. 2013;67:1.

Smith-Bindman R. Use of advanced imaging tests and the not-so-incidental harms of incidental findings. *JAMA Intern Med*. 2018;178:227–228.

Solberg LI. Improving medical practice: a conceptual framework. *Ann Fam Med*. 2007;5:251–261.

The Leapfrog Group. Leapfrog hospital safety grade. 2018. https://www.hospitalsafetygrade.org/.

US Department of Health and Human Services. 2017 National Healthcare Quality and Disparities Report. September 2018. AHRQ Pub. No. 18-0033-EF. https://www.ahrq.gov/research/findings/nhqrdr/nhqdr17/index.html.

US Senate. Hearings Before the permanent subcommittee on investigations, Committee on Government Operations, March 13 and 14, 1975. Prepaid health plans. US Government Printing Office; 1975.

Wachter R. *The Digital Doctor: Hope, Hype, and Harm at the Dawn of Medicine's Digital Age*. New York: McGraw Hill; 2015.

Willard-Grace R, Chen EH, Hessler D, et al. Health coaching by medical assistants to improve control of diabetes, hypertension, and hyperlipidemia in low-income patients: a randomized controlled trial. *Ann Fam Med*. 2015;13:130–138.

Yoon SS, Carroll MD, Fryar CD. Hypertension prevalence and control among adults: United States, 2011–2014. NCHS Data Brief, no. 220. Hyattsville, MD: National Center for Health Statistics. 2015. https://www.ncbi.nlm.nih.gov/pubmed/26633197.

Yoshihara H, Yoneoka D. National trends in the surgical treatment for lumbar degenerative disc disease. *Spine J*. 2015;15:265–271.

Population Health and Disease Prevention

US life expectancy rose from 50 years in 1900 to 80 years in 2010, a credit to both public health and medical efforts to decrease the toll of infectious and chronic diseases (Frieden, 2010). Between 1900 to 1940, the nation's public health efforts achieved a remarkable 97% reduction in the death rate for typhoid fever; 97% for diphtheria; 92% for infectious diarrhea; 91% for measles, scarlet fever, and whooping cough; and 77% for tuberculosis (Winslow, 1944). These accomplishments were largely due to preventive measures rather than better medical treatment. However, gains in life expectancy and quality were not universally shared: one's race-ethnicity and socioeconomic status are strongly related to shorter life expectancy, and these inequities have persisted—and even increased—over time. Moreover, life expectancy in the United States started to decline in 2014, reversing a longstanding historical trend (Woolf et al, 2018). This reversal accelerated with the arrival of the COVID-19 pandemic; in 2020, life expectancy in the United States was 77.3 years, the lowest it had been since 2003, with Latino, Black, and American Indian populations experiencing the greatest declines (Arias et al., 2021). The decline in life expectancy is attributable in part to inadequate investment in prevention.

WHAT IS PREVENTION?

The word "prevention" frequently brings to mind individual efforts to improve health, such as screening for health conditions, health education, or adopting a healthy lifestyle. These activities are part of a larger spectrum of prevention spanning individual and population efforts that the World Health Organization defined in 1998 as measures to "not only prevent the occurrence of disease, such as risk factor reduction, but also to arrest its progress and reduce its consequences once established" (Starfield et al., 2008). Prevention strategies may be applied to both infectious disease (such as measles, HIV, or COVID-19) and chronic disease (such as heart disease or diabetes).

INDIVIDUAL OR POPULATION?

Prevention may be viewed from two distinct perspectives: that of the individual (the medical model) and that of the population (the public health model) (Rose, 1985). The medical model seeks to identify high-risk individuals and offer them individual protection, often by counseling on such topics as smoking cessation or offering treatment. The public health approach seeks to reduce cardiovascular disease in the population as a whole, using such methods as restricting where people can smoke, requiring food vendors to post nutritional information, or building more walkable communities.

A coherent ideology underlies the medical model: for chronic disease, individuals play a major role in causing their own illnesses by such behaviors as smoking, drinking alcohol, and eating high-fat foods. It follows that chronic disease mortality rates can be reduced by persuading individuals to change their lifestyles. These statements are true, but do not tell the whole story. A 10% reduction in the serum cholesterol distribution of the entire population would do more to reduce the incidence of heart disease than a 30% reduction in the cholesterol levels of those relatively few individuals with counts greater than 300 mg/dL. Moreover, individual behaviors are shaped by their context and are difficult to modify without changing that context, as when intentions to eat healthfully are thwarted by the temptation of food the family cooks. As Rose explains:

> *Personal lifestyle is socially conditioned.... Individuals are unlikely to eat very differently from the rest of their families and social circle.... (Rose, 1992)*

This broader public health approach argues that modern industrial society creates the conditions leading to heart disease, cancer, stroke, and other major chronic diseases. Tobacco advertising; processed high-salt foods in "supersized" portions; easy availability of alcoholic beverages; societal stress; neighborhood safety issues deterring outdoor physical activity; communities designed for automobile travel;

and a markedly unequal distribution of wealth are the substrates upon which the modern epidemic of chronic disease has flourished. Such a worldview leads to an emphasis on societal rather than individual strategies for disease prevention (Fee & Krieger, 1993).

THE HEALTH IMPACT PYRAMID

The Health Impact Pyramid proposed by Dr. Thomas Frieden, a former director of the Centers for Disease Control and Prevention, provides a framework for uniting the medical model and public health approaches to prevention (Frieden, 2010).

The pyramid (Fig. 14–1) encompasses 5 levels, ranging from interventions addressing socioeconomic factors (Level 1) to individual education and counseling (Level 5). Interventions at the base of the pyramid have greater population impact and require less individual effort, but require greater political will. Interventions near the apex are less controversial but have limited impact and require

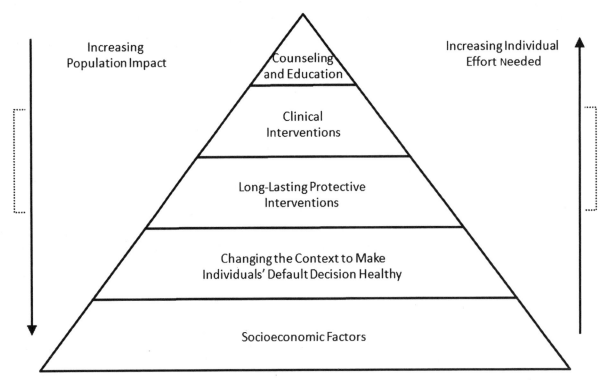

▲ **Figure 14–1.** The health impact pyramid. (*Source:* Frieden TR. A framework for public health action: the health impact pyramid. *Am J Public Health*. 2010;100:590–595.)

more individual effort. Interventions may be most powerful when they harness multiple levels of the Health Impact Pyramid.

At the base of the pyramid (Level 1), socioeconomic factors exert the strongest influence on the health of populations (Table 14–1). Historically, most of the increase in life expectancy between the nineteenth century and today was driven by improvements in living conditions, such as access to clean water, safe air, and adequate nutrition. In comparison, medical measures probably account for less than 5% of the decrease in mortality rates from infectious diseases during the twentieth century (McKinlay et al., 1989; McKeown, 1990). Improvements in socioeconomic conditions remain some of the most powerful levers to improve health. For example, providing financial help to families through tax policies (e.g., the Earned Income Tax Credit) improves birth weight, particularly for people with the greatest health inequities (Hoynes et al., 2015; Batra et al., 2022). Policies to support families or job creation programs to reduce unemployment may have a greater impact on preventing disease than specific public health programs or medical care services (Scott-Marshall & Tompa, 2011), but these require political will to implement.

Changes in the environment to make healthy choices the default option (Level 2) exert a powerful influence on behavior. Increased taxes on cigarettes reduce consumption (Chaloupka et al., 2019). Flouridation of water systems improves dental health for all users (CDC, 1999). Requiring vaccinations for school attendance increases rates of childhood vaccinations (Lee & Robinson, 2016). Building safe and walkable environments increases physical activity (Talen & Koschinsky, 2013). Helmet and seatbelt laws encourage their use and prevent motor vehicle fatalities (Shults et al., 2004; Mayrose, 2008). Like interventions in Level 1, efforts to make healthy options the default require political commitment.

HOW DOES HEALTH CARE FIT INTO PREVENTION?

In general, medical interventions fall within levels 3–5 (the top levels of the pyramid), and their reach is usually limited to people well-connected to health care—a shortcoming when a portion of a population lacks health care coverage or a medical home. In addition, health care frequently intervenes in a disease already in progress, which is less impactful (and more resource intensive) than preventing it in the first place. *Primary prevention* means averting the occurrence of a disease or injury (e.g., immunization against polio; laws requiring helmet use). *Secondary prevention* refers to early detection of a disease process and intervention to reverse or slow the progression of the condition (e.g., mammograms for early detection of breast cancer or antiretrovirals to slow or stop the progression of HIV infection).

The impact of medical interventions is amplified when health care organizations adopt a population-based approach. For example, a primary care practice might maintain a registry of enrolled patients and proactively reach out to those patients overdue for

Table 14–1. Levels of the Health Impact Pyramid

Level	Definition	Examples
Level 1: Socioeconomic factors	Reducing poverty, improving education	Earned income tax credit Universal education
Level 2: Changing the context to make individuals' default decisions healthy	Changing the environment in which a person lives to make their healthy choice easier	Water fluoridation Seatbelt laws and public health campaigns normalizing seatbelt use Taxes on cigarettes or sugary beverages Building walkable environments
Level 3: Long-lasting preventive interventions	One-time or infrequent protective interventions	Immunizations Colon cancer screening Long-acting contraception
Level 4: Clinical interventions	Medical intervention to reduce the burden of disease	Early recognition and treatment of cardiovascular disease
Level 5: Counseling and education	Information and education provided to individuals with the intention of changing health behaviors	Smoking cessation counseling Medical advice to lose weight

Source: Frieden TR. A framework for public health action: the health impact pyramid. *Am J Public Health.* 2010;100:590–595.

preventive services, such as vaccinations and cancer screening tests, without waiting for patients to schedule a preventive care visit. The Community-Oriented Primary Care approach goes further in bridging the medical and population health approaches (Geiger J, 2002). Primary care teams partner with communities to identify their health need priorities and develop community-based interventions to address these needs (Nutting, 1990). For example, a pediatrician might review data on her enrolled patients and find that many children are overweight. In addition to counseling individual families in her practice, the pediatrician would work with community members and agencies on broader public health interventions, such as advocating for improved school lunch programs or promoting consumption of water instead of sweetened beverages.

Reducing cardiovascular disease and the emergency response to the SARS-COV2 (COVID-19) pandemic provide examples of approaches to preventing disease.

MODELS OF PREVENTION: CARDIOVASCULAR DISEASE

Cardiovascular disease refers to several conditions affecting the heart and blood vessels, which can lead to heart attack, stroke, kidney failure, and other debilitating conditions. Cardiovascular disease is the number one cause of death and disability in the United States (Table 14–2). Key preventable risk factors for cardiovascular disease include hypertension, high cholesterol, smoking, unhealthy eating, and lack of physical activity. The medical model for cardiovascular disease secondary prevention involves early detection and treatment of hypertension and high cholesterol. Population-based primary prevention for cardiovascular disease (preventing the disease before it starts) includes smoking cessation; replacement of unhealthy foods with fruits, vegetables, and whole foods; and being more physically active. Prevention efforts have been a major contributor to the remarkable decrease in cardiovascular disease deaths since the 1950s, although significant differences persist in death rates by race and ethnicity (CDC, 2021a) (Fig. 14–2).

▶ The Medical Model Approach to Cardiovascular Disease

The medical model emphasizes identification and treatment of high-risk individuals with elevated

Table 14–2. Leading causes of death in the United States, 2019

All causes	2,855,000
Heart disease	659,000
Cancer	600,000
Unintentional injuries (accidents)	173,000
Chronic lower respiratory diseases	157,000
Cerebrovascular disease	150,000
Alzheimer's disease	121,000
Diabetes	88,000
Kidney disease	52,000
Pneumonia and influenza	50,000
Suicide	48,000
Top 3 contributors to mortality (2006)	
Tobacco	480,000
Diet and inactivity	460,000
Alcohol	88,000

Xu J, et al. Deaths: Final Data for 2019. National Vital Statistics Report, Vol 70, No 8, July 26, 2021. https://www.cdc.gov/nchs/data/nvsr/nvsr70/nvsr70-08-508.pdf.

cholesterol levels or blood pressure. Screening and treatment for high cholesterol and hypertension helped reduce deaths from cardiovascular disease, yet these efforts shared limitations common to medical model approaches. The medical approach, with its reliance on health care personnel and medications, is expensive, and 1 in 6 people with hypertension do not know they have high blood pressure (Park et al., 2018). People may not be able to afford medications, tolerate their side effects, or be convinced of the need to take medication regularly. Indeed, only about half of people prescribed a medication for hypertension or high cholesterol are taking it a year later (Maningat et al., 2013; Poulter et al., 2020). As a result, half of people with hypertension and 80% of people with high cholesterol do not have their conditions well controlled (Ford et al., 2010; Park et al., 2018). Medical interventions are most powerful when used as a secondary strategy in coordination with

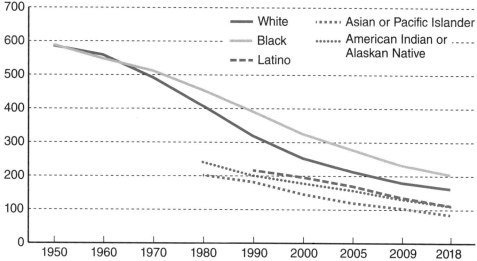

▲ **Figure 14–2.** Trends in age-adjusted mortality from heart disease in the United States, by race and ethnicity, 1950–2018. (*Source:* National Center for Health Statistics, National Vital Statistics System, Mortality Statistics, 2023. *Health, United States, 2020–2021.*)

population-based interventions that make healthy behaviors the easy choice (Hayward et al., 2010).

▷ Moving Upstream: A Population Health Approach to Cardiovascular Disease

A primary prevention approach to cardiovascular disease that reduces smoking and increases healthy eating and physical activity could improve health and quality of life while reducing medical expenditures.

Smoking

Following the 1964 release of the first Surgeon General's Report on the Health Consequences of Smoking, the proportion of US adults who smoke plummeted between 1965 and 2016: from 51% to 18% for men and 34% to 14% for women. These reductions in smoking prevalence avoided a projected 3 million deaths between 1964 and 2000—a major public health achievement (Warner, 1989). Although individually focused educational and nicotine-addiction treatment interventions played a role (operating at levels 4 and 5 of the pyramid), the most powerful influences were policy actions at the second level of the prevention

pyramid, such as cigarette taxes and prohibitions on indoor smoking. A 10% increase in the price of cigarettes reduces consumption by 4% (Chaloupka et al., 2019). Despite this overall reduction in smoking rates, inequities persist. Between 1974 and 2012, cigarette smoking declined only 40% among persons with lower levels of educational attainment, while it dropped 71% among the most educated (Health United States, 2017). In 2020, adults without a college degree were much more likely than those with a college degree to smoke cigarettes (Fig. 14–3). Twenty-seven percent of American Indian and Alaska Native adults smoke, compared with 12.5% of the overall US adult population. Disparities also exist by sexual orientation, with 16% of adults identifying as lesbian, gay, or transgender smoking compared with 12% of adults identifying as heterosexual (CDC, 2022b). Systematic marketing of tobacco and e-cigarettes by tobacco companies to vulnerable communities has partly fueled these disparities and harmful e-cigarette use is increasing, especially among youth (Glantz & Bareham, 2018; Soneji et al., 2019). Smoking continues to be the leading preventable cause of death in the United States (Health United States, 2017).

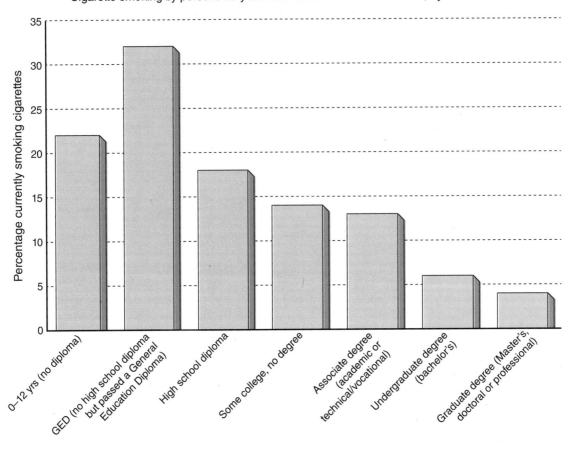

▲ **Figure 14–3.** Cigarette smoking by persons 25 years and older in the United States, by level of education. Percentages are age adjusted. (*Source:* Centers for Disease Control and Prevention 2018.)

Food Choices and Staying Active

Healthy eating and physical activity can reduce the incidence of cardiovascular disease (Pallazola et al., 2019; Kahn et al., 2002), yet fewer than half of adults in the United States meet CDC recommendations for physical activity and 90% do not meet dietary guidelines (Ussery et al., 2021). Sixty-nine percent of adults in the United States were classified as overweight or obese during 2013–2016, up from 56% in 1988 (Health United States, 2017). The food industry spends billions of dollars on advertising, a substantial portion of which promotes fast foods and sugary drinks (Harris et al., 2010). Moreover, low-income neighborhoods are more likely to be "food deserts" (lacking grocery stores or healthy food options) and to have lower walkability compared with higher income neighborhoods (Marshall et al., 2009; Walker et al., 2010).

Population health approaches include financially de-incentivizing unhealthy options and making healthy options more available (level 2 of the pyramid). Taxing sugary drinks may reduce consumption (Backholer & Baker, 2018). Reforms to the federal farm bill could increase support for sustainable farming of healthful fruits and vegetables while reducing subsidies for corn, which contributes to the flooding of the nation with low-cost, high-fructose corn sweeteners and other high-calorie processed foods (Pollan, 2007; Wallinga, 2010). Changing school lunch and food assistance programs to increase their healthy content, restricting food advertising directed at children, and eliminating school-based candy and soft-drink vending machines are effective ways to change the environment to promote healthy eating (Frieden et al., 2010b; Basu et al., 2014). Establishing grocery stores or farmer's markets in food deserts, stocking corner stores with fresh produce, and setting up community gardens reduce physical barriers to healthy foods and promote physical activity at the same time (Walker et al., 2010; Gary-Webb et al., 2018). Effective interventions to increase physical activity include creating safe public places and walkable communities (CDC, 2013). The last few decades have seen efforts to re-design public spaces in partnership with community residents, to ensure that changes are aligned with community needs, whether that be for walking trails, showers and changing spaces, or building sidewalks and safer bike lanes (Sallis et al., 1998). Population-based interventions such as these reach people who do not know they are at risk for cardiovascular disease.

MODELS OF PREVENTION: COVID-19

At the start of the COVID-19 pandemic in 2020, Jayden was a high school senior thrown abruptly into Zoom school. He worked as a checker in a grocery store part time. Jayden's mom Marilyn worked as a nurse in the hospital emergency department, so she quickly recognized the signs of COVID-19 infection when Jayden got sick early in the pandemic.

Compared to other high-income countries, the United States experienced one of the highest per capita death rates from COVID-19, due in part to a poorly funded public health infrastructure and fragmented and inconsistent response (Bilinski et al., 2023). During the first year of the pandemic, the primary tools to control infection were social distancing and masking. Initially, social distancing was enforced through the closure of businesses, schools, and places of gathering by public health mandate (CDC, 2022a), which proved successful in reducing deaths and alleviating strain on the health care system (Lyu & Wehby, 2020). These public health measures all lie at the second level of the prevention pyramid: public policies to change the context for behaviors that put people at risk for COVID-19.

Socioeconomic factors played a glaring role in producing inequities in COVID-19 (Fig. 14–4). People's wherewithal to distance varied by employment and housing conditions. Low-wage "essential workers," such as those in food, transportation, safety, and health care occupations, were far less able to work remotely than individuals working in technology, finance, or similar occupations, resulting in much higher rates of COVID-19 among essential workers (Gwynn, 2021). Similarly, infection was rampant in congregate living facilities, such as nursing homes and prisons (Terebuh et al., 2021), or in crowded or multi-generational housing (Almagro et al., 2020). As with other conditions, people with the greatest involuntary exposure to COVID-19 were often those with the least resources to manage quarantine and isolation (Khanijahani et al., 2021) and cope with financial hardship from business and school closures. These social and environmental factors largely explain the higher death rates from COVID-19 among Black, Latino, and American Indian groups in the United States relative to the White population (Mackey et al., 2021).

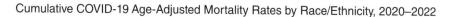

Cumulative COVID-19 Age-Adjusted Mortality Rates by Race/Ethnicity, 2020–2022

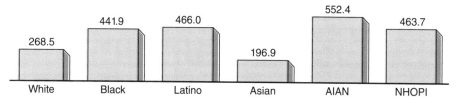

White	Black	Latino	Asian	AIAN	NHOPI
268.5	441.9	466.0	196.9	552.4	463.7

▲ **Figure 14–4.** COVID-19 deaths 2020–2022, by race & ethnicity. (*Kaiser Family Foundation, 2022.* https://www.kff.org/coronavirus-covid-19/issue-brief/covid-19-cases-and-deaths-by-race-ethnicity-current-data-and-changes-over-time/)

During this early phase of the pandemic, some preventive measures were implemented at the base of the pyramid to address socioeconomic factors, ranging from direct financial assistance to eviction moratoria. While these were temporary measures, they did in some cases have far-reaching impacts that affirm socioeconomic interventions as a prevention tool. For example, eviction moratoria reduced disruptions in health care coverage and access (Schwartz et al., 2022).

COVID-19 Vaccination

When COVID-19 vaccines became available, Marilyn was one of the first to be eligible because of her work in the emergency department. She immediately got vaccinated and over the coming months helped her family members navigate complex on-line appointment systems and get rides to get vaccinated. Her brother Roy remained skeptical and unvaccinated, and Marilyn worried about whether he might spread the virus to their aging parents. She was even more upset when Jayden adopted his uncle's views and refused the vaccine.

A second phase of prevention came with the widespread rollout of vaccines. By August 2021, 62% of adults in the United States had received their initial vaccination series (Centers for Disease Control and Prevention, 2021)—a remarkable scientific and public health achievement accomplished only 20 months after the first US case of COVID-19. As noted earlier in the chapter, vaccination is the prototypical long-lasting protective intervention situated at level 3 of the prevention pyramid. COVID-19 death rates were significantly lower in states with high vaccine uptake (Bilinski et al., 2023).

Yet uptake of the vaccine was highly variable across population groups. Initially, there were barriers to access for individuals at greatest risk. For example, navigating on-line appointment systems posed barriers to many older adults, low-income communities without internet access, and limited English proficiency populations. Vaccine sites were not always easily accessible by public transportation (Ndugga et al., 2021). Immigrants, who comprise a significant proportion of essential workers, worried about the impact on future eligibility for residency of receiving free government-sponsored vaccination (Artiga et al., 2021).

In addition, vaccine skepticism played a role in variable vaccination patterns. The reasons for vaccine skepticism range from broken relationships of trust due to racist mistreatment in science and medicine of historically marginalized groups, lack of access to culturally competent sources of information, pervasive misinformation, or low perception of risk (Quinn & Andrasik, 2021). Vaccine skepticism is as old as vaccines themselves. In the nineteenth century, Anti Vaccination Leagues formed in response to public mandates for smallpox vaccinations, rallying as many as 80,000–100,000 protesters in the Leicester Demonstration March of 1895 (Durbach, 2000). In 2019, the World Health Organization listed vaccine skepticism as one of the top 10 threats to global health (World Health Organization, 2019). Anti-vaccination disinformation has become prolific in social media (Wilson & Wiysonge, 2020). While vaccine skepticism spans the political spectrum of the United States, by late 2021, the strongest predictor of a lack of COVID-19 vaccination was political party affiliation (Palosky, 2021).

Requiring vaccination for schools or workplaces has been an important mechanism to increase vaccination rates. These requirements may be considered a blended-approach from the prevention pyramid of leveraging policies to change the context (level 2) to motivating people to receive a vaccine (level 3). Federal and state governments made efforts to require vaccination for health care workers or federal government employees. Almost immediately, objection to vaccine requirements became a rallying point, with 26 states led by Republican officials filing lawsuits in opposition (Musumeci, 2021). While the US Supreme Court ultimately allowed the health care worker vaccine mandate to take effect, on-going litigation has blocked most enforcement efforts for large employers or federal contractors (National Academy for State Health Policy, 2022).

COVID-19 Summary

The history of COVID-19 prevention may be seen as both a success story and a cautionary tale. COVID-19 precautions and immunizations have reduced deaths. Yet, an overreliance on the medical model and intervention at higher levels of the Health Impact Pyramid limited prevention from achieving its full potential.

The public health response to COVID-19 highlights the tension between collective actions at the bottom of the pyramid and individual actions at the top—a tension especially prominent when framed as a contest between government mandates and individual choice. Many emergency response pandemic interventions fell at level 2, "Changing the context to make individual's default decisions healthy," such as mandatory business and school closures and public masking or vaccination requirements. As fatigue and discontent with these measures grew, pressure mounted to move from mandatory policies to voluntary individual choice. In the highly partisan US political context, some political leaders found it advantageous to broadly oppose prevention measures (Bergengruen, 2022). Population-based measures to prevent cardiovascular disease have also often faced political resistance. One argument that proved successful for enactment of smoking bans in public places was similar to the case for COVID-19 era masking and vaccination—that an unhealthful behavior did not just put the individual at risk but jeopardized the health of others through exposure to second-hand smoke or the SARS-COV2 virus.

Individual medical treatments, while costlier and less effective than public health interventions, are less controversial. COVID-19 vaccination refusers sought medical treatment when infected, opting to receive monoclonal antibodies costing $2,000 a dose compared to the $20 cost of a vaccine freely distributed to the public (Mueller, 2021).

Counseling and Education, at the top level of the pyramid, becomes particularly important in a context of partisan conflict over public health measures and rapidly shifting scientific information, as occurred with COVID-19. Physicians and nurses are some of the most trusted sources of information about vaccines (Altman, 2021).

DOES PREVENTION SAVE MONEY?

Primary prevention using public health measures is often more cost-effective than prevention through medical care, largely because public health measures do not require millions of expensive one-to-one health care interactions. A systematic review of 52 population-based studies found a median return on investment of $14 dollars for every dollar invested in population level prevention (Masters et al., 2017). For example, higher cigarette taxes reduce the annual cost of tobacco-related disease and premature death, while at the same time yielding billions of dollars per year in tax revenues (Chaloupka et al., 2019).

For medical model-based prevention, some measures save money and some do not. Every dollar invested in measles, mumps, and rubella immunizations for children saves many more dollars in averted medical care costs. COVID-19 vaccination is probably cost-saving for older populations, but not younger ones (Kohli et al., 2021). Physician counseling on smoking cessation is a low-cost activity that can reduce the multibillion-dollar cost of caring for people with tobacco-related illness (Maciosek et al., 2017). In contrast, medical care to reduce cholesterol and high blood pressure does not result in significant savings to the health care system (US Government Accountability Office, 2014). Moreover, money saved by preventing disease X will ultimately be spent on the treatment of disease Y or Z, which will strike people spared from disease X.

CONCLUSION

While tremendous gains have been made in preventing infectious and chronic diseases in the past centuries, these gains are neither linear nor irreversible. New infectious diseases, prominently COVID-19, have threatened population health and demonstrated the fragility of our public health and health care systems (Trust for America's Health, 2021). The benefits of prevention have not been evenly distributed across society and prominent health inequities persist.

Many people working in medicine and public health believe that "prevention has broken down" because society has dedicated insufficient resources and commitment. In 2019, the United States spent $3.8 trillion on health care. Only 2.6% of this total was dedicated to government public health activities designed to prevent illness. Primary prevention through public health action can be powerfully effective in reducing the burden of human suffering. Further improvements in the health of society will likely require shifting investment to lower levels of the Health Impact Pyramid, focusing on social and environmental determinants of health, reducing the growing gap between rich and low-income, and spending a greater proportion of the health dollar on disease prevention.

REFERENCES

Almagro M, Coven J, Gupta A, Orane-Hutchinson A. Racial disparities in frontline workers and housing crowding during COVID-19. Sep 23, 2020. https://econpapers.repec.org/paper/fipfedmoi/88803.htm.

Altman D. Why doctors and nurses can be vital vaccine messengers. Kaiser Family Foundation. April 5, 2021.

Arias E, Tejada-Vera B, Ahmad F, Kochanek KD. Provisional life expectancy estimates for 2020. Report July 2021. https://stacks.cdc.gov/view/cdc/107201.

Artiga S, Ndugga N, Pham O. Immigrant access to COVID-19 vaccines. Issue brief. Kaiser Family Foundation. Jan 2021.

Backholer K, Baker P. Sugar-sweetened beverage taxes: the potential for cardiovascular health. Curr Cardiovasc Risk Rep. 2018;12:28.

Basu S, Seligman HK, Gardner C, Bhattacharya J. Ending SNAP subsidies for sugar-sweetened beverages could reduce obesity and type 2 diabetes. Health Aff (Millwood). 2014;33:1032–1039.

Batra A, Karasek D, Hamad R. Racial Differences in the Association between the U.S. Earned Income Tax Credit and Birthweight. Womens Health Issues. 2022;32(1):26–32.

Bergengruen V. How the anti-vaxx movement is taking over the right. 26 Jan 2022. Time. https://time.com/6141699/anti-vaccine-mandate-movement-rally/.

Bilinski A, Thompson K, Emanuel E. COVID-19 and excess all-cause mortality in the US and 20 comparison countries, June 2021–March 2022. JAMA. 2023;329:92–94.

Centers for Disease Control and Prevention (CDC). Ten great public health achievements—United States, 1900–1999. MMWR. 1999;48:241–243.

Centers for Disease Control and Prevention. More people walk to better health. 6 Aug 2013. https://www.cdc.gov/vitalsigns/walking/index.html.

Centers for Disease Control and Prevention. Tobacco related spending. 2018. https://www.cdc.gov/tobacco/data_statistics/fact_sheets/economics/econ.../index.htm.

Centers for Disease Control and Prevention. COVID Data Tracker. 2021. Webpage. https://covid.cdc.gov/covid-data-tracker/#datatracker-home.

Centers for Disease Control and Prevention. CDC Museum COVID-19 Timeline. 2022a. Website. https://www.cdc.gov/museum/timeline/covid19.html.

Centers for Disease Control and Prevention. Office on Smoking and Health. Burden of Cigarette Use in the U.S. 2022b.

Chaloupka FJ, Powell LM, Warner KE. The use of excise taxes to reduce tobacco, alcohol, and sugary beverage consumption. Annu Rev Public Health. 2019;40:187–201.

Durbach N. They might as well brand us: Working class resistance to compulsory vaccination in Victorian England. Soc Soc Hist Med. 2000;13:45–62.

Fee E, Krieger N. Thinking and rethinking AIDS: implications for health policy. Int J Health Serv. 1993;23:323–346.

Ford ES, Li C, Pearson WS, Zhao G, Mokdad AH. Trends in hypercholesterolemia, treatment and control among United States adults. Int J Cardiol. 2010;140(2):226–235.

Frieden TR. A framework for public health action: the health impact pyramid. Am J Public Health. 2010;100:590–595.

Gary-Webb TL, Bear TM, Mendez DD, Schiff MD, Keenan E, Fabio A. Evaluation of a mobile farmer's market aimed at increasing fruit and vegetable consumption in food deserts. Health Equity. 2018;2(1):375–383.

Geiger J. Community-oriented primary care: a path to community development. Am J Pub Health. 2002;92:1713–1716.

Glantz SA, Bareham DW. E-cigarettes: use, effects on smoking, risks, and policy implications. Ann Rev Public Health. 2018;39:215–235.

Gwynn RC. Health inequity and the unfair impact of the COVID-19 pandemic on essential workers. Am J Public Health. 2021;111:1459–1461.

Harris JL, Schwartz MB, Brownell KD. Evaluating fast food nutrition and marketing to youth. Fast Food Facts. 2010. https://www.fastfoodmarketing.org/media/FastFood-FACTS_Report_Summary_2010.pdf.

Hayward RA, Krumholz HM, Zulman DM, Timbie JW, Vijan S. Optimizing statin treatment for primary prevention of coronary artery disease. Ann Intern Med. 2010;152:69–77.

Health United States. US Department of Health and Human Services. Report. 2017. https://www.cdc.gov/nchs/data/hus/hus17.pdf.

Hoynes HW, Miller D, Simon D. Income, the Earned Income Tax Credit, and infant health. Am Econ J Econ Policy. 2015;7(1):172–211.

Kahn EB, Ramsey LT, Brownson RC, et al. The effectiveness of interventions to increase physical activity: a systematic review. Am J Prev Med. 2002;22(Suppl 1):73–107.

Khanijahani A, Iezadi S, Gholipour K, Azami-Aghdash S, Naghibi D. A systematic review of racial/ethnic and socioeconomic disparities in COVID-19. *Int J Equity Health.* 2021;20:1–30.

Kohli M, Maschio M, Becker D, Weinstein MC. The potential public health and economic value of a hypothetical COVID-19 vaccine in the United States. *Vaccine.* 2021; 39:1157–1164.

Lee C, Robinson JL. Systematic review of the effect of immunization mandates on uptake of routine childhood immunizations. *J Infect.* 2016;72:659–666.

Lyu W, Wehby GL. Shelter-in-place orders reduced COVID-19 mortality and reduced the rate of growth in hospitalizations. *Health Aff.* 2020;39:1615–1623.

Maciosek MV, LaFrance AB, Dehmer SP, et al. Updated priorities among effective clinical preventive services. *Ann Fam Med.* 2017;15:14–22.

Mackey K, Ayers CK, Kondo KK, et al. Racial and ethnic disparities in COVID-19–related infections, hospitalizations, and deaths a systematic review. *Ann Intern Med.* 2021;174:362–373.

Maningat P, Gordon BR, Breslow JL. How do we improve patient compliance and adherence to long-term statin therapy? *Curr Atheroscler Rep.* 2013;15(1):1–8.

Marshall JD, Brauer M, Frank LD. Healthy neighborhoods: walkability and air pollution. *Environ Health Perspect.* 2009; 117:1752–1759.

Masters R, Anwar E, Collins B, Cookson R, Capewell S. Return on investment of public health interventions: a systemic review. *J Epidem Comm Health.* 2017;71:827–834.

Mayrose J. The effects of a mandatory motorcycle helmet law on helmet use and injury patterns among motorcyclist fatalities. *J Saf Res.* 2008;39:429–432.

McKeown T. Determinants of health. In: Lee PR, Estes CL, eds. *The Nation's Health.* Boston, MA: Jones & Bartlett; 1990.

McKinlay JB, McKinlay SM, Beaglehole R. A review of the evidence concerning the impact of medical measures on recent mortality and morbidity in the United States. *Int J Health Serv.* 1989;19:181–208.

Mueller B. They shunned COVID vaccines but embraced antibody treatment. The New York Times, September 18, 2021.

Musumeci MB. Explaining the new COVID-19 vaccination requirement for health care provider staff. Kaiser Family Foundation Issue Brief, December 15, 2021.

National Academy for State Health Policy. Federal Vaccine Mandates and Legal Challenges. 2022. https://www.nashp.org/federal-vaccine-mandates-and-legal-challenges/.

Ndugga N, Artiga S, Pham O. How are states addressing racial equity in COVID-19 vaccine efforts. Issue brief. Kaiser Family Foundation Issue Brief, March 10, 2021.

Nutting PA, ed. *Community Oriented Primary Care: From Principle to Practice.* Albuquerque, NM: University New Mexico Press; 1990.

Pallazola VA, Davis DM, Whelton SP, et al. A clinician's guide to healthy eating for cardiovascular disease prevention. *Mayo Clin Proc Innov Qual Outcomes.* 2019;3(3):251–267.

Palosky C. Unvaccinated adults are now more than three times as likely to lean Republican than Democratic. News release. Kaiser Family Foundation. 16 Nov 2021.

Park S, Gillespie C, Baumgardner J, et al. Modeled state-level estimates of hypertension prevalence and undiagnosed hypertension among US adults during 2013–2015. *J Clin Hypertens.* 2018;20:1395–410.

Pollan M. You are what you grow. N Y Times Mag. April 22, 2007.

Poulter NR, Borghi C, Parati G, et al. Medication adherence in hypertension. *J Hypertens.* 2020;38:579–587.

Quinn SC, Andrasik MP. Addressing vaccine hesitancy in BIPOC communities—toward trustworthiness, partnership, and reciprocity. *N Engl J Med.* 2021;385:97–100.

Rose G. Sick individuals and sick populations. *Int J Epidemiol.* 1985;14:32–38.

Rose G. *The Strategy of Preventive Medicine.* Oxford: Oxford University Press; 1992.

Sallis JF, Bauman A, Pratt M. Environmental and policy interventions to promote physical activity. *Am J Prev Med.* 1998;15:379–397.

Schwartz GL, Feldman JM, Wang SS, Glied SA. Eviction, healthcare utilization, and disenrollment among New York City Medicaid patients. *Am J Prev Med.* 2022;62(2):157–164.

Scott-Marshall H, Tompa E. The health consequences of precarious employment experiences. *Work.* 2011; 38(4):369–382.

Shults RA, Elder RW, Sleet DA, Thompson RS, Nichols JL. Primary enforcement seat belt laws are effective even in the face of rising belt use rates. *Accid Anal Prev.* 2004;36(3):491–493.

Soneji S, Knutzen KE, Tan ASL, Moran MB, Yang J, Sargent J, Choi K. Online tobacco marketing among US adolescent sexual, gender, racial, and ethnic minorities. *Addict Behav.* 2019;95:189–196.

Starfield B, Hyde J, Gérvas J, Heath I. The concept of prevention: a good idea gone astray? *J Epidemiol Comm Health.* 2008;62(7):580–583.

Talen E, Koschinsky J. The walkable neighborhood: a literature review. *Int J Sustain Land Use and Urban Plan.* 2013;1(1).

Terebuh PD, Egwiekhor AJ, Gullett HL, et al. Characterization of community-wide transmission of SARS-CoV-2 in congregate living settings and local public health-coordinated response during the initial phase of the COVID-19 pandemic. *Influenza and Other Respir Viruses.* 2021;15:439–445.

The White House. National COVID-19 preparedness plan. https://www.whitehouse.gov/covidplan/.

Trust for America's Health. The Impact of Chronic Underfunding on America's Public Health System: Trends, Risks, and Recommendations, 2021. https://www.tfah.org/report-details/funding-report-2022/.

US Government Accountability Office, Health Prevention. Cost-effective services in recent peer-reviewed health care literature. 2014. www.gao.gov/products/GAO-14-789R.

Ussery EN, Omura JD, McCain K, Watson KB. Change in prevalence of meeting the aerobic physical activity guideline among us adults, by states and territories, 2011 and 2019. *J Phys Act Health.* 2021;18(S1):S84–S85.

Walker RE, Keane CR, Burke JG. Disparities and access to healthy food in the United States: a review of food deserts literature. *Health Place.* 2010 Sep 1:876–884.

Wallinga D. Agricultural policy and childhood obesity. *Health Aff (Millwood).* 2010;29:405–410.

Warner KE. Smoking and health: a 25-year perspective. *Am J Public Health.* 1989;79:141–143.

Wilson SL, Wiysonge C. Social media and vaccine hesitancy. *BMJ Global Health.* 2020;5(10):e004206.

Winslow CEA. Who killed Cock Robin? *Am J Public Health.* 1944;34:658–659.

Woolf SH, Chapman DA, Buchanich JM, Bobby KJ, Zimmerman EB, Blackburn SM. Changes in midlife death rates across racial and ethnic groups in the United States: systematic analysis of vital statistics. *BMJ.* 2018;362:k3096.

World Health Organization. Ten threats to global health in 2019. https://www.who.int/news-room/spotlight/ten-threats-to-global-health-in-2019.

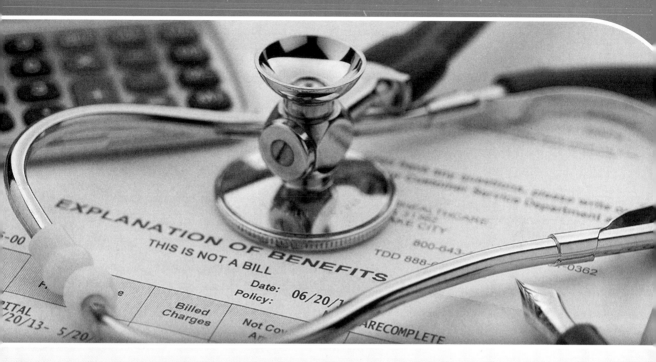

THE POLITICAL ECONOMY OF HEALTH CARE

Health Care in Four Nations

The financing and organization of medical care in high-income nations spans a broad spectrum. In most countries, the preponderance of medical care is financed or delivered (or both) in the public sector; in others, like the United States, most people both pay for and receive their care through private institutions.

In this chapter, we describe the health care systems of four nations: Germany, Canada, the United Kingdom, and Japan. Each of these nations resides at a different point on the international health care continuum. Examining their diverse systems may aid us in our search for an improved health care system for the United States.

Recall from Chapter 2 the four varieties of health care financing: out-of-pocket payments, individual private insurance, employment-based private insurance, and government financing. Germany, Canada, the United Kingdom, and Japan emphasize the last two modes of payment. Germany finances medical care through government-mandated, employment-based private insurance, though German private insurance is a world apart from that found in the United States. Canada and the United Kingdom feature government-financed systems. Japan's financing falls between the German method of financing and the government model of Canada and the United Kingdom. Regarding the delivery of medical care, the German, Japanese, and Canadian systems are predominantly private, while the United Kingdom's is a mixture of private and public delivery.

Although these four nations demonstrate great differences in their manner of financing and organizing medical care, in one respect they are identical: They all provide universal health care coverage, thereby guaranteeing to their populations financial access to medical services.

GERMANY

Health Insurance

Hans Deutsch is a bank teller living in Germany. He and his family receive health insurance through a sickness fund that insures other employees and their families at his bank and at other workplaces in his city. When Hans went to work at the bank, he was required by law to join the sickness fund selected by his employer. The bank contributes 7.3% of Hans's salary to the sickness fund, and 7.3% is withheld from Hans's paycheck and sent to the fund.

Germany was the first nation to enact compulsory health insurance legislation. Its pioneering law of 1883 required certain employers and employees to make payments to existing voluntary sickness funds, which would pay for the covered employees' medical care. Initially, only industrial wage earners with incomes less than $500 per year were included; the eligible population was extended in later years.

In 2019, 88% of Germans received their health insurance through the mandatory sickness funds, with 11% covered by voluntary insurance plans (Fig. 15–1). Some of the 109 sickness funds are organized by geographic area, some by employer or occupation, and some are nationally based.

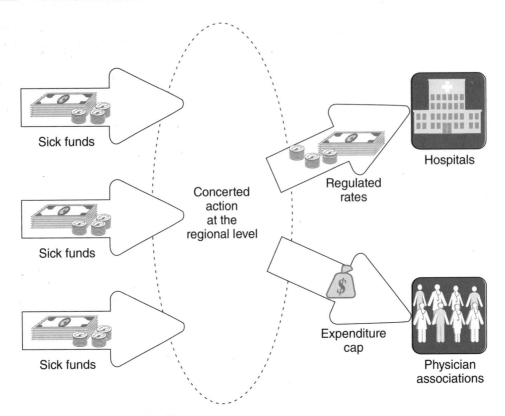

▲ Figure 15–1. The German national health insurance system.

In 2018, the proportion of earnings going to a sickness fund was set at 14.6%, with employers and employees each paying half. These contributions formerly went directly to the sickness funds, which are nonprofit, closely regulated entities that lie somewhere between the private and public sectors. Since 2009, employee and employer contributions are collected by a government-run health fund, which then distributes the money to health funds based on a risk-adjusted (more for older and sicker people) amount per insured person. The funds are not allowed to exclude people because of illness, or to raise contribution rates according to age or medical condition; that is, they may not use experience rating. The funds are required to cover a broad range of benefits, including hospital and physician services, prescription drugs, and dental, preventive, and maternity care. Hospital care and prescription drugs may require copayments; physician visits do not (Blumel & Busse, 2020).

Hans's father, Peter Deutsch, is retired from his job as a machinist in a steel plant. When he worked, his family received health insurance through a sickness fund set up for employees of the steel company. The fund was run by a board, half of whose members represented employees and the other half the employer. On retirement, Peter's family continued its coverage through the same sickness fund with no change in benefits. The sickness fund continues to pay approximately 60% of his family's health care costs (subsidized by the contributions of active workers and the employer), with 40% paid from Peter's retirement pension fund.

Hans has a cousin, Georg, who formerly worked for a gas station in Hans's city, but is now unemployed. Georg remained in his sickness fund after losing his job. His contribution to the fund is paid by the government. Hans's best friend at the bank was diagnosed with lymphoma and became permanently disabled and unable to work. He remained in the sickness fund, with his contribution paid by the government.

Upon retiring from or losing a job, people and their families retain membership in their sickness fund. Health insurance in Germany, as in the United States, is employment based, but German health insurance, unlike in the United States, must continue to cover its members whether or not they change jobs or stop working for any reason. Germany's health insurance system also covers long-term care.

Hans's Uncle Karl is an assistant vice president at the bank. Because of his high income, he is not required to join a sickness fund, but can opt to purchase private health insurance. Many higher-paid employees choose a sickness fund; they are not required to join the fund selected by the employer for lower-paid workers but can join one of 15 national "substitute" funds.

Eleven percent of Germans, those with higher incomes, choose voluntary private insurance. Private insurers pay higher fees to physicians than do sickness funds, often allowing their policyholders to receive preferential treatment.

In summary, Germany finances health care through a merged social insurance and public assistance structure (see Chapters 2 and 16 for discussion of these concepts), such that no distinctions are made between employed people who contribute to their health insurance, and unemployed people, whose contribution is made by the government.

Medical Care

Hans Deutsch develops chest pain while walking, and it worries him. He does not have a physician, and a friend recommends a general practitioner (GP), Dr. Helmut Arzt. Because Hans is free to see any ambulatory care physician he chooses, he indeed visits Dr. Arzt, who diagnoses angina pectoris—coronary artery disease. Dr. Arzt prescribes some medications and a healthy diet, but the pain persists. One morning, Hans awakens with severe, suffocating chest pain. He calls Dr. Arzt, who orders an ambulance to take Hans to a nearby hospital. Hans is admitted for a heart

attack and is cared for by Dr. Edgar Hertz, a cardiologist. Dr. Arzt does not visit Hans in the hospital. Upon discharge, Dr. Hertz sends a report to Dr. Arzt, who then resumes Hans's medical care. Hans never receives a bill.

German medicine maintains a separation of ambulatory care physicians and hospital-based physicians. Most ambulatory care physicians are prohibited from treating patients in hospitals, and most hospital-based physicians do not have private offices for treating outpatients. People often have their own primary care physician but are allowed to make appointments to see ambulatory care specialists without referral from the primary care physician. Forty-five percent of Germany's physicians are generalists compared with 33% in the United States. The German system tends to use a dispersed model of medical care organization (see Chapter 7), with little coordination between ambulatory care physicians and hospitals.

Paying Physicians and Hospitals

Dr. Arzt bills his regional association of physicians and receives a fee for each patient visit and for each procedure done during the visit, but is aware that total regional association payments are subject to a spending cap. If in the first quarter of the year, the physicians in his regional association bill for more patient services than expected, each fee is proportionately reduced during the next quarter. If the volume of services continues to increase, fees drop again in the third and fourth quarters of the year. Dr. Arzt's colleague Dr. Hertz, as a hospital physician, receives a salary and is not affected by the spending cap.

Ambulatory care physicians are required to join their regional physicians' association. Rather than paying physicians directly, sickness funds pay a global sum each year to the physicians' association in their region, which in turn pays physicians on the basis of a detailed fee schedule. These sums have been based on the number of patients cared for by the physicians in each regional association, but in 2007, a risk-adjustment factor was introduced that increases payments for populations with greater health problems. Physicians' associations, in an attempt to stay within their global budgets, can reduce fees if the volume of services delivered by their physicians is too high. Sickness funds pay hospitals on a basis similar to the diagnosis-related groups used in the US Medicare program. Included within this payment is the salary of hospital-based physicians (Blumel & Busse, 2020).

▶ Cost Control

The 1977 German Cost Containment Act created a body called Concerted Action, made up of representatives of the nation's health providers, sickness funds, employers, unions, and different levels of government. Concerted Action sets guidelines for physician fees, hospital rates, and the prices of pharmaceuticals and other supplies. Based on these guidelines, negotiations are conducted at state, regional, and local levels between the sickness funds in a region, the regional physicians' association, and the hospitals to set physician fees and hospital rates that reflect Concerted Action guidelines (Gusmano et al., 2020). Since 1986, not only have physician fees been controlled, but as described in the above vignette about Dr. Arzt, the total amount of money flowing to physicians has been capped. As a result of these efforts, Germany's health expenditures as a percentage of the gross domestic product are increasing more slowly than in the United States (Table 15–1).

CANADA

▶ Health Insurance

The Maple family owns a small grocery store in Outer Snowshoe, a tiny Canadian town. Grandfather Maple has a heart condition for which he sees Dr. Rebecca North, his family physician, regularly. The rest of the family is healthy and goes to Dr. North for minor problems and preventive care, including children's immunizations. Neither as employers nor as health consumers do the Maples worry about health insurance. They receive a plastic card from their provincial government and show the card when they visit Dr. North.

The Maples do worry about taxes. The federal personal income tax, the goods and services tax, and the various provincial taxes take a significant amount of family income. But the Maples would never let anyone take away their health insurance system.

In 1947, the province of Saskatchewan initiated the first publicly financed universal hospital insurance program in North America. Other provinces followed suit, and in 1957, the Canadian government passed the Hospital Insurance Act, which was fully implemented by 1961. Hospital, but not physician, services were covered. In 1963, Saskatchewan again took the lead and enacted a medical insurance plan for physician services. The Canadian federal government passed universal medical insurance in 1966. The Canada Health Act of 1984 enumerates the responsibilities of the federal and provincial governments in providing universal health care.

Canada has a tax-financed, public, single-payer health care system. In each Canadian province, the single payer is the provincial government (Fig. 15–2), with funding of the provincial programs coming from both federal and provincial tax revenues. During the 1970s, federal taxes financed 50% of health services,

Table 15–1. Total health expenditures as a percentage of gross domestic product (GDP), 1970–2021

	1970	1980	1990	2000	2010	2021
Germany	5.5	7.9	8.3	10.3	11.0	12.8
United Kingdom	4.5	5.8	6.0	7.0	8.5	11.9
Canada	7.2	7.4	8.9	8.8	10.6	11.7
Japan	4.1	6.5	6.0	7.7	9.2	11.1
United States	7.4	9.2	11.9	13.4	16.4	17.8

Sources: Commonwealth Fund, U.S. Health Care from a Global Perspective, 2022. https://www.commonwealthfund.org/publications/issue-briefs/2023/jan/us-health-care-global-perspective-2022; OECD Health Statistics, 2019, www.oecd.org>health-data.

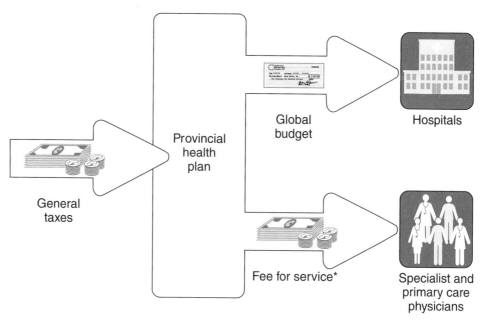

▲ **Figure 15–2.** The Canadian national health insurance system. *Some primary care physicians are paid capitation or salary.

but the federal share has since declined and in 2017/18 constituted 24% of provincial health program expenditures (Allin et al., 2020). Provincial taxes vary in type from province to province and include income taxes, payroll taxes, and sales taxes. Some provinces, for example, British Columbia and Alberta, charge a health care premium—essentially an earmarked tax—to finance a portion of their health budgets.

Unlike Germany, Canada has severed the link between employment and health insurance. Regardless of income bracket, employment status, or age, every Canadian receives the same health insurance. No Canadian would even imagine that leaving, changing, retiring from, or losing a job has anything to do with health insurance. In Canada, no distinction is made between the two public financing mechanisms of social insurance (in which only those who contribute receive benefits) and public assistance (in which people receive benefits based on need rather than on having contributed). Everyone contributes through the tax structure and everyone receives benefits.

The benefits provided by Canadian provinces are broad, including hospital, physician, and ancillary services, with no deductibles or copayments. Most provinces have public prescription drug coverage

programs for specific populations, such as seniors, low-income families, and children. Some charge premiums and co-pays, often income-related. Most provinces also provide limited long-term care benefits. In 2016, 21% of lower income Canadians reported cost-related access problems compared with 50% in the United States (Commonwealth Fund, 2021).

The Canadian health care system is unique in its prohibition of private health insurance for coverage of services included in the provincial health plans. Hospitals and physicians that receive payments from the provincial health plans are not allowed to bill private insurers for such services, thereby avoiding the preferential treatment of privately insured patients that occurs in many health care systems. Canadians may purchase private health insurance policies, sometimes through employment, for gaps in provincial health plan coverage, such as pharmaceutical benefits, home care, vision and dental care, and private hospital rooms.

▶ **Medical Care**

Grandfather Maple has had intermittent sensations of palpitations in his chest for a few weeks. He calls Dr. North, who tells him to come right over.

An electrocardiogram reveals rapid atrial fibrillation, an abnormal heart rhythm. Because Mr. Maple is tolerating the rapid rhythm, Dr. North starts treatment in the office with a blood thinner to prevent a stroke and metoprolol to gradually slow his heart rate, tells him to return the next day, and writes out a referral slip to see Dr. Jonathan Hartwell, a cardiologist in a nearby small city.

Dr. Hartwell arranges a stress echocardiogram at the local hospital to evaluate Mr. Maple's arrhythmia, finds evidence of coronary ischemia and recommends a coronary angiogram and possible coronary artery bypass surgery. Because Mr. Maple's condition is not urgent, Dr. Hartwell arranges for his patient to be placed on the waiting list at the University Hospital in the provincial capital 50 miles away. One month later, Mr. Maple awakens at 2 AM in a cold sweat, gasping for breath. His daughter calls Dr. North, who urgently sends for an ambulance to transport Mr. Maple to the University Hospital. There Mr. Maple is admitted to the coronary care unit, his condition is stabilized, and he undergoes emergency coronary artery bypass surgery the next day. Ten days later, Mr. Maple returns home, complaining of pain in his incision but otherwise feeling well.

In 2017, half of Canadian physicians were family physicians (contrasted with the United States, where only 33% of physicians are generalists). Canadians have free choice of physician, though family physicians can close their lists and not accept new patients. As a rule, Canadians see their family physician for routine medical problems and visit specialists only through referral by the family physician. Specialists are allowed to see patients without referrals, but only receive the higher specialist fee if they specify the referring primary care physician in their billing; for that reason, most specialists will not see patients without a referral. Unlike the European model of separation between ambulatory and hospital physicians, Canadian family physicians are allowed to care for their patients in hospitals. Because of the close scientific interchange between Canada and the United States, the practice of Canadian medicine is similar to that in the United States; the differences lie in the financing system and the greater use of primary care physicians. The treatment of Mr. Maple's heart condition is not significantly different from what would occur in the United States, with the exception that high-tech procedures such as cardiac surgery and magnetic resonance imaging (MRI) scans are regionalized in a limited number of facilities and performed far less frequently than in the United States. In 2017, Canada had 10 MRI scanners per million inhabitants compared with 37.5 in the United States. In 2016, Canada performed 66 coronary artery bypass graft surgeries per 100,000 population per year compared with 82 in the United States.

For Canadians, prompt access to some types of services is more difficult than for people in the United States. Canadians on average wait longer for elective operations than do insured people in the United States. In 2018, between 60% and 80% of patients in Canada scheduled for elective hip replacement received their operations within 6 months. For urgent surgery such as hip fracture repair, 80% to 90% receive surgery within 2 days. Waits vary greatly among provinces; in Ontario and Quebec which make up 60% of Canada's population, elective wait times are shorter (Canadian Institute for Health Information, 2018). Access to primary care has recently become a challenge for some Canadians, particularly in low-income areas. Canadian primary care clinicians are experiencing the same stresses described for the United States in Chapter 7. Fewer Canadian medical students are choosing family medicine and many experienced physicians are thinking of closing their practice (Kiran, 2022).

Canada's universal insurance program has created a fairer system for distributing health services. Canadians are much less likely than their counterparts in the United States to report experiencing financial barriers to medical care. Nonetheless, serious inequities in care remain for low-income families despite universal insurance coverage, particularly for indigenous populations (Martin et al., 2018).

▶ Paying Physicians and Hospitals

For Dr. Rebecca North, collecting fees is a simple matter. Each week she electronically bills the provincial government, listing the patients she saw and the services she provided. Within a month, she is paid in full according to a fee schedule. Dr. North wishes the fees were higher, but loves the simplicity of the billing process. Her staff spends 2 hours per week on billing, compared with the 30 hours of staff time her friend Dr. South in Michigan needs for billing purposes.

Dr. North is less happy about the global budget approach used to pay hospitals. She often begs the hospital administrator to hire more physical therapists, to speed up the reporting of laboratory results, and to institute a program of diabetic teaching. The administrator responds that he receives a fixed payment from the provincial government each year, and there is no extra money.

Until relatively recently, almost all physicians in Canada—family physicians and specialists—were paid on a fee-for-service basis, with fee levels negotiated between provincial governments and provincial medical associations (Fig. 15–2). Physicians participating in the provincial programs must accept the government rate as payment in full and cannot bill patients directly for additional payment. Because fee-for-service payment emphasizes volume over quality of care and makes cost control difficult (see Chapter 12), Canadian provinces are experimenting with alternative forms of payment such as salary or capitation, particularly for family physicians. In 2017–2018, 73% of physician payments were fee-for-service and 27% were alternative payment models (Canadian Institute for Health Information, 2019).

Canadian hospitals, most of which are private nonprofit institutions, negotiate a global budget with the provincial government each year. Hospitals have no need to prepare the itemized patient bills that are so administratively costly in the United States. Hospitals must receive approval from their provincial health plan for new capital projects such as the purchase of expensive new technology or the construction of new facilities. Canada also regulates pharmaceutical prices and provincial plans maintain formularies of drugs approved for coverage.

▶ Cost Control

In contrast to the United States, the Canadians have found a way to deliver comprehensive care to their entire population at far less cost. In 1970, the year before Canada's single-payer system was fully in place,

Canada and the United States spent approximately the same proportion of their gross domestic products on health care—7.2% and 7.4%, respectively. By 1990, Canada's health expenditures had risen to 9% of the gross domestic product, compared with 12% for the United States. In 2021, Canada dedicated 11.7% of its gross domestic product to health care while the United States reached 17.8% (Table 15–1). The differences in cost between the United States and Canada are primarily accounted for by four items: (1) administrative costs, which are more than 300% greater per capita in the United States; (2) more widespread use of expensive high-tech services in the United States; (3) cost per patient day in hospitals; and (4) physician fees and pharmaceutical prices, which are much higher in the United States (Woolhandler et al., 2003; Reinhardt, 2008; Squires & Anderson, 2015).

While 2021 Canadian per capita health care costs ($5,370) were far lower than those in the United States ($10,943), Canada became concerned with cost increases in the 1990s, when Canadian provinces instituted caps on physician payments similar to those used in Germany (Barer et al., 1996). However, the Canadian federal government's fiscal austerity policies of the 1990s appear to have shaken the public's traditionally high level of confidence in the Canadian health care system. In a 2021 comparison of overall health system performance, the United States ranked last and Canada ranked second to last among 11 developed nations (Commonwealth Fund, 2021). While two-thirds of Canadians are satisfied with their public insurance system, about one-quarter of Canadians worry that access to health services may deteriorate over time.

THE UNITED KINGDOM

▶ Health Insurance

Roderick Pound owns a small bicycle repair shop in the north of England; he lives with his wife and two children. His sister Jennifer is a lawyer in Scotland. Roderick's younger brother is a student at Oxford, and their widowed mother, a retired saleswoman, lives in London. Their cousin Anne is totally and permanently disabled from an automobile accident. A distant relative, a French citizen, recently arrived to help care for Anne.

Simply by virtue of existing on the soil of the United Kingdom—whether employed, retired, disabled, or a foreign visitor from Europe—each of the Pound family members is entitled to receive tax-supported medical care through the National Health Service (NHS).

In 1911, Great Britain established a system of health insurance similar to that of Germany. Approximately half the population was covered, and the insurance arrangements were highly complex, with contributions flowing to "friendly societies," trade union and employer funds, commercial insurers, and county insurance committees. In 1942, the world's most renowned treatise on social insurance was published by Sir William Beveridge. The Beveridge Report proposed that Britain's diverse and complex social insurance and public assistance programs, including retirement, disability and unemployment benefits, welfare payments, and medical care, be financed and administered in a simple and uniform system. One part of Beveridge's vision was the creation of a national health service for the entire population. In 1948, the NHS began.

The great majority of NHS funding comes from taxes. As in Canada, the United Kingdom completely separates health insurance from employment, and no distinction exists between social insurance and public-assistance financing. There are no deductibles or co-payments except for prescription drugs, which are waived for children, older adults, and low-income families. Long-term care and dental care are partially covered. Unlike Canada, the United Kingdom allows private insurance companies to sell health insurance for services also covered by the NHS. Almost 11% of the population purchase private insurance or have private insurance provided as an employment benefit. Private insurance may be used to pay for care at private hospitals and allows patients to "hop over" the queues that exist for some NHS services and receive expedited treatment at private facilities. People with private insurance are also paying taxes to support the NHS (Thorlby, 2020) (Fig. 15–3).

▶ Medical Care

Dr. Timothy Broadman is an English GP, whose list of patients numbers 1,750. Included on his list is Roderick Pound and his family. One day, Roderick's son broke his leg playing soccer. He was brought to the NHS district hospital by ambulance

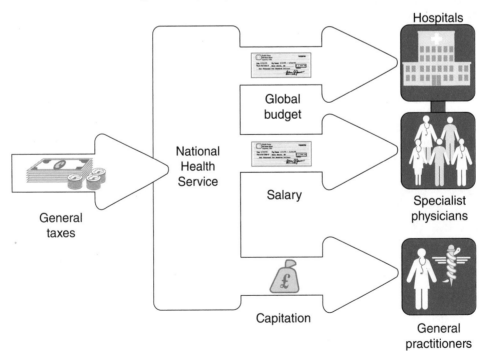

▲ Figure 15–3. The British National Health Service: traditional model.

and treated by Dr. Pettibone, the hospital orthopedist, without ever seeing Dr. Broadman.

Roderick's mother has severe degenerative arthritis of the hip, which Dr. Broadman cares for. A year ago, Dr. Broadman sent her to Dr. Pettibone to be evaluated for a hip replacement. Because this was not an emergency, Ms. Pound required a referral from Dr. Broadman to see Dr. Pettibone. The orthopedist examined and x-rayed her hip and agreed that she needed a hip replacement, but not on an urgent basis. Ms. Pound has been on the waiting list for her surgery for more than 6 months. Ms. Pound has a wealthy friend with private health insurance who got her hip replacement within 3 weeks from Dr. Pettibone, who has a private practice in addition to his employment with the NHS.

Most primary medical care is delivered through GPs. The NHS formalized a gatekeeper system by which specialty and hospital services (except in emergencies) are available only by referral from a GP. Every person in the United Kingdom who wants to use the NHS must be enrolled on the list of a GP. There is free choice of GP (unless the GP's list of patients is full), and people can switch from one GP's list to another. Sixty percent of GPs are self-employed and GP practices are evolving from small offices to larger groups. The average list size is 1,400 patients per GP (Thorlby, 2020).

Whereas the creation of the NHS in 1948 left primary care essentially unchanged, it revolutionized Britain's hospital sector. As in the United States, hospitals had mainly been private nonprofit institutions or were run by local government; most of these hospitals were nationalized and arranged into administrative regions. Because the NHS unified the United Kingdom's hospitals under the national government, it was possible to institute a true regionalized plan (see Chapter 7).

Patient flow in a regionalized system tends to go from GP (primary care for common illnesses) to local hospital (secondary care for more serious illnesses) to regional or national teaching hospital (tertiary care for complex illnesses). Traditionally, most specialists have had their offices in hospitals. As in Germany, GPs do not provide care in hospitals. GPs have a tradition of working closely with social service agencies in the community, and home care is highly developed in the United Kingdom.

▶ Paying Physicians and Hospitals

Dr. Timothy Broadman does not think much about money when he goes to his surgery (office) each morning. He receives a payment from the NHS to cover part of the cost of running his office, and every month he receives a capitation payment for each of the 1,750 patients on his list. Ten percent of his income has been coming from extra fees he receives when he gives vaccinations to the kids; does Pap smears, family planning, and other preventive care; and makes home visits after hours. He also receives additional payments from the pay-for-performance system for GPs.

Since early in the twentieth century, the major method of payment for British GPs has been capitation (see Chapter 4), accounting for 60% of GP payment. Fifteen percent of physician payment is fee-for-service, as an encouragement to provide certain preventive services and home visits during nights and weekends. Consultants (specialists) are salaried employees of the NHS, although some consultants are allowed to see privately insured patients on the side, whom they bill fee-for-service. Hospitals receive global budgets from the NHS.

In 2004, a major new payment mode began for GPs: pay for performance (P4P) (see Chapter 13), known in the United Kingdom as the Quality and Outcomes Framework (QOF). NHS management negotiated the program with the British Medical Association (BMA), and the success of the negotiations was in large part because of the government's policy of increasing payment to GPs, whose average income rose by 60% from 2002 to 2007, with GP incomes approaching those of hospital specialists (Doran & Roland, 2010). The NHS and BMA agreed on dozens of clinical indicators measuring quality for preventive services, common chronic illnesses, and access to care. Physician practices were awarded points for GPs who performed well on these measures with each point worth a sum of money. In 2005, GP practices achieving maximum quality could increase earnings by approximately $77,000 per physician, though the size of performance-related payments has since declined (Roland & Campbell, 2014) and by 2014, GP incomes had slid back to their pre-QOF level (Roland & Guthrie, 2016).

In the first year of the program, quality appeared to improve, largely due to nurse-run chronic disease management. An analysis of performance improvement prior to and following the introduction of P4P suggests that performance had been increasing before P4P, but that quality increased slightly faster after P4P for some chronic conditions. A key quality measure, prompt access to GP appointments, has been worsening. In 2014, financial incentives were removed from some of the quality indicators, resulting in quality reductions for the measures with financial incentives removed with no change in measures with incentives maintained. Scotland abolished the QOF altogether in 2016 (Minchin et al., 2018).

Cost Control

Health expenditures in the United Kingdom accounted for 7.0% of the gross domestic product (GDP) in 2000, far below the US figure of 13.4%. Believing that the NHS needed more resources, the government of Prime Minister Tony Blair infused the NHS with a major increase in funds. Between 1999 and 2004, the number of NHS physicians increased by 25%. In addition, the QOF channeled the equivalent of several billion new dollars into physician practices. By 2021, health expenditures as a proportion of the GDP had risen to 11.9% (Table 15–1). Under subsequent governments, the NHS has scaled back its funding, creating stress throughout the NHS. Queues have lengthened for some nonemergency consultant visits and elective surgeries.

Two major factors allow the United Kingdom to keep its health care costs relatively low: the power of the governmental single payer to limit budgets and the mode of payment of physicians. While Canada also has a single payer of health services, it traditionally paid most physicians fee-for-service. In contrast, the United Kingdom relies chiefly on capitation and salary to pay physicians; payment can more easily be controlled by limiting increases in capitation payments and salaries. Moreover, because consultants (specialists) are NHS employees, the NHS can restrict the number of consultant slots. Overall, the United Kingdom controls costs by controlling the supply of personnel and facilities; for example, in 2017, the United Kingdom had 7.2 MRI scanners per million population compared with the US rate of 37.5 (OECD, 2019).

The United Kingdom is often viewed as a nation that rations certain kinds of health care. In fact, primary and preventive care are not rationed, and average waiting times to see a GP in the United Kingdom are similar to those for people in the United States seeking medical appointments (Schneider et al., 2017).

Reforms of the English National Health Service

Since 1991, England has diverged from the classic NHS model and implemented a series of structural changes. Currently, GPs are required to belong to one of the 191 local "clinical commissioning groups" (Fig. 15–4). These groupings of GPs use these funds to pay for primary care and buy specialty care for their patients.

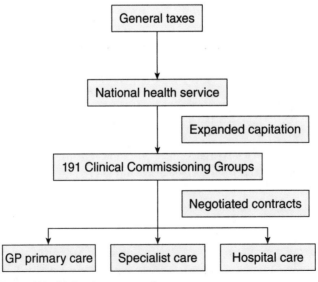

▲ Figure 15–4. The British National Health Service: recent reforms.

The formerly strict regionalization of specialist and hospital services has been weakened as GPs and patients have some choice in which specialists and hospitals will provide their care. Hospitals are organized into trusts which contract with local commissioning groups to provide services. Critics of these reforms have questioned whether the revised structures in England are superior to the traditional structure in Scotland and Wales.

JAPAN

▶ Health Insurance

Akiko Tanino works in the accounting department of the Mazda car company in Hiroshima. Like all Mazda employees, she is enrolled in the health insurance plan directly operated by Mazda. Each month, a percentage of Akiko's salary is deducted from her paycheck and paid to the Mazda health plan. Mazda makes an additional equal payment to its health plan for Akiko.

Akiko's father Takeshi recently retired after working for many years as an engineer at Mazda. When he retired, his health insurance changed from the Mazda company plan to the community-based health insurance plan administered by the municipal government where he lives. Mazda makes payments to this health insurance plan to help pay for the health care costs of the company's retirees. In addition, the health insurance plan requires that Takeshi pay the plan a premium indexed to his income.

Akiko's brother Kazuo is a mechanic at a small auto repair shop in Tokyo. He is automatically enrolled in the government-managed health insurance plan operated by the Japanese national government. Kazuo and his employer each contribute equal percentages of Kazuo's salary to the government plan.

Although Japanese society has a cultural history distinct from the other nations discussed in this chapter, its health care system draws heavily from European and North American traditions. Similar to Germany, Japan's modern health insurance system is rooted in an employment-linked social insurance program. Japan first legislated mandatory employment-based

social insurance for many workers in 1922. The system was gradually expanded until universal coverage was achieved in 1961 with passage of the National Health Insurance Act (Fig. 15–5).

Every large employer is required to operate its own self-insured plan for employees and dependents, known as "society-managed insurance" plans. About 1,400 of these plans exist. The boards of directors of society plans comprise 50% employee and 50% employer representatives. Employees and their dependents are required to enroll in their company's society plan, and the employee and the employer must contribute a premium to fund the society. Society-managed insurance plans cover 59% of the Japanese population.

Other sectors of the population are required to enroll in two other types of insurance plans funded by individual contributions plus national and municipal tax moneys. Employees and dependents in smaller companies, the self-employed, unemployed, and retirees are enrolled in Citizens Health Insurance Plans (27% of the population). Individuals age 75 or above are insured by Health Insurance for the Elderly plans (13% of the population). Seventy percent of the population choose to obtain private health insurance which supplements the public insurance covered.

All plans are required to provide standard comprehensive benefits, including payment for hospital and physician services, prescription drugs, maternity care, and dental care. In addition, in 2000 Japan implemented a long-term insurance plan, financed by general tax revenues and an earmarked income tax. Except for children, older adults, and those with low incomes, all plans require cost-sharing at the point of service, with patients paying 30% of the costs of their care and the health insurance plan paying 70% (Matsuda, 2020).

In summary, Japan—like Germany—builds on an employment-based social insurance model, using additional general tax subsidies to create a universal insurance program. Compared with Germany, the national and local governments in Japan are more involved in directly administering health plans.

▶ Medical Care

Takeshi Tanino's knee has been aching for several weeks. He makes an appointment at a clinic operated by an orthopedic surgeon. At the clinic Takeshi has a medical examination, an x-ray of the knee, and is scheduled for regular physical

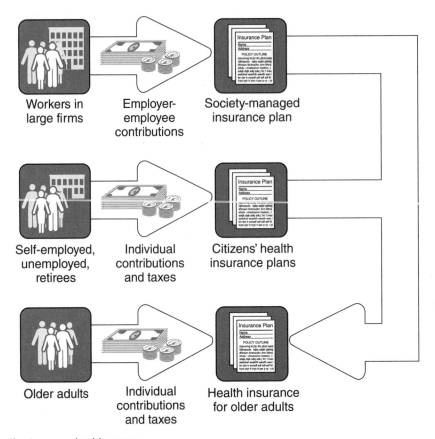

Workers in large firms — Employer-employee contributions — Society-managed insurance plan

Self-employed, unemployed, retirees — Individual contributions and taxes — Citizens' health insurance plans

Older adults — Individual contributions and taxes — Health insurance for older adults

▲ **Figure 15–5.** The Japanese health system.

therapy. During the examination, the orthopedist notes that Takeshi's blood pressure is high and recommends that Takeshi see an internist at a different clinic about this problem.

Six months later, Takeshi develops a cough and fever. He makes an appointment at the medical clinic of a nearby hospital run by Dr. Suzuki, is diagnosed with pneumonia, and is admitted to the medical ward. He is treated with intravenous antibiotics for 2 weeks and remains in the hospital for an additional 2 weeks after completing antibiotics for further intravenous hydration and nursing care.

Health plans place no restrictions on choice of hospital and physician and do not require preauthorization before using medical services. Most medical care is provided in three types of settings: (1) independent clinics, each owned by a physician and staffed by the physician and other employees, with many clinics

also having small inpatient wards; (2) small hospitals with inpatient and outpatient departments, owned by a physician with employed physician staff; and (3) larger public and private hospitals with outpatient and inpatient departments and salaried physician staff. Larger hospitals offer a wide range of specialties while smaller hospitals and clinics have a more limited selection of specialty departments. Care is delivered in a specialty-specific manner, with only a few organizations using a primary care-oriented gatekeeper model (Matsuda, 2017).

Physician entrepreneurship is a strong element in the organization of health care in Japan. Many clinics and small hospitals are family-owned businesses founded and operated by independent physicians, often passed down within a family from one generation to another. Many physicians expanded their clinics to become small hospitals; larger hospitals are often operated by the government. The distinction between clinics and hospitals in Japan is not as great as in most nations. Clinics are permitted to operate inpatient beds and only become classified as hospitals when they have more than 20 beds. Although many physician-owned clinics and hospitals are modest facilities, others are larger institutions offering a wide array of outpatient and inpatient services featuring the latest biomedical technology, electronic medical records, and automated dispensing of medications.

Rates of hospital admission and surgery are relatively low in Japan; yet when hospitalized, patients remain unusually long compared with most developed nations. Average length of stay was 16 days in 2019 compared with 6 days in the United States.

Paying Physicians and Hospitals

One month after returning home from the hospital, Takeshi Tanino develops stomach pain that awakens him several nights. He makes an appointment at a general medical clinic run by Dr. Sansei. Dr. Sansei performs an endoscopy, which reveals gastritis. Dr. Sansei prescribes a proton pump inhibitor and arranges for Takeshi to return to the clinic every 4 weeks for the next 6 months. Takeshi's stomach ache improves after a few days of using the medication. At each follow-up visit, Dr. Sansei questions Takeshi about his symptoms and dispenses a new 4-week supply of medications.

In the past, insurance plans paid both physicians and hospitals on a fee-for-service basis. In 2003, a per diem hospital payment based on diagnosis was introduced while physicians continue to be paid fee-for-service. The government strictly regulates physician fees, hospital payments, and medication prices, which are low by US standards, and also attempts to control the volume of expensive services. Services such as MRI scans that had shown large increases in volumes have had substantial cuts in fees (Ikegami & Anderson, 2012). Physicians make up for low fees with high volume, at times seeing 60 patients per day. In 2017, the number of physician visits per capita was approximately 13, compared with 4 for the United States. Physicians are permitted to directly dispense medications, not just to prescribe them, and make a profit from the sale of pharmaceuticals, and many physician visits are solely for the purpose of refilling medications.

Recently, pharmacists have begun to fill an increasing number of prescriptions (Matsuda, 2020).

Cost Control

Health care costs in Japan were 11.1% of GDP in 2021, up from 7.7% in 2000. Concerns are mounting due to Japan's demographics. The health care system relies heavily on employer-employee contributions and thus requires a large employed population. But with a low birth rate and the longest life expectancy in the world, Japan's population is aging faster than that of other developed nations. The proportion of Japanese older than 65 years was 30% in 2021 compared with about 16% for the United States.

Through its fee schedule, the government has kept medical prices low, which is the main cost-containment strategy. The stresses resulting from Japan's demographic reality make for an uncertain future.

CONCLUSION

Key issues in evaluating and comparing health care systems are access to care, level of health expenditures, public satisfaction with health care, and the overall quality of care as expressed by the health of the population. Germany, Canada, the United Kingdom, and Japan provide universal financial access to health care through government-run or government-mandated programs. These four nations have controlled health care costs more successfully than has the United States (Tables 15–1 and 15–2), though all four face challenges in containing their spending.

Table 15–2. Per capita health spending in US dollars, 2019

Germany	$6,518
United Kingdom	$4,500
Canada	$5,370
Japan	$4,691
United States	$10,943

Source: Organisation for Economic Co-operation and Development, Health at a Glance, 2021. https://www.oecd-ilibrary.org/sites/ae3016b9-en/1/3/7/index.html?itemId=/content/publication/ae3016b9-en&_csp_=ca413da5d44587bc56446341952c275e&itemIGO=oecd&itemContentType=book

In 2020, data from international surveys of 11 developed nations showed that the United States ranked last in overall health system performance. Adults in the United States were much more likely than adults in Germany, the United Kingdom, and Canada to report problems with access to medical services due to costs (Fig. 15–6) (Commonwealth Fund, 2021).

Crossnational comparisons of health care quality are treacherous since it is difficult to disentangle the impacts of social factors and medical care on the health status of the population. But such comparisons can convey rough impressions of whether a health care system is functioning at a reasonable level of performance. From Table 15–3, it is clear that the United States has an infant mortality rate higher than Germany, the United Kingdom, and Japan, with the Japanese rate being the lowest. Japan also has the highest male and female life expectancy rates at birth. The life expectancy rate at age 65 is believed to measure the impact of medical care more than it measures underlying socioeconomic influences. Even by this standard, the United States ranks below the other four nations (Table 15–3).

Just as epidemiologic studies often derive their most profound insights from comparisons of different populations (see Chapter 14), research into health services can glean insights from the experience of other nations. As the United States confronts the challenge of achieving universal access to care at an affordable cost,

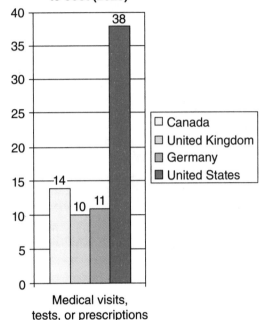

% of people who had access problems due to cost (2020)

Canada, United Kingdom, Germany, United States

Medical visits, tests, or prescriptions

▲ **Figure 15–6.** Problems accessing medical services due to costs. (Commonwealth Fund. Mirror Mirror 2021: Health Care in the U.S. Compared to Other High Income Countries. August 4, 2021.)

lessons may be learned from examining how other nations have addressed this challenge.

Table 15–3. Health outcome measures

	Infant Mortality, per 1,000 Live Births, 2021	Life Expectancy at Birth (years), 2021		Life Expectancy at Age 65 (years), 2021	
		Men	Women	Men	Women
Germany	3.1	78.7	83.5	18.0	21.2
United Kingdom	3.6	78.4	82.4	18.0	20.6
Canada	4.5	79.5	84.0	19.4	22.1
Japan	1.8	81.6	87.7	20.1	24.9
United States	5.4	74.2	79.9	17.0	19.8

[a]Data from the Organisation for Economic Co-operation and Development, 2021. www.oecd.org. https://data.oecd.org/healthstat/life-expectancy-at-birth.htm

REFERENCES

Barer ML, Lomas J, Sanmartin C. Re-minding our Ps and Qs: medical cost controls in Canada. *Health Aff (Millwood)*. 1996;15(2):216–234.

Blumel M, Busse R. International Health Care System Profiles. Germany. Commonwealth Fund, June 2020. https://www.commonwealthfund.org/international-health-policy-center/countries/germany.

Allin S, Marchildon G, Peckham A. International Health Care System Profiles: Canada. Commonwealth Fund, 2020. https://www.commonwealthfund.org/international-health-policy-center/countries/canada.

Canadian Institute for Health Information. Physicians in Canada, 2018. CIHI 2019. https://www.cihi.ca/en/physicians-in-canada.

Canadian Institute for Health Information. Access Data and Reports, 2018. https://www.cihi.ca/en.

Commonwealth Fund. Mirror Mirror 2021: Health Care in the U.S. Compared to Other High Income Countries. August 4, 2021.

Doran T, Roland M. Lessons from major initiatives to improve primary care in the United Kingdom. *Health Aff (Millwood)*. 2010;29:1023–1029.

Gusmano MK, Laugesen M, Rodwin VG, Brown LD. Getting the price right: how some countries control spending in a fee-for-service system. *Health Aff (Millwood)*. 2020;39:1867–1874.

Ikegami N, Anderson GF. In Japan, all-payer rate setting under tight government control has proved to be an effective approach to containing costs. *Health Aff (Millwood)*. 2012;31:1049–1056.

Kiran T. Keeping the front door open: ensuring access to primary care for all in Canada. *CMAJ*. 2022;194:E1555–1556.

Martin D, Miller AP, Quesnel-Vallée A, Caron NR, Vissandjée B, Marchildon GP. Canada's universal health-care system: achieving its potential. *Lancet*. 2018;391:1718–1735.

Matsuda R. The Japanese Health Care System. In Commonwealth Fund. International Profiles of Health Care Systems. 2017. https://www.commonwealthfund.org/publications/fund-reports/2017/may/international-profiles-health-care-systems.

Matsuda R. International Health Care System Profiles: Japan. Commonwealth Fund, 2020. https://www.commonwealthfund.org/international-health-policy-center/countries/japan.

Minchin M, Roland M, Richardson J, Rowark S, Guthrie B. Quality of care in the United Kingdom after removal of financial incentives. *N Engl J Med*. 2018;379:948–957.

Organisation for Economic Co-operation and Development (OECD). Health Statistics, 2019. https://www.oecd.org/OECD › health › health-data.

Reinhardt U. Why does US health care cost so much? Economix. November 14, 2008. http://economix.blogs.nytimes.com.

Roland M, Campbell S. Successes and failures of pay for performance in the United Kingdom. *N Eng J Med*. 2014;370:1944–1949.

Roland M, Guthrie B. Quality and Outcomes Framework: what have we learnt? *BMJ*. 2016;354:i4060.

Schneider EC, Sarnak DO, Squires D, Shah A, Doty MM. Mirror Mirror 2017: International Comparison Reflects Flaws and Opportunities for Better US Health Care. Commonwealth Fund, July 2017.

Squires D, Anderson C. US Health Care from a Global Perspective. Commonwealth Fund, October 2015.

Thorlby R. International Health System Profiles: England. June 5, 2020. Commonwealth Fund. https://www.commonwealthfund.org/international-health-policy-center/countries/england.

Woolhandler S, Campbell T, Himmelstein DU. Costs of health care administration in the United States and Canada. *N Engl J Med*. 2003;349:768–775.

Health Care Reform and National Health Insurance

For more than 100 years, reformers in the United States have argued for the passage of a national health insurance program, a government guarantee that every person is financially covered for basic health care. Finally in 2010, the United States took a major, though incomplete, step forward toward universal health insurance with the passage of the Affordable Care Act (ACA). However, in 2021, 27 million people remained uninsured (Chapter 3), a number likely to grow during the following few years.

The subject of national health insurance has seen six periods of intense activity, alternating with times of political inattention. From 1912 to 1916, 1946 to 1949, 1963 to 1965, 1970 to 1974, 1991 to 1994, and 2009 to 2019, it was the topic of major national debate. In 1916, 1949, 1974, and 1994, national health insurance was defeated and temporarily consigned to the nation's back burner. Guaranteed health coverage for two groups—older adults and some people in low-income bracket—was enacted in 1965 through Medicare and Medicaid. In 2010, the passage of the ACA or "Obamacare" expanded coverage to millions of uninsured people. National health insurance means the guarantee of health insurance for all the nation's residents—what is commonly referred to as "universal coverage." Much of the focus, as well as the political contentiousness, of national health insurance proposals concerns how to pay for universal coverage. National health insurance proposals may also address provider payment and cost containment.

The controversies that erupt over universal health care coverage become simpler to understand if one returns to the four basic modes of health care financing outlined in Chapter 2: out-of-pocket payment, individual private insurance, employment-based private insurance, and government financing. There is general agreement that out-of-pocket payment does not work as a sole financing method for costly contemporary health care. National health insurance involves the replacement of out-of-pocket payments by one, or a mixture, of the other three financing modes.

Under government-financed national health insurance plans, funds are collected by a government or quasigovernmental fund, which in turn pays hospitals, physicians, and other health care providers. Under private individual or employment-based national health insurance, funds are collected by private insurance companies, which then pay providers of care.

Historically, health care financing in the United States began with out-of-pocket payment and progressed through individual private insurance, then employment-based insurance, and finally government financing for Medicare and Medicaid (see Chapter 2). In the history of US national health insurance, the chronologic sequence is reversed. Early attempts at national health insurance legislation proposed government programs; private employment-based national health insurance was not seriously entertained until 1971, and individually purchased universal coverage was not suggested until the 1980s (Table 16–1). Following this historical progression, we shall first discuss government-financed national health insurance, followed by private employment-based and then individually purchased coverage. The ACA represents a pluralistic approach that draws on all three of these financing models: government financing, employment-based private insurance, and individually purchased private insurance.

Table 16–1. Attempts to legislate national health insurance

1912–1919	American Association for Labor Legislation
1946–1949	Wagner–Murray–Dingell bill supported by President Truman
1963–1965	Medicare and Medicaid passed as a first step toward national health insurance
1970–1974	Kennedy and Nixon proposals
1991–1994	A variety of proposals introduced, including President Clinton's Plan
2010	Patient Protection and Affordable Care Act signed into law by President Obama

GOVERNMENT-FINANCED NATIONAL HEALTH INSURANCE

▷ The American Association for Labor Legislation Plan

In the early 1900s, 25% to 40% of people who became sick did not receive any medical care. In 1915, the American Association for Labor Legislation (AALL) published a national health insurance proposal to provide medical care, sick pay, and funeral expenses to lower-paid workers—those earning less than $1,200 a year—and to their dependents. Thus, the first national health insurance proposal in the United States was a government-financed program (Starr, 1982).

In 1910, Edgar Peoples worked as a clerk for Standard Oil, earning $800 a year. He lived with his wife and three sons. Under the AALL proposal, Standard Oil and Mr. Peoples would each pay $13 per year into the regional fund, with the state government contributing $6. The total of $32 (4% of wages) would cover the Peoples family.

The AALL's road to national health insurance followed the example of European nations, which often began their programs with lower-paid workers and gradually extended coverage to other groups in the population. Key to the financing of national health insurance was its compulsory nature; mandatory payments were to be made on behalf of every eligible person, ensuring sufficient funds to pay for people who fell sick. This first attempt at national health insurance failed (Starr, 1982).

▷ The Wagner–Murray–Dingell Bill

In 1943, Democratic Senators Robert Wagner of New York and James Murray of Montana, and Representative John Dingell of Michigan introduced a health insurance plan based on the social security system enacted in 1935. Employer and employee contributions to cover physician and hospital care would be paid to the federal social insurance trust fund, which would in turn pay health providers. The Wagner–Murray–Dingell bill had its lineage in the New Deal reforms enacted during the administration of President Franklin Delano Roosevelt.

In the 1940s, Edgar Peoples' daughter Elena worked in a General Motors plant manufacturing trucks to be used in World War II. Elena earned $3,500 per year. Under the 1943 Wagner–Murray–Dingell bill, General Motors would pay 6% of her wages up to $3,000 into the social insurance trust fund for retirement, disability, unemployment, and health insurance. An identical 6% would be taken out of Elena's check for the same purpose. One-fourth of this total amount ($90) would be dedicated to the health insurance portion of social security. If Elena or her children became sick, the social insurance trust fund would reimburse their physician and hospital.

Edgar Peoples, in his seventies, would also receive health insurance under the Wagner–Murray–Dingell bill, because he was a social security beneficiary.

Elena's younger brother Marvin was permanently disabled and unable to work. Under the Wagner–Murray–Dingell bill he would not have received government health insurance unless his state added unemployed people to the program.

As discussed in Chapter 2, government-financed health insurance can be divided into two categories. Under the social insurance model, only those who pay into the program, usually through social security contributions, are eligible for the program's benefits. Under the public assistance (welfare) model, eligibility is based on a means test; those below a certain income may receive assistance. In the welfare model, those who benefit may not contribute, and those who contribute (usually through taxes) may not benefit (Bodenheimer & Grumbach, 1992). The Wagner–Murray–Dingell bill, like the AALL proposal, was a social insurance proposal. Working and retired families were eligible because they made social security contributions. The permanently unemployed were not eligible.

In 1945, President Truman, embracing the Wagner–Murray–Dingell legislation, became the first US president to champion national health insurance. After Truman's surprise election in 1948, the AMA succeeded in a massive campaign to defeat the Wagner–Murray–Dingell bill. In 1950, national health insurance returned to obscurity (Starr, 1982).

Medicare and Medicaid

In the late 1950s, fewer than 15% of older adults had health insurance (see Chapter 2) and a strong social movement clamored for the federal government to come up with a solution. The Medicare law of 1965 took the Wagner–Murray–Dingell approach to national health insurance, narrowing it to people 65 years and older. Medicare was financed through social security contributions, federal income taxes, and individual premiums. Congress also enacted the Medicaid program in 1965, a public assistance or "welfare" model of government insurance that covered a portion of the low-income population. Medicaid was paid for by federal and state taxes.

In 1966, at age 66, Elena Peoples was automatically enrolled in the federal government's Medicare Part A hospital insurance plan, and she chose to sign up for the Medicare Part B physician insurance plan by paying a $3 monthly premium to the Social Security Administration. Elena's son, Tom, and Tom's employer helped to finance Medicare Part A; each paid 0.5% of wages (up to a wage level of $6,600 per year) into a Medicare trust fund within the social security system. Elena's Part B coverage was financed in part by federal income taxes and in part by Elena's monthly premiums. In case of illness, Medicare would pay for many of Elena's hospital and physician bills.

Elena's disabled younger brother, Marvin, age 60, was too young to qualify for Medicare in 1966. Marvin instead became a recipient of Medicaid, the federal–state program for certain groups of low-income people. When Marvin required medical care, the state Medicaid program paid the hospital, physician, and pharmacy, and a substantial

portion of the state's costs were picked up by the federal government.

Medicare is a social insurance program, requiring individuals or families to have made social security contributions to gain eligibility to the plan. Medicaid, in contrast, is a public assistance program that does not require recipients to make contributions but instead is financed from general tax revenues. Because of the rapid increase in Medicare costs, the social security contribution has risen substantially. In 1966, Medicare took 1% of wages, up to a $6,600 wage level (0.5% each from employer and employee); by 2019, the payments had risen to 2.9% of all wages, higher for wealthy people. The Part B premium has jumped from $3 per month in 1966 to $164.90 per month in 2023, higher for wealthy people.

The 1970 Kennedy Bill and the Single-Payer Plan of the 1990s

Many people believed that Medicare and Medicaid were a first step toward universal health insurance. European nations started their national health insurance programs by covering a portion of the population and later extending coverage to more people. Medicare and Medicaid seemed to fit that tradition. Shortly after Medicare and Medicaid became law, Senator Edward Kennedy of Massachusetts, and Representative Martha Griffiths of Michigan drafted legislation to cover the entire population through a national health insurance program. The 1970 Kennedy–Griffiths Health Security Act followed in the footsteps of the Wagner–Murray–Dingell bill, calling for a single federally operated health insurance system that would replace all public and private health insurance plans.

Under the Kennedy–Griffiths 1970 Health Security Program, Tom Peoples, who worked for Great Books, a small book publisher, would continue to see his family physician as before. Rather than receiving payment from Tom's private insurance company, his physician would be paid by the federal government. Tom's employer would no longer make a social security contribution to Medicare (which would be folded into the Health Security Program) and would instead make a larger contribution of 3% of wages up to a wage level of $15,000 for each employee. Tom's employee contribution *was set at 1% up to a wage level of $15,000. These social insurance contributions would pay for approximately 60% of the program; federal income taxes would pay for the other 40%.*

Tom's Uncle Marvin, on Medicaid since 1966, would be included in the Health Security Program, as would all residents of the United States. Medicaid would be phased out as a separate public assistance program.

The Health Security Act went one step further than the AALL and Wagner–Murray–Dingell proposals: It combined the social insurance and public assistance approaches into one unified program. In part because of the staunch opposition of the AMA and the private insurance industry, the legislation went the way of its predecessors: political defeat.

In 1989, Physicians for a National Health Program offered a new government-financed national health insurance proposal. The plan came to be known as the "single-payer" program, because it would establish a single government fund within each state to pay hospitals, physicians, and other health care providers, replacing the multipayer system of private insurance companies (Himmelstein & Woolhandler, 1989). Several versions of the single-payer plan were introduced into Congress in the 1990s, each bringing the entire population together into one health care financing system, merging the social insurance and public assistance approaches (Table 16–2). The California Legislature passed a single-payer plan in 2006 and 2008, but the proposals were vetoed by the Governor.

THE EMPLOYER-MANDATE MODEL OF NATIONAL HEALTH INSURANCE

In response to Democratic Senator Kennedy's introduction of the 1970 Health Security Act, President Nixon, a Republican, countered with a plan of his own, the nation's first employment-based, privately administered national health insurance proposal. For 3 years, the Nixon and Kennedy approaches competed in the congressional battleground; however, because most of the population was covered under private insurance, Medicare, or Medicaid, there was relatively little public pressure on Congress. In 1974, the momentum for national health insurance collapsed, not to be seriously revived until the 1990s. The essence of the Nixon

Table 16–2. Categories of national health insurance plans

1. Government-financed health insurance plans	Money is collected through taxes or premiums by a public or quasipublic fund that pays health care providers
2. Employer-mandated private health insurance plans	The government requires employers to pay for all or part of private health insurance policies for their employees
3. Voluntary employer-based private health insurance	Some employers voluntarily offer health insurance to their employees, with government subsidies to employers
4. Individual private health insurance plans with government subsidies	The government offers private health insurance to individuals, with subsidies for lower-income people
5. Hybrid plans	Government-financed insurance for older adults and people in low-income bracket, employer-based private insurance for some employees, and individual private insurance for those without government or employer-based insurance

proposal was the employer mandate, under which the federal government requires (mandates) employers to purchase private health insurance for their employees.

Tom Peoples' cousin Blanche was a receptionist in a physician's office in 1971. The physician did not provide health insurance to his employees. Under Nixon's 1971 plan, Blanche's employer would be required to pay 75% of the private health insurance premium for his employees; the employees would pay the other 25%.

Blanche's boyfriend, Al, had been laid off from his job in 1970 and was receiving unemployment benefits. He had no health insurance. Under Nixon's proposal, the federal government would pay a portion of Al's health insurance premium.

No longer was national health insurance equated with government financing. Employer mandate plans preserve and enlarge the role of the private health insurance industry rather than replacing it with tax-financed government-administered plans. The Nixon proposal changed the entire political landscape of national health insurance, moving it toward the private sector.

Between 1980 and 2010, the number of people in the United States without health insurance rose from 25 million to about 50 million (see Chapter 3). Approximately three-quarters of the uninsured were employed or dependents of employed persons. In response to this crisis, President Clinton submitted legislation to Congress in 1993 calling for universal health insurance through an employer mandate. The proposal failed.

A variation on the employer mandate type of national health insurance is the voluntary approach. Rather than requiring employers to purchase health insurance for employees, employers are given incentives such as tax credits to cover employees voluntarily. The attempt of some states to implement this type of voluntary approach failed to significantly reduce the numbers of uninsured workers.

THE INDIVIDUAL-MANDATE MODEL OF NATIONAL HEALTH INSURANCE

In 1989, a new species of national health insurance appeared, sponsored by the conservative Heritage Foundation: the individual mandate. Just as many states require motor vehicle drivers to purchase automobile insurance, the Heritage plan called for the federal government to require all US residents to purchase individual health insurance policies. Tax credits would be made available on a sliding scale to individuals and families who cannot afford health insurance premiums (Butler, 1991). Under the most ambitious versions of the individual mandate, employer-sponsored insurance and government-administered insurance would be dismantled and replaced by a universal, individual mandate program. Ironically, the individual insurance mandate shares at least one feature with the single-payer, government-financed approach to universal coverage: Both would sever the connection between employment and health insurance, allowing portability and continuity of coverage as workers moved from one employer to another or became self-employed.

Tom Peoples received health insurance through his employer, Great Books. Under an individual mandate plan, Tom would be legally required to purchase health insurance for his family. Great Books could offer a health plan to Tom and his coworkers but would not be required to contribute anything to the premium. If Tom purchased private health insurance

for his family at a cost of $10,000 per year, he would receive a tax credit of $4,000 (i.e., he would pay $4,000 less in income taxes). Tom's Uncle Marvin, formerly on Medicaid, would be given a voucher to purchase a private health insurance policy.

With individual mandate health insurance, the tax credits may vary widely in their amount depending on characteristics such as household income and how much of a subsidy the architects of individual mandate proposals build into the plan. Under most proposals, a family might receive a $4,000 tax credit for a $10,000 premium, subsidizing less than half of the premium's cost. Another version of individual health insurance expansion is the voluntary concept, supported by President George W. Bush during his presidency. Uninsured individuals would not be required to purchase individual insurance but would receive a tax credit if they chose to purchase insurance. The tax credits in the Bush plan were small compared to the cost of most health insurance policies, with the result that these voluntary approaches would have convinced few uninsured people to purchase coverage.

The Massachusetts Individual Mandate Plan of 2006

Nearly 20 years after the Heritage Foundation's individual mandate proposal, Massachusetts enacted a state-level health coverage bill implementing the nation's first individual mandate. The Massachusetts plan, enacted under Republican Governor Mitt Romney, mandated that every state resident must have health insurance meeting a minimum standard set by the state or pay a penalty. The law provided state subsidies for purchase of private health insurance coverage to individuals with incomes below 300% of the federal poverty level if they were not covered by Medicaid or through employment-based insurance. The law did not eliminate existing employer-based or government insurance programs for those already covered by those mechanisms.

Following enactment of the Massachusetts Plan, the uninsurance rate among adults in the state dropped from 14% in 2006 to 3.7% in 2014 (Skopec & Long, 2015). Some residents of Massachusetts continued to have trouble affording private insurance even with some degree of state subsidy, and the high levels of cost-sharing allowed under the minimum benefit standards left many insured individuals with substantial out-of-pocket payments. The Massachusetts Plan set the stage for a national plan enacted under the sponsorship of Barack Obama after his election as President in 2008.

THE PLURALISTIC REFORM MODEL: THE AFFORDABLE CARE ACT OF 2010

Following a year-long bitter debate, the Democrat-controlled House of Representatives and Senate passed the Affordable Care Act (ACA) without a single Republican vote in favor. President Obama, on March 23, 2010, signed the most significant health legislation since Medicare and Medicaid in 1965 (Morone, 2010). Although the ACA was attacked as "socialized medicine" and a "government takeover of health care," its policy pedigree derives much more from the proposals of a Republican President (Nixon), a Republican Governor (Romney), and a conservative think tank (the Heritage Foundation) than from the single-payer national health insurance tradition of Democratic Presidents Roosevelt and Truman. The pluralistic financing model of the ACA included individual and employer mandates for private insurance and an expansion of the publicly financed Medicaid program (see Chapter 2).

In 2013, Mandy Must, a single mother of 2 children working for a small shipping company in Houston that did not offer health insurance benefits, was uninsured. In 2014, Mandy earned $35,000 per year and was required by the ACA to obtain private insurance coverage. She received a federal subsidy of $9,000 toward her purchase of an individual insurance policy with an annual premium cost of $12,000.

Mandy's older sister Dorothy Woent was a self-employed accountant with no dependents living in Dallas and earning $48,000 a year. She did not have health insurance, and at her income level was not eligible for a federal subsidy to purchase an individual insurance policy. She would have to pay $5,500 annually to purchase a qualifying health plan that included a $5,000 annual deductible. In 2014, Dorothy was in good health and having trouble paying the mortgage on her house. She decided not to enroll in a health insurance plan and instead paid a $695 fine to the federal

government for not complying with the ACA's individual mandate. In 2019, she was relieved to learn that these fines had been discontinued.

In 2013, Walter Groop worked full-time as a salesperson for a large department store in Miami which did not offer health insurance benefits to its workers. In 2014, he began to apply for an individual policy to meet the requirements of the ACA, but his employer informed him that the department store would start contributing toward group health insurance coverage for its employees to avoid paying penalties under the ACA.

In 2013, Job Knaught had been an unemployed construction worker in Chicago for over 18 months and, aside from an occasional odd job, had no regular source of income. Because he did not have disabilities, he did not qualify for Medicaid prior to the ACA despite having a low income. In 2014, Job became eligible for Illinois' expanded Medicaid program.

As a result of the ACA, the number of uninsured Americans dropped from about 50 million in 2010 to 27 million in 2021 (see Chapter 3). Yet the ACA has weathered recurring storms since its enactment.

▶ 2017–2019: Undermining the ACA

From 2011 to 2017, the Republican-controlled House of Representatives voted 70 times to repeal all or parts of the law. The final legislative attempt to cripple the ACA was a bill passed in the House in the summer of 2017. In a dramatic 2 AM July 27, 2017, 51–49 vote in the Senate, moderate Republican Senator John McCain, soon to die from brain cancer, cast the deciding vote to save the ACA.

One legislative effort to undermine the ACA succeeded: the December 2017 passage of the Tax Cuts and Jobs Act eliminated the tax penalty to be paid by uninsured persons who failed to enroll in an individual health insurance plan. This effectively ended the individual insurance mandate because the requirement to purchase health insurance could no longer be enforced. As a result, healthy people whose enrollment is important to keep down insurance premiums will increasingly forgo health insurance which could make insurance less affordable.

When the 2018 election gave Democrats control over the House of Representatives, legislative efforts to repeal the ACA ended. However, in June 2012, the Supreme Court ruled that the ACA could not require states to expand their Medicaid programs, making Medicaid expansion optional. Most states with Republican governors and/or Republican-controlled legislatures refused to expand Medicaid, leaving millions of low-income Americans uninsured. Fifty-five percent of the public had a favorable opinion of the ACA in March, 2022, with 42% unfavorable.

2017–2019: Resurgence of the Single-Payer Concept

Because Medicare, private insurance, and the ACA were increasingly burdening their enrollees with high deductibles and copayments, many political figures in the Democratic Party were proclaiming that the ACA is only a first step and now was the time to take the next step toward government-financed health insurance. In 2019, the single-payer concept took on a more popular name: Medicare for All, since the public overwhelmingly supports Medicare. Under this proposal, the entire population would become enrolled in the Medicare program over time, perhaps starting the process by reducing the Medicare eligibility age from 65 to 55. In April 2019 public opinion polling, 56% favored Medicare for All with 38% opposed. However, the proposal died because most people want to retain the choice to keep their private insurance, which a pure Medicare for All plan would not allow (Kaiser Family Foundation, 2019).

The COVID Pandemic Temporarily Strengthens the ACA

Under the ACA, premium subsidies are provided for individuals and families with incomes between 100% and 400% of the federal poverty level ($27,750 to $111,000 for a family of four in 2022). However, the insurance plans available under the ACA had substantial deductibles and copayments. The American Rescue Plan Act of 2021, enacted during the COVID-19 pandemic, temporarily increased premium subsidies and added subsidies for many middle-income individuals and families with incomes above 400% of the federal policy level. The onerous ACA deductibles were also reduced. The Inflation Reduction Act of 2022 extended these changes through 2025. After 2025, the return to the original ACA provisions—with insurance premiums rising—will have a serious impact on health care affordability for millions of people.

SECONDARY FEATURES OF NATIONAL HEALTH INSURANCE PLANS

The primary distinction among national health insurance approaches is the mode of financing: government versus employment-based versus individual-based health insurance, or a mixture of all three. But while the overall financing approach is the headline news of reform proposals, details in the fine print are important in determining whether a universal coverage plan will be able to deliver true health security to the public (Table 16–3). What are some of these secondary features?

Benefit Package

An important feature of any health plan is its benefit package. Most national health insurance proposals cover hospital care, physician visits, laboratory, x-rays, physical and occupational therapy, pharmacy, and

Table 16–3. Features of national health insurance plans

Primary Feature	
How the plan is financed	Government, employer, or individual?
Secondary Features	
Benefit package	Which services are covered?
Patient cost-sharing	Will there still be considerable amounts of out-of-pocket payments in the form of patient share of premiums, and deductibles and copayments at the point of service?
Effect on existing programs	Do Medicare, Medicaid, and private insurance arrangements continue in their current form or are they largely dismantled?
Cost containment	Are cost controls introduced, and, if so, what type of controls?
Delivery system reform	Is only health care financing addressed, or does the plan call for changes in the organization and structure for delivering care?

other services usually emphasizing acute care. Mental health services were often not fully covered, a situation in part addressed by the Mental Health Parity Act of 1996 and Mental Health Parity and Addiction Equity Act of 2008 which apply to group private health insurance plans. Neither the ACA nor most previous reform proposals include comprehensive benefits for dental care, long-term care, or complementary medicine services such as acupuncture.

Patient Cost-Sharing

Patient cost-sharing involves payments made by patients at the time of receiving medical care. It is sometimes broadened to include the amount of health insurance premium paid directly by an individual. The breadth of the benefit package influences the amount of patient cost-sharing: the more the services are not covered, the more the patients must pay out of pocket. Many plans impose patient cost-sharing requirements on covered services, usually in the form of deductibles (a lump sum each year), coinsurance payments (a percentage of the cost of the service), or copayments (a fixed fee, e.g., $20 per visit or per prescription). In general, single-payer proposals restrict cost-sharing to minimal levels, financing most benefits from taxes. In comparison, the individual mandate provisions of the ACA have generally included high levels of cost-sharing. Critics have argued that this degree of out-of-pocket payment raises questions about whether the "Affordable" Care Act (ACA) is a misnomer and that people of modest incomes are seriously underinsured. The arguments against cost-sharing as a cost-containment tool are discussed in Chapter 12.

Effects on Medicare, Medicaid, and Private Insurance

Any national health insurance program must interact with existing health care programs, whether Medicare, Medicaid, or private insurance plans. Single-payer proposals make far-reaching changes: Medicaid and private insurance are eliminated in their current form and melded into a single insurance program that resembles a Medicare-type program for all Americans. The most sweeping versions of individual mandate plans would dismantle both employment-based private insurance and government-administered insurance programs.

Employer mandates, which extend rather than supplant employment-based coverage, have the least effect on existing dollar flows in the health care system, as do pluralistic models such as the ACA that preserve and extend existing financing models.

Cost Containment

By increasing access to medical care, national health insurance has the capacity to cause a rapid rise in national health expenditures, as did Medicare and Medicaid (see Chapter 2). By the 1990s, policymakers recognized that access gains must be balanced with cost control measures.

National health insurance proposals have vastly disparate methods of containing costs (see Chapter 12). As noted above, individual- and employment-based proposals tend to use patient cost-sharing as their chief cost-control mechanism. In contrast, government-financed plans look to global budgeting and regulation of fees to keep expenditures down. Single-payer plans, which concentrate health care funds in a single public insurer, can more easily establish a global budgeting approach than can approaches with multiple private insurers.

Proposals that build on the existing pluralistic financing model of US health care, such as the ACA, face challenges in taming the unrelenting increases in health expenditures endemic to a fragmented financing system. An item contributing to the demise of President Bill Clinton's health reform proposal was a measure to cap annual increases in private health insurance premiums. President Obama rejected such a regulatory approach in developing the ACA. Overall, health insurance expansion has failed to curb rising costs.

Reform of Health Care Delivery

Throughout the history of US national health insurance proposals, reformers viewed their primary goal as modifying the methods of financing health care to achieve universal coverage. Addressing how providers were paid often emerged as a closely related consideration because of its importance for making universal coverage affordable. However, intervening in health care delivery did not feature prominently in reform proposals. Reformers were loath to antagonize the

AMA and hospital associations by challenging professional sovereignty over health care organization and delivery. Even advocates of single-payer reform in the United States looked to the lessons of government insurance in Canadian provinces, where until recently government took great pains to focus on insurance financing and payment rate regulation and not on care delivery reform.

WHICH FINANCING MODEL FOR NATIONAL HEALTH INSURANCE PLAN IS BEST?

Historically, in the United States, the government-financed single-payer road to national health insurance is the oldest and most traveled of the three approaches. Advocates of government financing cite its universality: Everyone is insured in the same plan simply by virtue of being a US resident. Its simplicity creates a potential cost saving: The 15–25% of health expenditures spent on administration could be reduced, thus making available funds to extend health insurance to the uninsured (Chapter 11). Employers would be relieved of the burden of providing health insurance to their employees. Employees would regain free choice of physician, choice that is being lost as employers are choosing which health plans (and therefore which physicians) are available to their employees. Health insurance would be delinked from jobs, so that people changing jobs or losing a job would not be forced to change or lose their health coverage. Single-payer advocates, citing the experience of other nations, argue that cost control works only when all health care moneys are channeled through a single mechanism with the capacity to set budgets (Woolhandler & Himmelstein, 2019). While opponents accuse the government-financed approach as an invitation to bureaucracy, single-payer advocates point out that private insurers have average administrative costs of 14%, far higher than government programs such as Medicare with its 2% administrative overhead. A cost-control advantage intrinsic to tax-financed systems in which a public agency serves as the single payer for health care is the administrative efficiency of collecting and dispensing revenues under this arrangement.

Single-payer detractors charge that one single government payer would have too much power over people's health choices, dictating to physicians and patients which treatments they can receive and which

they cannot, resulting in waiting lines and the rationing of care. Millions of people would lose the private insurance that they like. Opponents also state that the shift in health care financing from private payments (out of pocket, individual insurance, and employment-based insurance) to taxes would be unacceptable in an antitax society. Moreover, the United States has a long history of politicians and government agencies being overly influenced by wealthy private interests, and this has contributed to making the public mistrustful of the government.

The employer mandate approach—requiring all employers to pay for the health insurance of their employees—is seen by its supporters as the most logical way to raise enough funds to insure the uninsured without massive tax increases (though employer mandates have been called hidden taxes). Because most people younger than 65 years now receive their health insurance through the workplace, it may be less disruptive to extend this process rather than change it.

The conservative advocates of individual-based insurance and the liberal supporters of single-payer plans both criticize employer mandate plans, saying that forcing small businesses—many of whom do not insure their employees—to shoulder the fiscal burden of insuring the uninsured is inequitable and economically disastrous; rather than purchasing health insurance for their employees, many small businesses may simply lay off workers, thereby pitting health insurance against jobs. Moreover, because millions of people change their jobs in a given year, job-linked health insurance is administratively cumbersome and insecure for employees, whose health security is tied to their job. Finally, critics point out that under the employer mandate approach, "Your boss, not your family, chooses your physician"; changes in the health plans offered by employers often force employees and their families to change physicians, who may not belong to the health plans being offered.

Advocates of the individual mandate assert that their approach, if adopted as the primary means of financing coverage, would free employers of the obligation to provide health insurance, and would grant individuals a stable source of health insurance whether they are employed, change jobs, or become disabled. While opponents argue that low-income families would be unable to afford the mandatory purchase of health insurance, supporters claim that income-related subsidies (as in the ACA) are a fair and effective method to assist such families.

The individual mandate approach is criticized as inefficient, with each family having to purchase its own health insurance. To enforce a requirement that every person buy coverage could be even more difficult for health insurance than for automobile insurance. Moreover, to reduce the price of their premiums, many families would purchase high-deductible plans with high cost-sharing, leaving lower- and middle-income families with unaffordable out-of-pocket costs.

CONCLUSION

Historically, trends in health insurance coverage in the United States in the modern era can be divided into three phases. The first phase, occurring between the 1930s and mid-1970s, saw a large increase in the proportion of Americans with health insurance due to the growth of employment-based private health insurance and the 1965 passage of Medicare and Medicaid. The second phase marks a reversal of this trend; between 1980 and 2010, the number of uninsured people in the United States grew from 25 to about 50 million due to a sharp decrease in the number of people with private health insurance. The number of uninsured peaked in 2010—the year the ACA was signed into law—heralding the third phase during which the number of uninsured decreased to 27 million between 2010 and 2021. The United States may be heading into an unfortunate fourth historical phase with relentless insurance premium and deductible increases and tightening Medicaid eligibility (Rosenbaum et al., 2023).

The concept of national health insurance rests on the belief that everyone should contribute to finance health care and everyone should benefit. People who pay more than they benefit are likely to benefit more than they pay years down the road when they face an expensive health problem. In the years during and after the passage of the ACA, national health insurance took center stage in the United States with fierce debate over "Obamacare." This debate revealed a wide gulf between those who believe that all people should have financial access to health care and those who do not share this belief. In 2023, it is unclear which of those two beliefs holds sway in the United States.

REFERENCES

Bodenheimer T, Grumbach K. Financing universal health insurance: taxes, premiums, and the lessons of social insurance. *J Health Polit Policy Law*. 1992;17:439–462.

Butler SM. A tax reform strategy to deal with the uninsured. *JAMA*. 1991;265:2541–2544.

Himmelstein DU, Woolhandler S. A national health program for the United States: a physicians' proposal. *N Engl J Med*. 1989;320:102–108.

Kaiser Family Foundation. Tracking Public Opinion on National Health Plan. April 24, 2019.

Morone J. Presidents and health reform: from Franklin D. Roosevelt to Barack Obama. *Health Aff (Millwood)*. 2010;29:1096–1100.

Rosenbaum S, Collins SR, Musumeci M, Somodevilla A. Unwinding continuous Medicaid enrollment. *N Engl J Med*. 2023;388(12):1061–1063.

Skopec L, Long SK. Findings from the 2014 Massachusetts Health Insurance Survey, May 2015. SHADAC › sites › default › files › MA_2014_HH_findings.

Starr P. *The Social Transformation of American Medicine*. New York, NY: Basic Books; 1982.

Woolhandler S, Himmelstein DU. Single-payer reform—"Medicare for all". *JAMA*. 2019;321:2399–2400.

The Business of US Health Care

As this book enters its closing chapters, we step back from the details of US health care to view the system as a larger whole. We examine the economics driving accelerating changes in the configuration and business of health care. Market forces shape health care in the United States to a much larger degree than in most other high-income nations. Even when government administers a public insurance program such as Medicare, for-profit corporations capture portions of that market; examples include commercial insurers operating Medicare Advantage plans (see Chapter 2) or the two giant corporations owning 60% of kidney dialysis centers, for which Medicare is the main payer. We begin this chapter by defining the major actors in the health care economy. We then pick up on a theme from Chapter 8: the growing horizontal and vertical integration of health care organizations. We use an economic lens to examine this integration as a form of market consolidation which health care companies use to amass greater market power. We also describe a newer actor on the scene: investors in for-profit health care enterprises.

THE MAJOR ACTORS

The health care sector of the nation's economy is a four trillion dollar system that finances, organizes, and provides health care services for the people of the United States. Traditionally, four major actors have roles on this stage (Table 17–1).

1. The *purchasers* supply the funds. These include individual health care consumers, businesses that pay for the health insurance of their employees, and the government, which pays for care through public programs such as Medicare and Medicaid. All purchasers of health care are ultimately individuals, because individuals finance businesses by purchasing their products and fund the government by paying taxes. Nonetheless, businesses and the government assume special importance as the nation's *organized* purchasers of health care.

2. The *insurers* receive money from the purchasers and pay the providers. Traditional insurers take money from purchasers (individuals or businesses) and pay providers when policyholders require medical care. Yet some insurers are the same as purchasers; the government can be viewed as an insurer or purchaser in the Medicare and Medicaid programs, and businesses that self-insure their employees can similarly occupy both roles.

3. The *providers* include health systems, hospitals, medical groups, home care agencies, nursing homes, pharmacies, and individual caregivers such as physicians, nurses, pharmacists, and behavioral health professionals.

4. The *suppliers* include the pharmaceutical, medical supply, computer, and virtual care industries, which manufacture medications, equipment, supplies, electronic health records, and health care apps used by patients and providers.

To these four traditional actors must now be added a fifth actor: corporate shareholders and private equity investors. As all four of the traditional actors become increasingly owned and operated by commercial enterprises, shareholders and investors are now major

Table 17–1. The major actors

Purchasers
Individuals
Employers
Government
Insurers
Providers
Health systems
Hospitals
Nursing homes
Home care agencies
Pharmacies
Clinicians (physicians, nurse practitioners, and physician assistants)
Nurses, pharmacists, behaviorists, and other caregivers
Suppliers
Pharmaceutical companies
Pharmacy benefit managers (PBMs)
Medical supply companies
Electronic medical record vendors
Investor shareholders
Shareholders of for-profit corporations
Private equity firms

players on the health care stage with their own set of interests.

Insurers, providers, suppliers, and their owners make up the health care industry. Each dollar spent on health care represents an expense to the purchasers and income to the health care industry. In the past, purchasers viewed this expense as an investment, money spent to improve the health of the population and thereby the economic and social vitality of the nation. But over the past 50 years, conflict has intensified between the purchasers and the health care industry: The purchasers wish to reduce, and the health care industry to increase, the number of dollars spent on health care. This conflict has see-sawed over time, sometimes purchasers and more often the health care

industry having the upper hand (Table 17–2). There is now rapid consolidation within each of the actors as well as blurring of boundaries, as the actors create trans-sector conglomerates and health care enters a mega-consolidation phase.

MARKET CONSOLIDATION

In Chapter 8, we discussed the evolution of the health care system from a cottage industry of small independent physician practices, pharmacies, and community hospitals to one featuring many large, integrated health care delivery organizations. We discussed some of the drivers of this evolution, including the belief that group practice and vertically integrated systems might deliver more coordinated and higher-quality care, and generational changes in the workforce with more physicians desiring to be employed rather than run their own small business. But another major factor has been driving this evolution: the desire for market power. Simply put, the greater the share of a market an entity controls, the greater leverage it has to be a price setter rather than price taker in negotiations with payers and purchasers and to otherwise shape the business of health care to its financial advantage.

▶ Provider Consolidation

Chapter 8 introduced the concepts of horizontal and vertical integration, which could also be called horizontal and vertical consolidation. Horizontal consolidation—that is, consolidation within a particular sector—came first: by 2001, 65% of hospitals were members of multihospital systems or networks (Bazzoli, 2004). Hospital consolidation intensified in the ensuing two decades and by 2020, the 10 largest health systems controlled nearly one-quarter of the market (Meyer, 2022). Many cities have only two or three competing hospital systems with enough market power to demand large price increases from insurers.

Small physician practices also consolidated into larger practices and physician groups, particularly single-specialty groups. In 2020, 43% of physicians worked in single-specialty groups compared with 26% in multi-specialty groups (Kane, 2021). In many metropolitan areas, almost all specialist physicians have joined one of the few groups in that specialty, giving them major clout to extract high payment rates

Table 17–2. Historical overview of US health care

1945–1970: provider–insurer pact

Independent hospitals and small private practices

Many private insurers

Providers tended to dominate the insurers, especially in Blue Cross and Blue Shield

Purchasers (individuals, businesses, and, after 1965, government) had relatively little power

Payments for providers were generous

The 1970s: tensions develop

Purchasers (especially government) become concerned about costs of health care

Under pressure from purchasers, insurers begin to question generous payments of providers

The 1980s: revolt of the purchasers

Purchasers (business joining government) become very concerned with rising health care costs

Attempts are made to reduce health cost inflation through Medicare DRGs, fee schedules, capitated HMOs, and selective contracting

The 1990s: breakup of the provider–insurer pact

Spurred by the purchasers, selective contracting spreads widely as a mechanism to reduce costs

Price competition is introduced

Large integrated health networks are formed

Large physician groups emerge

Insurance companies dominate many managed care markets

For-profit institutions increase in importance

Insurers gain increasing power over providers, creating conflict and ending the provider–insurer pact

The new millennium: resurgence of provider and supplier power

HMOs fade in importance

Hospitals consolidate into hospital systems, forcing insurers to pay them more

Insurers respond by consolidating, with a few large national insurers dominating many markets

Many specialists form single-specialty groups

Specialists move profitable procedures out of hospitals into specialist-owned centers

Pharmaceutical companies and pharmacy benefit managers earn huge profits

Less uninsurance and more underinsurance

The present: mega-consolidation

Cross-sector consolidation brings insurers, providers, and suppliers together into huge conglomerates

from insurers. Although multispecialty groups, which include primary care physicians, have tended to have the best scores on quality report cards, they have not grown in part because many specialist physicians do not want to share their high incomes with primary care physicians (Casalino et al., 2004; Mehrotra et al., 2006; Urwin & Emanuel, 2019). Similar horizontal consolidation has occurred for pharmacies, with small community pharmacies bought up by huge pharmacy chains. CVS and Walgreens together control between 50% and 75% of the drugstore market in each of the country's 14 largest metropolitan areas.

Horizontal consolidation spawned vertical consolidation. Large hospital systems needed physicians. The traditional dispersed hospital-physician model, described in Chapter 8, allowed physicians to admit patients to more than one hospital, which gave physicians power over hospitals. The best way for hospital systems to guarantee a steady flow of patient admissions was to acquire physicians as employees (vertical consolidation) or to make exclusive contracts with them (virtual consolidation). Integrated provider systems now dominate the market. Health systems can be defined as groups of commonly owned or managed entities including at least 1 general acute care hospital and 50 physicians. In 2018, 51% of physicians and 72% of hospitals were affiliated with one of the 637 health systems in the United States, with 91% of all general acute hospital beds in these systems (Furukawa et al., 2020).

As noted in Chapter 8, there is little evidence that provider consolidation has overall resulted in better quality of care (Greaney, 2018). But this consolidation has increased costs. As hospital systems and large physician groups gained an upper hand in negotiations with health plans, costs accelerated. Insurance premiums for family coverage went from an average of $6,000 per year in 2000 to over $22,000 in 2022. One recent national study found that prices paid to health system physicians and hospitals were 12–26% higher for physician services and 31% higher for hospital services than prices paid to physicians and hospitals, respectively, that were not part of integrated systems (Beaulieu et al., 2023). Health systems have sufficient market power to reduce competition, increase health spending, and influence federal and state health policy in ways that do not clearly benefit patients (Casalino, 2023).

Consolidation in many regions is at a tipping point, with near monopolistic control by some provider organizations raising concerns about anti-competitive behavior violating anti-trust laws. In 2019, the large hospital system Sutter Health settled a suit for $575 million in response to allegations that its dominant market share in many regions of California increased health care costs for consumers. Under the Biden Administration, the Federal Trade Commission

has begun to take a more active role in challenging hospital consolidation (Bonta, 2021). In 2022, four separate proposed hospital mergers and acquisitions were called off after the Federal Trade Commission filed lawsuits to block these transactions (Meyer, 2022). Hospital systems have also come under criticism for closing many small rural hospitals that are considered unprofitable but are key anchors of health services for rural communities.

▶ Insurer Consolidation

To counter provider consolidation, large insurers have bought up smaller ones and merged with one another. Three huge for-profit insurers—Anthem, UnitedHealthcare, and Aetna—dominate many markets: 73% of metropolitan areas have highly concentrated insurance markets and 46% have one insurer with over 50% market share. In a number of states, one insurer dominates the market with over 70% market share. Insurer consolidation may successfully counter provider market power. However, the financial benefit may not be shared with the patients enrolled in the insurance plan but simply be retained by the insurer as additional profit. For example, in 2022, UnitedHealthcare's profits increased by 16% over 2021, reaching $20.6 billion, while hospital profit margins declined (Shryock, 2022; Pifer, 2023). Insurer market concentration is associated with increases in premium prices.

▶ Supplier Consolidation

Pharma, consisting of pharmaceutical manufacturers and pharmacy benefit managers, is a huge supplier actor that we have only briefly touched on in previous chapters.

Pharmaceutical Manufacturers

In 1988, prescription drugs accounted for 5.5% of national health expenditures, and 71% of drug costs were paid out of pocket by individuals. By 2020, prescription drug costs had risen to 10% of total health expenditures, with 82% of these costs covered by employers, insurers, and governmental purchasers. The growing expense of pharmaceuticals for older adults became a major national issue, resulting in the passage of Medicare Part D in 2003 and portions of the Inflation Reduction Act of 2022.

Companies developing a new brand-name drug enjoy a patent for 20 years from the date the patent application is filed, during which time no other company can produce the same drug. Once the patent expires, generic drug manufacturers can compete by selling the same product at lower prices. To fend off this competition, brand-name manufacturers can use delaying tactics that extend the patent (Tribble, 2018). In 2016, the patent on the anti-inflammatory medication Humira—priced at $50,000 a year—was expiring. Through legal exploitation of the patent system, Humira's manufacturer blocked competitors from entering the market. For the next six years, the drug's price rose by 60%, making Humira the most lucrative product in pharmaceutical history. Many patients had to forgo treatment due to the cost (Robbins, 2023).

Even with these tactics, 90% of drugs prescribed in 2020 were generic. Yet brand-name manufacturers have been acquiring generic companies and generic companies have been merging with one another. The volume of these mergers and acquisitions skyrocketed from 2013 to 2016 (Gagnon & Volesky, 2017). One outcome of this consolidation has been price increases for generic drugs; even so, generics continue to be far less costly than their brand-name counterparts.

For years, large pharmaceutical companies have been among the most profitable industries in the United States, in recent years earning an average of 13.8% profits compared with 7.7% for large non-pharmaceutical companies (Ledley et al., 2020). The pharmaceutical industry argues that high drug prices are justified by its expenditures on research and development of new drugs. Yet in 2020, 7 of the 10 largest drug companies spent more on marketing than on research (AHIP, 2021). For some pharmaceutical companies, the returns paid to shareholders are as much as four times the amount invested in research (Milani, 2019). Unlike many nations, the US government has not imposed regulated prices on drugs as a result of drug industry lobbying (Scutti, 2019). Responding to widespread public anger about drug prices, the Inflation Reduction Act of 2022 mandates that the government negotiate the prices of 10 Medicare prescription drugs starting in 2026 with more drugs to come in ensuing years (Kaiser Family Foundation, 2023).

Pharmacy Benefit Managers

Contributing to the cost of medications is an entity that most health care consumers have never heard of. Pharmacy benefit management companies (PBMs), which appeared in the late 1960s, have become formidable players in the pharmaceutical supply chain. Insurers contract with PBMs to handle their drug benefit. PBMs in turn contract with both pharmaceutical companies as suppliers and with pharmacies as providers of medications. Despite being largely invisible to patients, PBMs play a complex but influential role in determining what drugs will be available to a patient at what price.

Mega Pharmaceutical Company developed Sugarlow, a new diabetes drug and set the list price as $1,000 for a month supply of 60 pills. Because many excellent, low-cost diabetes drugs had been on the market for decades, Mega spent $300 million advertising Sugarlow on TV and another $150 million persuading doctors on its benefits.

Mega made a deal with Super PBM, a big pharmacy benefits manager company, to place Sugarlow as number 1 on the formularies of the largest insurance companies and Medicare Part D plans—which increased the odds that doctors would prescribe the medication. To pay Super PBM for giving Sugarlow such a favorable formulary placement, Mega offered a rebate to Super PBM of $200 for every 60 pills sold through Super PBM; pharmacies would receive a discount from $1,000 to $800 for the pills and Super PBM could keep the $200. Mega and Super PBM made large profits within the first year of Sugarlow being on the market as Sugarlow became one of the most widely prescribed diabetic drugs. Mega soon increased the price of Sugarlow to $1,200 for a month supply for pharmacies not using Super PBM.

Insurers (including Medicare Part D plans) have given PBMs the authority to decide whether a particular medication will be on the insurer's formulary and thereby covered by insurance. Getting on formularies is crucial for manufacturers because medications not on formularies will not sell. To persuade PBMs to place their drugs on insurers' formularies, drug companies reduce the drug's price as a discount paid to the PBM.

These discounts, which add up to billions of dollars annually, have turned PBMs into highly profitable companies. Moreover, PBMs are paid by insurers to reimburse pharmacies for medications the insurer's patients obtain, yet PBMs pay pharmacies less than what they receive from insurers; this "spread" also increases PBM profits. In 2022, 3 PBMs—CVS Caremark, Express Scripts, and United Healthcare's Optum—controlled 80% of the PBM market.

Digital and Information Technology

In the digital era, among the fastest growing health care suppliers have been vendors of electronic medical records (EMRs). In 2008, only 9% of hospitals had EMRs. By 2016, 96% had adopted EMRs. During the same period, EMR use in physician offices increased from 17% to 78% (ONC, 2023). Over this period the number of EMR vendors decreased from more than 1,000 to about 400. The two largest vendors (Epic and Cerner) now control more than 80% of the hospital EMR market (Scarborough, 2022). Advocates of consolidation have argued that this trend facilitates sharing of electronic patient data when organizations use different EMRs. Similar trends have occurred in the broader information technology market, such as Microsoft's dominance in personal computer operating system software. But as in other instances of health care consolidation, this concentration of the market among a few huge corporations has raised concerns about anti-competitive, oligopolistic power in setting prices.

INVESTOR-OWNED HEALTH CARE AND THE QUEST FOR PROFITABILITY

▶ For-Profit Corporations

The trend of consolidation has coincided with a rise of for-profit corporations in the health care industry. For-profit corporations are ones that have investor shareholders who financially benefit by receiving dividends or a share of corporate profits. Managers of these corporations have a fiduciary obligation to maximize financial return to shareholders. Historically, for-profit corporations predominated in certain sectors of the health industry such as pharmaceutical manufacturers and other suppliers. Most large for-profit health

care enterprises operate as public corporations, meaning that shares of their stock are traded on financial exchanges open to any willing investor. As noted in Chapter 2, a largely nonprofit health insurance sector transitioned in the late twentieth century to become one dominated by for-profit insurers as many formerly nonprofit Blue Cross and Blue Shield insurance plans converted to for-profit status. The provider sector, however, until relatively recently continued to largely consist of small self-owned businesses and nonprofit organizations. In the early 1990s, for-profit hospital chains formed by acquiring formerly nonprofit community hospitals. Although slowly gaining market share, for-profit hospitals are still a minority at 24% of US hospitals. For-profit enterprises currently own most hospices, nursing homes, dialysis clinics, imaging facilities, and home care agencies.

The distinction, however, between for-profit and nonprofit health care organizations has narrowed over the years. Nonprofit hospitals first formed as local charitable organizations, many sponsored by religious organizations, providing considerable amounts of care free of charge to low-income patients. Because of this, government granted these institutions exemption from certain obligations such as paying property taxes. For huge, horizontally integrated hospital systems, these tax exemptions now amount to tens of millions of dollars annually for each system and billions of dollars for all US nonprofit hospitals combined. Although these organizations do not pay profits to shareholders, they nonetheless strive to generate robust margins, that is, revenues in excess of expenses. Hospitals use these margins to build new facilities, purchase new equipment and technology, and generously compensate their executive officers. The amount of charity care has steadily fallen—now about 2% on average for nonprofit hospitals as a percent of total expenses—as many hospitals aggressively bill even low income patients and hire collection agencies to use tactics such as garnishing wages to force patients to pay medical bills. Hospital systems are coming under increasing scrutiny to justify their tax-exempt status (Silver-Greenberg & Thomas, 2022).

In contrast to hospitals, physician practices started not as nonprofit organizations but as self-owned businesses. A physician's income was essentially the margin between practice revenues and expenses. Over time, some physicians found ways to be more entrepreneurial to increase their incomes. For example, individual physicians or small physician partnerships began operating their own ambulatory centers focusing on highly reimbursed procedures that traditionally were performed in hospitals, such as cataract surgery, orthopedic procedures, colonoscopies, and CT or MRI studies. Physicians earn income from both the professional services they directly provide and the fees billed by the ambulatory facility that they own. Physician ownership of imaging centers has been found to be associated with greater referral of patients for imaging services, increasing costs and exposing patients to unnecessary radiation (Relman, 2009; Young et al., 2020). For physicians working in medical groups, groups were typically structured as professional corporations with physician partners as the sole shareholders and margins distributed among the partners.

Private Equity

A new actor has joined traditional corporate shareholders as investors on the health care stage: private equity. Private equity is a different model of investor owners than the traditional form of shareholders of a publicly traded for-profit corporation. As described by one analyst:

> "Private equity firms pool money from investors, ranging from wealthy people to college endowments and pension funds. They use that money to buy into businesses they hope to flip at a sizable profit, usually within three to seven years, by making them more efficient and lucrative (Schulte, 2022)."

In an accelerating development, private equity firms are investing in start-up physician groups and buying physician practices, especially practices not yet owned by hospital-dominated systems. For physicians, private equity investors may have appeal as a way to obtain an infusion of capital to purchase expensive items such as an electronic medical record, acquire office space in desirable locations, and hire clinicians and staff during the ramp up phase of a new medical group. The promise of stable income in an employed position is an attractor for some physicians to join such practices. Equity firms in turn expect rapid growth, economic efficiencies, and an ability to command high fees. They aim to sell their

shares within a few years at many times the dollar value of their original investment (Ikram et al., 2021).

Private equity firms initially focused on single specialty practices. For example, in 2018, the private equity firm Blackstone acquired Team Health, one of the nation's largest employers of emergency medicine physicians. Team Health has arrangements with more than 3,400 hospitals across the country to provide physician staffing for their emergency departments. In recent years Team Health has paid tens of millions of dollars in settlements in response to allegations of overbilling insurance plans and patients (McLaren, 2017). Private equity has bought many anesthesiology, gastroenterology, and dermatology practices. Studies have shown that following private equity acquisition, practices raise fees, up-code charges, and increase the volume of services of questionable value to patients (Shah et al., 2023). Some venture capital firms have invested in primary care start-ups that they perceive to have profitable business models due to innovative concierge (e.g., One Medical) or care management (e.g., Oak Street Health) approaches (Shah et al., 2023). Private equity is also investing billions in virtual health care tech start-ups.

Private equity's role in hospital investment and ownership has often been one of trying to turn around a financially distressed facility and make it profitable, and then sell it to a buyer or cash in on its assets. Following private equity acquisition, hospital charges increase and care of Medicaid patients decreases (Bruch et al., 2020). In one highly publicized case, in 2018 a private equity firm bought Hahnemann Hospital in Philadelphia, one of the nation's oldest hospitals, located in a low-income neighborhood and serving many patients from marginalized populations. After cost-cutting manuevers and attempts to boost productivity and revenues failed to eliminate operating deficits, the private equity firm closed Hahnemann Hospital in 2019. Patients were left without a coordinated plan to find new medical homes. A private equity firm that had contributed to financing the acquisition had its investment repaid in full, plus 10% interest (Pomorski, 2021).

MEGA-CONSOLIDATION

This chapter began by introducing the major actors on the health care stage (Table 17–1), and we added a new actor: corporate shareholders and private equity investors. It used to be clear who was a purchaser, an insurer, a provider, or a supplier. This is becoming no longer true. In the past, consolidation took place within each actor's sphere: insurers buying other insurers, hospitals merging into multi-hospital systems, hospitals buying physician practices or private equity aggregating physician practices. By 2020, the lines separating the actors became blurred as trans-sector vertical consolidations altered the health care landscape. Actors are merging with one another and non-health companies are entering the health care world.

▶ Trans-sector Consolidation

CVS Health and Aetna

In 2007, the pharmacy chain CVS acquired Caremark, a large PBM, to become CVS Health. Caremark had posed a threat to brick-and-mortar pharmacies with its mail-order pharmacy business. Today, CVS Caremark is one of the nation's largest PBMs, steering patients to CVS pharmacies, including calling patients using independent drug stores to encourage them to switch to CVS (Candisky, 2018). A decade later, CVS Health turned its sights to an even bigger actor, purchasing Aetna, the nation's third largest health insurer, for $69 billion in 2018. This trans-sector vertical consolidation means that the millions of Aetna policyholders are preferentially directed to CVS's 9,600 pharmacies and mail-order supplier and the 1,100 walk-in clinics located at its pharmacies. CVS and its competitor Walgreens together control between 50% and 75% of the drugstore market in each of the country's 14 largest metropolitan areas, but pharmacy chains like CVS are worried that Amazon will start a lower-cost mail-order prescription business; Aetna could prevent its policyholders from choosing such an Amazon option. More recently, CVS Health has entered the business of delivering medical and not just pharmacy services, purchasing Oak Street Health, a primary care group focused on caring for patients in Medicare Advantage plans, along with other medical groups and home health providers.

Walgreens, Cigna, and Medical Groups

Walgreens has in turn responded with its own trans-sector consolidation, partnering in 2022 with Cigna, a major health insurance company, to purchase large medical practices. Walgreens' ambition to provide medical services grew from operating some walk-in clinics co-located with its pharmacies to purchasing large medical groups with a much wider array of urgent care, primary care, and specialty practices. Walgreens and Cigna together now own medical practices at 680 different sites across the United States (Landi, 2022). Cigna also purchased one of the largest PBMs, Express Scripts, in 2018, following in the steps of CVS's purchase of the Caremark PBM.

From Blue Cross to Anthem to Elevance Health

Health insurance companies other than Cigna have moved from being strictly payers to also becoming providers by acquiring medical practices. In 2011, Anthem, the second largest health insurer, acquired CareMore, a large health system focused on seniors with complex chronic conditions. In 2020, Anthem acquired Beacon Health Options, a behavioral health provider. Anthem changed its name in 2022 to Elevance Health to convey a new identity as something more than just an insurance plan. What was initially established by hospital and physician provider organizations as nonprofit Blue Cross-Blue Shield insurance plans, and then consolidated into the national for-profit Anthem insurance corporation, has come full circle in the modern age of mergers and acquisition by buying up physician groups and creating the huge payer-provider conglomerate Elevance Health.

UnitedHealthcare and Optum

The insurance company that has been most aggressive in its trans-sector consolidation is UnitedHealthcare, the nation's largest health insurer. Buried inside UnitedHealthcare is Optum, a rapidly growing health services company that has been referred to as "the biggest health system you have never heard of." In 2017, UnitedHealthcare acquired the DaVita Medical Group for $4.9 billion and placed it in the Optum unit. DaVita had previously engineered a major horizontal consolidation, acquiring 300 clinics, outpatient surgicenters, and urgent care centers. Optum has subsequently purchased hundreds of additional ambulatory surgery centers, urgent care centers, and medical groups. By 2022, Optum was employing more physicians than Kaiser

Permanente, with about one in fifteen physicians in the United States working for Optum and its subsidiaries. Optum also operates its own PBM. Another division of Optum provides population health management, analytics, and other services to care providers, insurance plans, and government entities.

Non-Health Companies Moving into Health Care

Corporations with longstanding presence in health care are not the only actors driving consolidation through mergers and acquisitions. In 2022, Amazon purchased One Medical, a primary care system with 188 offices in 29 communities; this purchase afforded a large return on investment for early investors in One Medical. Many observers expect Amazon to pursue additional health care acquisitions. In 2021, Microsoft bought Nuance Communications, a pioneer in speech recognition and artificial intelligence technology, used by many physician practices and hospitals.

CONCLUSION

For private actors in the health care industry, health care has always been a business. Even before the advent of huge, for-profit entities in health care, providers — whether an independent physician, a pharmacist-owned retail pharmacy, or a community hospital — have acted on economic self-interest as well as on an ethos of professionalism and service. The economist Robert Evans has suggested that the very term non-profit for hospitals is a misnomer, and that these organizations should be called "not only for profit" to acknowledge their attention to financial margin (Evans, 1984).

If health care has always been a business, it is now big business. An ever-greater share of the health care industry is owned and controlled by shareholders and investors rather than by the people delivering care. Even non-profit entities operate in a market environment compelling them to "grow or die;" small fish health care organizations are consumed by the big fish of huge conglomerates that amass market power. Horizontal consolidation of hospitals and vertical integration of hospitals acquiring physician practices has caused many local areas to be dominated by one or two powerful health systems. Horizontal insurance company mergers have led to similar domination by

a few insurance giants. The recent conglomeration of health care with cross-sector vertical integration of insurers, providers, and suppliers is producing a health care landscape populated by fewer, and much larger, companies. The long historical trend from the 1–2 doctor practice and neighborhood drug store to the mega-corporation is nearing its apogee. Yet for patients, the irony is that a consolidated system continues to bring an experience of fragmented care: primary care is challenged while specialty services abound; vertically integrated health systems don't consistently deliver more coordinated care; the few large insurance companies offer a dizzying array of insurance products; pharmaceutical drug delivery by three huge PBMs is complicated by confusing pricing and copays. Patients continue to be challenged as health care costs rise and as individuals bear a greater share of those costs.

The drive to make money—whether for physicians, for-profit and non-profit hospitals, insurers, pharmaceutical companies, or health care conglomerates—increasingly determines what happens in health care. This drive is intensified by the growing role of finance capital in health care. Although private equity may help seed innovation in small start-up health care companies, it brings with it a philosophy that views health care organizations as assets to buy, optimize profitability, and then sell, rather than as long-term investment in the health of the community. The commitment of all health care professionals to the ethical principles of beneficence, nonmaleficence, patient autonomy, and distributive justice is tested on a daily basis in the profit-oriented environment of twenty-first century health care in America.

Chapter 1 introduced the concept that *the United States is spending too much money on health care and getting too little health.* The inequities in health and health care discussed in Chapter 5 are related to the growing income inequality in American society. The top 10% of earners received 50% of the nation's total income in 2017 compared with 33% in 1965 (Saez, 2019). The top 10% also controls three-quarters of all the wealth in the United States (Khullar & Chokshi, 2018). Not only is there growing concentration of wealth in the United States, but wealthy individuals are consuming a larger share of health care services. Following enactment of Medicare and Medicaid, the average annual health care expenditures per capita for the poorest 20% of people in the United States increased to a level above that for high-income individuals—consistent with the greater health care needs among people with low income. In recent years, average health care expenditures have flipped back to the pre-Medicare and Medicare pattern, with the wealthiest 20% of people in the United States now consuming more health care than individuals in lower income groups. Health care must be understood in this broader context of winners and losers in the US economy. One can rightly ask who benefits from the US approach to the business of health care.

REFERENCES

AHIP. New Study: In the Midst of COVID-19 Crisis, 7 out of 10 Big Pharma Companies Spent More on Sales and Marketing than R&D. Oct, 2021. https://www.ahip.org/news/articles/new-study-in-the-midst-of-covid-19-crisis-7-out-of-10-big-pharma-companies-spent-more-on-sales-and-marketing-than-r-d.

Bazzoli GJ. The corporatization of American hospitals. *J Health Polit Policy Law*. 2004;29:885–905.

Beaulieu ND, Chernew ME, McWilliams JM, et al. Organization and performance of US health systems. *JAMA*. 2023;329:325–335.

Bonta R. Attorney General Bonta announces final approval of $575 million settlement with Sutter Health resolving allegations of anti-competitive practices. August 21, 2021.

Bruch JD, Gondi S, Song Z. Changes in hospital income, use, and quality associated with private equity acquisition. *JAMA Intern Med*. 2020;180:1428–1435.

Candisky C. Three CVS actions raise concerns for some pharmacies, consumers. *The Columbus Dispatch*. April 15, 2018.

Casalino LP, Pham H, Bazzoli G. Growth of single-specialty medical groups. *Health Aff (Millwood)*. 2004;23(2):82–90.

Casalino LP. Health systems—the present and the future. *JAMA*. 2023;329:293–2294.

Evans RG. *Strained Mercy*. Toronto: Butterworths; 1984.

Furukawa MF, Kimmey L, Jones DJ, Machta RM, Guo J, Rich EC. Consolidation of providers into health systems increased substantially, 2016-18. *Health Aff (Millwood)*. 2020;39:1321–1325.

Gagnon M-A, Volesky KD. Merger mania: mergers and acquisitions in the generic drug sector from 1995 to 2016. *Global Health*. 2017;13:62–68.

Greaney TL. The new health care merger wave: does the "vertical, good" maxim apply? *J Law Med Ethics*. 2018;46(4):918–926.

Ikram U, Aung K-K, Song Z. Private equity and primary care: lessons from the field. *NEJM Catalyst*. November 19, 2021.

Kaiser Family Foundation. Explaining the prescription drug provisions in the Inflation Reduction Act. January 24, 2023.

Kane CK. Recent changes in physician practice arrangements: private practice dropped to less than 50 percent of physicians in 2020. AMA Economic and Health Policy Research, May 2021. https://www.ama-assn.org/system/files/2021-05/2020-prp-physician-practice-arrangements.pdf.

Khullar D, Chokshi DA. Health, income and poverty: where we are and what could help. *Health Affairs Policy Brief*. October 4, 2018.

Landi H. Walgreens' Village MD inks $9B deal to buy Summit Health, making the largest physician deal of the year. *Fierce Healthcare*, November 7, 2022.

Ledley FD, McCoy SS, Vaughan G, Cleary EG. Profitability of large pharmaceutical companies compared with other large public companies. *JAMA*. 2020;323:834–843.

McLaren ML. $11M Whistleblower award on TeamHealth $60M overbilling Medicare & Medicaid at IPC Healthcare. *Whistleblower News Review*, February 27, 2017.

Mehrotra A, Epstein AM, Rosenthal MB. Do integrated medical groups provide higher-quality medical care than individual practice associations? *Ann Intern Med*. 2006;145:826–833.

Meyer H. Biden's FTC has blocked 4 hospital mergers and is poised to thwart more consolidation attempts. *Kaiser Health News*, July 18, 2022.

Milani K. Profit over patients. Roosevelt Institute, 2019.

ONC (Office of the National Coordinator for Health Information Technology). National Trends in Hospital and Physician Adoption of Electronic Health Records. 2023.

Pifer R. UnitedHealth, flush off 2022 momentum, eyes membership, value-based growth. Health Care Dive, January 13, 2023.

Pomorski C. The death of Hahnemann Hospital. *The New Yorker*, May 31, 2021.

Relman AS. The health reform we need and are not getting. *New York Rev Books*. 2009;56(11):38–40.

Robbins R. How a drug company made $114 billion by gaming the U.S. patent system. *New York Times*, January 28, 2023.

Saez E. Striking it richer: the evolution of top incomes in the United States. *UC Berkeley*. 2019. https://eml.berkeley.edu/~saez/saez-UStopincomes-2017.pdf.

Scarborough N. EHRs Ranked by Market Share. Healthgrades for Professionals, July, 2022.

Schulte F. Sick profit: investigating private equity's stealthy takeover of health care across cities and specialties. *Kaiser Health News*, November 14, 2022.

Scutti S. Big Pharma spends record millions on lobbying amid pressure to lower drug prices. *CNN*. January 24, 2019. https://www.cnn.com/2019/01/23/health/phrma-lobbying-costs-bn/index.html.

Shah S, Rooke-Ley H, Fuse Brown EC. Corporate investors in primary care: profits, progress and pitfalls. *N Engl J Med*. 2023;288:99–101.

Shryock T. Hospital profits decline. *Medical Economics*, May 11, 2022.

Silver-Greenberg J, Thomas K. They were entitled to free care, hospitals hounded them to pay. *New York Times*, December 15, 2022.

Tribble SJ. Drugmakers play the patent game to lock in prices, block competitors. *Kaiser Health News*. October 2, 2018.

Urwin JW, Emanuel EJ. The relative value scale update committee: time for an update. *JAMA*. 2019;322:1137–1138.

Young GJ, Flaherty S, Zepeda ED, Mortele KJ, Griffith JL. Effects of physician experience, specialty training, and self-referral on inappropriate diagnostic imaging. *J Gen Intern Med*. 2020;35:1661–1667.

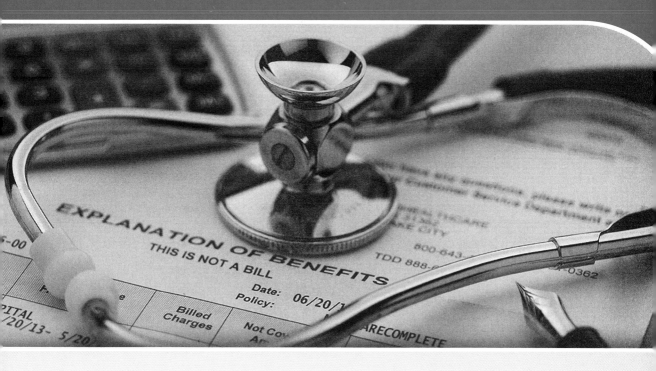

SECTION VI

CONCLUSION AND STUDY GUIDE

Conclusion: Tensions and Challenges

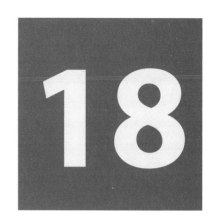

The perfect health care system is like perfect health—a noble aspiration but one that is impossible to attain. In the preceding chapters, we have discussed many fundamental issues and principles involved in formulating health care policy. A recurrent theme has been the notion that "magic bullets" are hard to come by. Policy changes may offer a degree of relief for a pressing problem, such as inadequate access to care, but frequently also give rise to various side effects, such as stimulating increased health care costs.

All health care systems face the same challenges: improving health and health equity, controlling costs, prioritizing allocation of resources, enhancing the quality of care, and distributing services fairly. These challenges require the management of various tensions that pull at the health care system (O'Neil & Seifer, 1995). The goal of health policy is to find the points of equilibrium that produce the optimal system of health care (Table 18–1).

Dr. Madeleine Longview is chief resident in critical care medicine and supervises the intensive care unit of a large municipal hospital. It's 5:30 am, and the intensive care unit team has finally stabilized the condition of a 15-year-old admitted the previous evening with gunshot wounds to the abdomen and chest. Dr. Longview sits by the nursing desk and surveys the other patients in the unit: a 91-year-old woman admitted from a nursing home with sepsis from a urinary tract infection, a 50-year-old man with shock lung caused by drugs ingested in a suicide attempt, and a 32-year-old

woman with lupus erythematosus who is rejecting her second kidney transplant. Dr. Longview feels personally responsible for the care of every one of these patients. She tells herself that she will do her best to help each of them survive.

As Dr. Longview gazes out of the windows of the intensive care unit, the apartment houses surrounding the hospital take shape in the breaking dawn. She wonders: Which block will be the scene of the next drive-by shooting or episode of domestic abuse? Which window shade hides a homebound older adult lying on the floor dehydrated and unable to move, waiting for someone to find him and bring him to the emergency department? Which one of the unvaccinated kids in the neighborhood will one day be rushed into the unit limp with meningitis? In which room is someone lighting up the first cigarette of the day? Dr. Longview somehow feels responsible for all those patients-to-be, as well as for the patients lying in the hospital beds around her. After these sleepless nights on duty, the doubts about the value of all the work she does in the intensive care unit creep into her thoughts. She has visions of shutting down the unit and putting all the money to work hiring public health nurses in the community, or maybe just paying for a better grammar school in the neighborhood. But then what would happen to the patients needing her care right now?

One of the most basic tensions affecting physicians and other caregivers is the tension between caring for the

Table 18–1. Major tensions in health care

Health of the individual patient	Health of the population
Tertiary care	Primary care
Acute care	Chronic and preventive care
Cost unawareness in medical practice	Cost awareness
Unlimited expectations for care	Affordability of care
Individual physician	Organized health care team
Professional management	Corporate management
Market-based health care	Government regulation
Inequity in distribution of health services and costs	Fair distribution
Health disparities	Health equity

Source: Adapted from O'Neil E, Seifer S. Health care reform and medical education: forces towards generalism. *Acad Med.* 1995;70(1 suppl):S37–S43.

individual patient and caring for the larger community or population. Many of the most important decisions to be made in health policy—decisions such as allocating health care resources, addressing the social drivers of health and illness, and augmenting activities in prevention and public health—depend on broadening the practitioner's view to encompass the population health perspective. The challenge for physicians and other clinicians will be to make room for this broader perspective while preserving the ethical duty to care for the individual patients under their charge.

Like Dr. Longview, the health care system as a whole will continue to struggle over finding the proper balance between the provision of acute care services and preventive and chronic care services, as well as striking the right balance between the levels of tertiary and primary care. Few observers would encourage Dr. Longview to succumb to her despair, close all the intensive care units, and expel all the critical care subspecialists from the health care system. Yet most would agree that health care in the United States has drifted too far away from the primary care end of the tertiary care–primary care axis.

Dr. Tom Ransom has performed what he believes to be a reasonably thorough workup for Zed's intermittent abdominal cramping and constipation,

including a detailed history and physical examination, blood tests, and abdominal ultrasound—all of which were normal. When Dr. Ransom tells Zed that they will have to work together to manage Zed's symptoms, starting with eating less fast food and more fruits and vegetables, Zed tells Dr. Ransom that he wants one more test, an abdominal CT scan. Zed says that he had a cousin with similar symptoms who was eventually diagnosed with advanced-stage lymphoma after complaining of pain for over a year.

Dr. Ransom is in a quandary. He believes it extremely unlikely that Zed has serious pathologic changes in his abdomen that will be detected on CT scan. He could order the scan, but then there's the issue of the cost. He can't recall whether Zed is covered by a fee-for-service plan or by one of the health plans with an alternative payment model that puts Dr. Ransom and his medical group at financial risk for all radiologic tests ordered. He starts to look at the medical record to check Zed's coverage but feels a pang of guilt that he should allow these economic considerations to intrude into his clinical judgment.

The desire (and in many instances, expectation) of patients to receive all potentially beneficial care, and the unwillingness of these same individuals in their role as purchasers to spend unlimited amounts to finance health care, creates a strain for all caregivers and systems of care. Health professionals are being called upon to incorporate considerations of costs when making clinical decisions. Debate will continue about the best ways to encourage clinicians to be more accountable for the costs of care in a manner that is socially responsible and does not unduly intrude on the clinician's ability to serve the individual patient. Is it necessary to use payment methods that place physicians at financial risk for their treatment decisions in order to control costs? Are more global methods available to induce physicians and other caregivers to practice in a more cost-conscious manner? If Zed does not get a CT scan, does that constitute painless or painful cost control?

On the eve of his retirement, Dr. Melvin Steadman reminisces with his son, Dr. Kevin Steadman.

The elder Dr. Steadman has practiced as a solo pediatrician for more than 40 years in the same town. The only boss he has known in his professional life has been himself. He has served as president of the local medical society, helped spearhead efforts to build a special children's wing of the local hospital, and antagonized several of his colleagues when he pushed for a change in hospital policy that required physicians to attend extra continuing medical education courses in order to maintain their hospital privileges. Mel swore that he'd never retire; but he also swore that he'd never let the insurance companies "tell me how to practice medicine." He has refused to sign any managed care contracts. Facing a dwindling supply of patients, Mel has decided to call it quits.

His son Kevin is also a pediatrician, working as a staff physician for a large for-profit multispecialty group that recently opened up an office in town. Kevin remembers the many nights when his father didn't get home from work until after he had gone to bed. Kevin's work hours are more regular at the group practice, and he is on call for only one weekend every 2 months. He considers his father's approach to medicine old-fashioned in many ways—excessively paternalistic toward patients and irrationally scornful of the pediatric nurse practitioners who work with Kevin. He does, however, envy his father's professional independence. Just this week, the group practice notified Kevin that he would have to divide his time between his current office and a new site that would soon open in a suburban mall. His schedule will be limited to 10-minute drop-in appointments at the new site, rather than the style of practice that promotes a sense of continuity, one that allows him to get to know his patients over time.

A system of health care formerly managed according to a professional model by independent practitioners is being pulled toward a corporate model of care featuring large organizations managed by executives and administrators. As the role of corporate entities expands, traditional responsibilities toward patients and local communities are vying with new obligations to shareholders. Power relationships are changing, with health care conglomerates challenging the dominance of the medical profession. A shift toward multidisciplinary group practice may provide more opportunity for health care professionals to work collegially and implement new approaches to quality improvement to elevate the competence of all health care providers. At the same time, a competitive, for-profit health care environment increasingly dominated by large investor-owned conglomerates is heightening tension between health care as a common good and as a business enterprise.

Aurora can't wait any longer in the crowded county hospital emergency department. She's already been there for 6 hours, and no one has seen her. Her lower abdomen still hurts, but she figures she'll just have to put up with it for a few days. Having a low income, no insurance, and no legal documents, she doesn't have much choice; where else could she go? Aurora has two young children at home who need to be put to bed. In half an hour, their father has to get to his night job as a security officer. As she enters her apartment, she collapses, the pregnancy in her fallopian tube having ruptured, producing internal hemorrhage. Her husband frantically dials 911, praying that his wife won't die.

Over the years, one tension within the US health care system that has been far from reaching a point of satisfactory equilibrium is the achievement of a basic level of fairness in the distribution of health care services and the burden of paying for those services. The Affordable Care Act took a step toward resolving that tension. But because financial barriers remain for millions of people, both insured and uninsured, not all patients benefit from early detection of potentially curable cancers, patients with chronic diseases are hospitalized because of lack of timely primary care, hypertensive patients forego the medications that might avert strokes and kidney failure, and babies are born prematurely and spend their first weeks of life in a neonatal intensive care unit. People in lower income households pay a greater proportion of their income for health care than do more affluent people.

People providing and receiving care in the United States must work together to achieve a brighter future for the nation's health care system. Changing the future will require that people look beyond their immediate self-interest to view the common good of a health care system that is accessible, affordable, and of high quality for all. A heightened level of public discourse will be needed, with a populace that is better informed and more actively engaged in shaping the future of their health care system. Concepts in health policy will need to be discussed and debated in a manner that connects with the daily realities experienced by patients and caregivers. Physicians and other health care professionals have the opportunity to help shape the future of health care in the United States. With leadership and foresight among the community of health care professionals, our nation may yet achieve a system that allows the most honorable features of the healing professions to flourish.

REFERENCE

O'Neil E, Seifer S. Health care reform and medical education: forces towards generalism. *Acad Med.* 1995;70:S37.

Questions to Assess Understanding

CHAPTER 2: PAYING FOR HEALTH CARE

1. What are the four modes of financing health care?
2. How does the money flow for each of the four modes?
3. Which of the four modes consumes the largest proportion of national health expenditures?
4. Is the sum total of health care financing regressive, progressive, or proportional?
5. Who is eligible for Medicare Part A?
   a. People 65 and over who have paid into Social Security for 10 years
   b. People under 65 who have been totally and permanently disabled for 24 months
   c. People with certain diseases such as end-stage kidney disease
   d. All of the above.
6. Who is eligible for insurance subsidies or tax credits under the Affordable Care Act?
   a. All people with incomes below the Federal Poverty Level.
   b. Uninsured people between 100 and 400 percent of the Federal Poverty Level.
   c. All people age 65 or over.
7. In all but 10 states (2023), all people and families below 138% of the Federal Poverty Level are eligible for Medicaid. True or False
8. Counties in states that expanded Medicaid under the ACA have lower mortality rates than counties in states that have not expanded Medicaid. True or False
9. All people who are uninsured are unemployed. True or False

CHAPTER 3: HEALTH INSURANCE AND ACCESS TO CARE

1. Which one of the following modes of health care financing is used by the largest number of people in the United States?
   a. Out-of-pocket payments
   b. Individual private insurance
   c. Employment-based private insurance
   d. Public insurance
2. About how many people in the United States had no health insurance in 2021?
   a. 15 million
   b. 21 million
   c. 27 million
   d. 33 million
3. Uninsured people have poorer access to health care and poorer health outcomes than people with insurance? True or False
4. What is a deductible? Give an example.
5. What is a co-payment?
6. What is underinsurance? Give an example.
7. Between 2010 and 2020, the number of uninsured people increased but the number of underinsured people went down. True or False

CHAPTER 4: PAYING HEALTH CARE PROVIDERS

1. Explain each mode of physician payment: fee-for-service, episode-of-illness, capitation, and salary.
2. What is per diem payment to a hospital?
3. What is DRG payment under Medicare?
4. Why should capitation payments be risk-adjusted?

CHAPTER 5: HEALTH EQUITY

1. For each of the following, indicate whether it is an example of either:
   - Interpersonal racism that contributes to a *health care* inequity.
   - Systemic/structural racism that contributes to a *health care* inequity.
   - Interpersonal racism that contributes to a *health* inequity that is not mediated by a health care inequity (that is, an example of how racism may directly and adversely affect health).
   - Systemic/structural racism that contributes to a *health* inequity that is not mediated by a health care inequity.
   a. Immigrant populations in many parts of the United States had difficulty accessing COVID vaccinations due to processes that required online access to schedule appointments, scheduling information that was only in English, and mass vaccination drive-in sites that were difficult to reach without an automobile.
   b. A medical resident notices that their attending is more likely to ask patients of color than White patients to submit a urine sample to test for drug use. When he asks about this, the attending frowns and say, "Is that right? I don't think I treat people differently because of their color." He asks his quality improvement division to produce a report on drug testing sorted by patient race-ethnicity, which shows that the resident is correct about much higher rates of drug testing for the attending physician's Black and Latino patients.
   c. A Black woman has a stroke at age 56. She confides in the nurse caring for her in the hospital that she has experienced stress for many years due to working at a job site where she feels subjected to frequent microaggressions from her supervisors and believes that less qualified White co-workers have been unfairly promoted to higher paying positions.
   d. A Latino man grew up in a racially segregated neighborhood and attended a public high school with mostly Latino students, with spending per student 30% lower than the spending per student at the high school in a nearby suburb serving mostly White students. He dropped out of high school and has been working for the past 15 years in minimum wage jobs. He has poorly controlled type 2 diabetes and his diet mainly consists of inexpensive highly processed foods.

2. On average, a person in the United States with an income four times the poverty level will live how many years longer than a person with an income below the poverty level?
   a. 2 years
   b. 5 years
   c. 7 years
   d. 10 years

3. Which of the following statements are TRUE (more than one may be true):
   a. Prior to the Supreme Court's ruling in Dobbs vs. Jackson Women's Health Organization, most pregnancy terminations (abortions) were fully covered by private or government insurance plans.
   b. Until 1973, the American Psychiatric Association's Diagnostic Manual categorized homosexuality as a sociopathic personality disturbance.
   c. Transgender youth are no more likely to attempt suicide than their counterparts who do not identify as transgender or non-gender conforming.
   d. Racial-ethnic inequities in health are almost completely accounted for by income and related social class disparities between marginalized racial groups and White populations.

CHAPTER 6: MEDICAL ETHICS AND RATIONING OF HEALTH CARE

1. Describe the four principles of medical ethics.
2. Mr. Jones wants a CT scan because he is worried about a mild pain in his chest. His nurse practitioner does not order the scan because she is able to diagnose and treat the pain without a CT scan and CT scans subject patients to a risk of cancer. Is care being rationed? Why or why not?
3. The hospital, which has empty beds, turns away Ms. Robinson because she does not have insurance. Is care being rationed? Why or why not?
4. Do policies to control costs always involve rationing? Give an example.

CHAPTER 7: HOW HEALTH CARE IS ORGANIZED—I: PRIMARY, SECONDARY, AND TERTIARY CARE

1. Match each of the following to its level of care: primary care, secondary care, or tertiary care.
    a. A hospitalist physician working on a general medical ward of a hospital
    b. A pediatric nurse practitioner caring for a panel of patients at a community health center
    c. A liver transplant surgeon working at an academic health center
    d. An obstetrician staffing a labor unit at a community hospital
    e. A registered nurse working in a neurosurgery intensive care unit
    f. A family physician working at a rural health center
2. List Starfield's four pillars of primary care: key tasks that provide a functional definition of primary care.
3. Dr. Evans works at an emergency department at a county hospital. Her emergency department is the first stop for a lot of families who work during the day, though they see a different provider every time. She takes care of pretty much everything, from fevers to broken bones or strokes. And she spends a lot of time coordinating care with skilled nursing facilities, pharmacies, specialists, and primary care.

Based on Dr. Starfield's principles, is Dr. Evans a primary care provider?
4. Using the Ecology of Medical Care framework, list the following in order of their prevalence in a month among a typical population of adults, from most prevalent to least prevalent.

    a. Visit to an emergency department
    b. Visit to a primary care physician's office
    c. Hospitalization
    d. Visit to a complementary or alternative medical care provider
    e. Experiencing at least one symptom

CHAPTER 8: HOW HEALTH CARE IS ORGANIZED—II: HEALTH DELIVERY SYSTEMS

1. For each of the following, indicate whether it is an example of horizontal integration, vertical integration, or both horizontal and vertical integration.
    a. A community hospital acquires two additional hospitals in the same metropolitan area.
    b. A rural hospital assumes control of the local rural health primary care clinic and also creates a home nursing agency serving its catchment area.
    c. Two moderately sized physician-owned medical groups merge to form a large multispecialty medical group.
    d. A multihospital system and a large physician medical group merge to create a new health system corporation with a dozen hospital facilities and 2,000 employed physicians working at 100 ambulatory care sites.
2. Identify at least three differences between the Kaiser-Permanente model of organizational integration and "virtual" models of integration such as network model HMOs and preferred provider organizations (PPOs).
3. Which of the following statements are TRUE (more than one may be true):

    a. As of 2018, half of physicians and about three-quarters of all hospitals in the United States are part of an integrated health system.

b. Although the proportion of physicians working in physician-owned practices is declining over time, as of 2020, the majority of physicians in the United States still worked in practices that were physician-owned.

c. Research shows that structurally integrated health care organizations in the United States consistently provide better quality of care and better patient experience of coordinated care than more dispersed models of care.

d. More than 30 million people in the United States receive care at community health centers.

CHAPTER 9: THE HEALTH CARE WORKFORCE AND THE EDUCATION OF HEALTH PROFESSIONALS

1. Which one of these entities licenses health professionals for clinical practice?
   a. The Federal Government Bureau of Health Professions
   b. State licensing boards
   c. Profession-run specialty boards
2. Which of these professions currently require a doctoral-level degree for entry into the profession?
   a. Physician
   b. Nurse practitioner
   c. Physician assistant
   d. Pharmacist
   e. Social worker
3. a. Define the meaning of health profession *diversity index* and how it is measured for a profession. b. Consider the following health professional groups: nurses, nurse practitioners, physicians, physician assistants, and pharmacists. Do any of these professions have a diversity index greater than 1.0 for Black, Latino, or American Indian workers?
4. What percentage of medical students in the United States come from families in the highest 20% of household income?
   a. 25%
   b. 35%
   c. 50%
   d. 60%

5. A high proportion of health workers in the United States are experiencing burnout. Specify at least three *organizational* strategies (that is, interventions to change the work environment in contrast to individual-worker focused strategies) that a health care organization could implement to reduce burnout.

CHAPTER 10: LONG-TERM CARE

1. List five ADLs.
2. List five IADLs.
3. Which of these statements is TRUE (more than one may be true)?
   a. Medicare pays for most of the costs of long-term care.
   b. Medicaid is the largest funder of long-term care.
   c. Few people have private long-term care insurance because it is too expensive and only partially covers the costs.
4. Which of these statements is FALSE (more than one may be false): Unpaid family caregivers
   a. Include about 5 million people.
   b. Are mostly men.
   c. Generally find their work stressful.
   d. Provide about $100 million per year in unpaid labor.
5. Nursing home residents who are people of color have poorer quality than White nursing home residents. True or False

CHAPTER 11: PAINFUL VERSUS PAINLESS COST CONTROL

1. Give an example of a medical intervention that lies on the steeper portions of the cost–benefit curve, and an intervention that lies on the flatter portions.
2. What does "painless cost control" refer to? Give examples of painless cost control. Are these painless for everyone?
3. Give an example demonstrating the equation $C = P \times Q$
4. Which of these statements is TRUE (more than one may be true)
   a. In 2020, the United States spent $4.1 billion on health care.

b. In 2020, health care costs for the average person in the United States were $5,000.

c. The United States spent almost 20% of gross domestic product on health care in 2020.

CHAPTER 12: MECHANISMS FOR CONTROLLING COSTS

1. Where does the money flow in a financing transaction?

2. Where does the money flow in a payment transaction?

3. Match each of the following with one of the mechanisms for controlling costs—regulatory financing controls, competitive financing controls, regulatory payment controls, competitive payment controls:
   a. Reducing taxes going to the Medicaid program
   b. Employers contract only with health plans that keep costs down
   c. Medicare reduces its fee for physicians doing cataract surgery

4. Patient cost-sharing is a highly effective way to reduce US health expenditures. True or False

5. Patient cost-sharing is an example of painless cost control. True or False

CHAPTER 13: QUALITY OF HEALTH CARE

1. Health care quality in the United States is characterized by (choose one)
   a. Uniformly high quality
   b. Uniformly low quality
   c. Examples of both high and low quality
   d. Quality has markedly improved since 2010

2. Which of these statements is TRUE (more than one may be true)?
   a. Fee-for-service payment encourages overuse (providing too much care) which can harm quality.
   b. Capitation payment encourages overuse which can harm quality.
   c. Hospitals that perform more cardiac surgeries have better outcomes for those surgeries than hospitals that perform fewer cardiac surgeries.

3. What is peer review and is it highly effective in improving quality?

4. Do electronic medical records improve quality and do they have any downsides?

5. Hospital pay for performance programs may increase payment for high quality hospitals and reduce payment for lower quality hospitals. Do these increase quality?

6. Measuring variations in practice patterns and health outcomes to identify and spread better practices. Does this method of continuous quality improvement improve quality?

CHAPTER 14: POPULATION HEALTH AND DISEASE PREVENTION

1. US life expectancy has risen steadily until the present. True or False

2. Give an example of the medical model and of the public health model for reducing tobacco use.

3. What is the Health Impact Pyramid?

4. Which part of the Pyramid has the greatest impact on the health of populations?

5. What is primary prevention? Give an example.

6. What is secondary prevention? Give an example.

7. Why was the mortality rate for COVID substantially higher among Black, Latino, Asian, and American Indian than among White populations in the United States?

8. Vaccine skepticism was a new phenomenon in the COVID pandemic. True or False

CHAPTER 15: HEALTH CARE IN FOUR NATIONS

1. You are a secretary in a large company in Germany, Canada, United Kingdom, or Japan. How is your health care paid for in Germany, Canada, United Kingdom, or Japan?

2. If you developed a urinary tract infection, what would you do in Germany, Canada, United Kingdom, or Japan?

3. You are a general practitioner in Germany, Canada, United Kingdom, or Japan. How are you paid?

4. You are a hospital administrator in Germany, Canada, United Kingdom, or Japan. How is your hospital paid?

CHAPTER 16: HEALTH CARE REFORM AND NATIONAL HEALTH INSURANCE

1. What are the three basic models of national health insurance?
2. What is Medicare for All? Give one argument in favor and one argument opposed.
3. What are two advantages of de-linking health insurance from employment?
4. What is the difference between the social insurance vs. public assistance models of financing government health insurance? Give an example of programs using each of these models.

CHAPTER 17: THE BUSINESS OF US HEALTH CARE

1. Name the five major actors in the health care economy. Only one of the actors wants to reduce health care expenditures; which actor is this?
2. What is a health system?
3. What is market power and why do health industry companies want it?
4. What percent of acute hospital beds are affiliated with a consolidated health system: 20%, 40%, 70%, or 90%?
5. Prices paid to hospitals in health systems, compared with prices to hospitals not belonging to a health system, are higher, the same, or lower.
6. In the last 30 years, the percent of national health expenditures going to pharmaceutical companies has increased from 5% to 10%. True or False
7. Large pharmaceutical companies earn about the same level of profits as large non-pharmaceutical companies. True or False
8. Describe what a private equity firm is.
9. What are some impacts of a private equity firm buying a physician group?

Appendix: Answers to Questions in Chapter 19

CHAPTER 2: 1 and 2. Out-of-pocket payments (individual to provider), individual private insurance (individual to health plan to provider), employment-based private insurance (employer and employee to health plan to provider), government financing (government to health plan to provider). 3. Government financing. 4. Regressive. 5. d. 6. b. 7. True. 8. True. 9. False.

CHAPTER 3: 1. c. 2. c. 3. True. 4. Patients pay the first $500 or $1000 each year. 5. Patients pay $20 for each physician visit. 6. Health insurance that leaves large expenses that patients have to pay, for example, Medicare. 7. False.

CHAPTER 4: 1. A fee for each service, like doctor visit or lab test. Episode of illness, one sum is paid for all services during an illness. Capitation, one payment for each patient's care during a month. Salary, a physician receives a $150,000 for a year's work. 2. A sum paid for each day the patient is in the hospital. 3. A hospital receives one payment for a patient's hospital stay; payments vary by diagnosis. 4. Physicians receive more payment for patients who are sicker so that they won't refuse to see very sick patients.

CHAPTER 5: 1. a. Systemic racism, health care inequity; b. Interpersonal racism, health care inequity; c. Interpersonal racism, health inequity; d. Systemic racism, health inequity. 2. c. 3. b.

CHAPTER 6: 1. Beneficence, helping people in need, Nonmaleficence, do no harm. Autonomy is the right

of people to make their own decisions. Justice means treating everyone fairly. 2. No, because the scan will not be beneficial. 3. No, because there is no limitation of resources. 4. No, for example reducing unneeded administrative costs.

CHAPTER 7: 1. a. Secondary; b. Primary; c. Tertiary; d. Secondary; e. Tertiary; f. Primary. 2. First contact care, comprehensive, continuity, coordinated. 3. No, because there is no continuity of care. 4. e, b, d, a, c.

CHAPTER 8: 1. a. Horizontal; b. Vertical; c. Horizontal; d. Horizontal and Vertical. 2. KP owns the hospitals and physicians versus HMO/PPO contracting with hospitals and physicians; KP pays hospitals' global budgets; KP pays physicians' salary. 3. a and d are true.

CHAPTER 9: 1. b. 2. a and d. 3. a. Percentage of practitioners in a racial-ethnic group relative to their % of US working age population. b. No. 4. c. 5. Reduce the number of patients per provider; reduce documentation burden; better team-based care.

CHAPTER 10: 1. Eating, dressing, bathing, toileting, and getting in or out of bed. 2. Housework, meal preparation, grocery shopping, transportation, and taking medications. 3. b, c. 4. a, b, d. 5. True.

CHAPTER 11: 1. Vaccination, smoking cessation counseling versus new unneeded MRI scanner. 2. Reducing excess administrative costs, ordering fewer unnecessary CT scans. These may be painful for people profiting from, or being employed by, those services. 3. Cost of hospital stay is per diem payment (price) times number of days (quantity). 4. c.

CHAPTER 12: 1. From individuals, employers, government to health plans. 2. From health plans (public or private) to providers. 3. a. Regulatory financing control; b. Competitive financing control; c. Regulatory payment control. 4. False. 5. False.

CHAPTER 13: 1. c. 2. a, c. 3. Evaluation of practitioners by other practitioners in same specialty; not highly effective. 4. May improve quality but increase the burden of documentation for clinicians. 5. No significant quality increase. 6. Yes.

CHAPTER 14: 1. False. 2. Medical model: cessation counseling; public health model: increase cigarette taxes. 3. A framework for uniting medical and public health approaches. 4. Base of pyramid. 5. Averting occurrence of a disease; vaccination. 6. Early detection or intervention to slow disease progression; mammograms. 7. Those populations were often essential workers who came in contact with people with COVID. 8. False.

CHAPTER 15: 1. Germany: your company's sick fund pays; Canada: the provincial government pays; UK: the government (National Health Service) pays; Japan: your company's plan pays. 2. All four countries: see family physician. 3. Germany: fee-for-service; Canada: mostly fee-for-service but some provinces have capitation; UK: capitation; Japan: fee-for-service. 4. Germany: DRG; Canada and UK: global budget; Japan: per diem.

CHAPTER 16: 1. Individual private insurance, employment-based private insurance, government-financed insurance. 2. Entire population insured through Medicare would create universal insurance with lower administrative costs, but Medicare could ration services. 3. You don't lose insurance if you lose your job, and employer could no longer choose your insurance plan and thereby choose your doctor. 4. Social insurance: only those who contribute receive benefits (Medicare); public assistance: you don't have to contribute to receive benefits (Medicaid).

CHAPTER 17: 1. Purchasers, insurers, providers, suppliers, and corporate shareholders/investors. Only purchasers want to reduce costs. 2. Organizations including at least one hospital and 50 physicians. 3. The share of the business that a company has; it increases ability to raise prices and profits. 4. 90%. 5. Higher. 6. True. 7. False. 8. Pools money from investors, buys control of businesses, sells the business at a sizable profit. 9. Higher prices to insurance companies and patients, making clinicians see more patients, increasing burnout, cutting out Medicaid patients.

Index

Note: Page numbers followed by f refer to figures; page numbers followed by t refer to tables.